Surgery
For UKMLA and Medical Exams

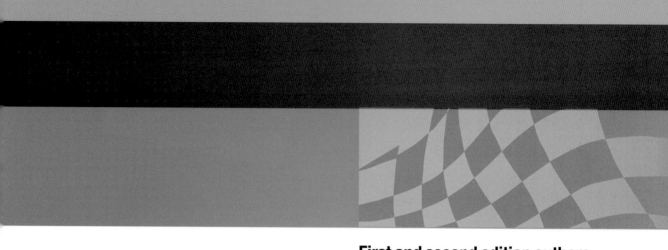

First and second edition authors

Helen Sweetland

Kevin Conway

James Cook

Third edition author

Angeliki Kontoyannis

4th Edition
CRASH COURSE

SERIES EDITOR
Philip Xiu
MA (Cantab), MB BChir, MRCP, MRCGP, MScClinEd, FHEA, MAcadMEd, RCPathME
Honorary Senior Lecturer
Leeds University School of Medicine
PCN Educational Lead
Medical Examiner
Leeds Teaching Hospital Trust
Leeds, UK

FACULTY ADVISOR
Giles Davies
MBBS, BSc, MD, FRCS (Gen Surg)
Oncoplastic Breast Surgeon
Director of Breast Surgery BUPA Cromwell Hospital
London, UK

Surgery
For UKMLA and Medical Exams

Hester Lacey
MBBS, MA, MAcadMEd
University Hospitals Sussex NHS Foundation Trust
Brighton, UK

ELSEVIER

Notices

Practitioners and researchers must always rely on their own experience and knowledge in evaluating and using any information, methods, compounds or experiments described herein. Because of rapid advances in the medical sciences, in particular, independent verification of diagnoses and drug dosages should be made. To the fullest extent of the law, no responsibility is assumed by Elsevier, authors, editors or contributors for any injury and/or damage to persons or property as a matter of products liability, negligence or otherwise, or from any use or operation of any methods, products, instructions, or ideas contained in the material herein.

ISBN: 978-0-443-11571-4

Content Strategist: Trinity Hutton
Content Project Manager: Taranpreet Kaur
Design: Miles Hitchen
Marketing Manager: Deborah Watkins
Illustration Manager: Nijantha Priyadharshini

Printed in India

Last digit is the print number: 9   8   7   6   5   4   3   2   1

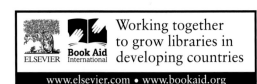

Working together to grow libraries in developing countries

www.elsevier.com • www.bookaid.org

Series editor's foreword

With great honour and pride, we present the latest edition of the *Crash Course* series. This series has traversed a journey of nearly a quarter-century, stemming from the vision of Dr. Dan Horton-Szar, and his legacy continues to walk with us on this pathway of knowledge.

The series has been popular with students worldwide, selling over **1 million copies** and being translated into more than **8 languages**, reinforcing our commitment to global learning.

We remain extremely grateful for your unwavering trust. The series has once again been refreshed and fully upgraded in accordance with the rapidly changing medical guidelines, ensuring the content is comprehensive, accurate and fully up-to-date.

This latest series continues our tradition of integrating clinical practice with basic medical sciences, tailored meticulously for today's medical undergraduate curriculum. A central highlight of this instalment is our emphasis on high-yield exam content designed specifically for the UKMLA curriculum.

The addition of the **Rapid UKMLA Index** at the beginning of the book enhances this offering, serving as a valuable aid to students to track their exam preparation efficiently. We have also revised all self-assessment questions to align with the single best answer format in line with the latest UKMLA examination style. We have also added *High-Yield Association Tables*. These are essential tools designed to aid students in recognizing clinical patterns and acing vignette-style exam questions. By condensing complex medical scenarios into digestible, manageable insights, these tables ensure efficient learning. They connect symptoms, diagnosis and treatment, bolstering understanding and confidence in tackling the rigorous UKMLA exams. This comprehensive approach makes these tables an indispensable asset in your exam preparations.

Utilizing student feedback, we have strived to maintain the core principles of this series: delivering precise and readable text that brings together depth and clarity. The authors are experienced junior doctors who successfully navigated these exams recently, ensuring practical and tested guidance. A team of expert faculty advisors from across the United Kingdom ensures the content's accuracy, making it resilient and reliable.

As we turn a new chapter with the latest edition, we honour the past, cherish the present, and embrace the promise of the future. We wish you every success in your journey of learning and growth and hope that this series adds value to your life, both as students and as future medical professionals.

Philip Xiu

Prefaces

Author

The creativity, problem solving, and innovation exemplified by the surgical specialities have been a source of endless fascination and my passion for many years. When revising for my own medical finals, I was surprised by the lack of comprehensive, high-quality resources for surgical content. This inspired and motivated me to produce exactly what I had been looking for.

Following a system-based approach, covering anatomy, physiology, history taking, differential diagnoses, examination, and essential diseases and disorders, this volume of Crash Course Surgery provides an all-in-one guide to acing surgical topics in written and practical medical finals. Integration of core anatomy and physiology provides readers with a solid foundation to appreciate the pathophysiology of disease. Incorporating differential diagnoses and relevant investigations, initial assessment and management flowcharts, and key radiological imaging aims to support the transition from student to doctor by providing a quick reference guide relevant to presenting complaints and conditions seen in clinical practice. An expanded, diversified self-assessment section finally ensures readers can determine they have the knowledge to feel confident assessing and managing surgical patients.

I hope this volume will be a valuable resource and will support others in pursuing their surgical careers.

Hester Lacey

Faculty advisor

The Crash Course series has been an essential handbook for doctors in training for many years and the latest edition brings together and integrates the rapid advances in medical research and drug development. Keeping the series relevant and engaging, whilst providing clear learning objectives, has always been and remains a key focus. Key aspects of learning for example communication skills and self-assessment tools are highlighted and the compact format allows students to dip in and out whilst providing sufficient depth of knowledge and detail for the series to be used as a comprehensive revision tool. We hope the balance between detail and ease of reference will allow the crash course series to be a valuable companion aid to success in future examinations.

Giles Davies

Acknowledgements

To Mum, Tom and Washington, for their love, support and unwavering belief. And to Phil, for being a fantastic mentor and taking a chance on me!

We would like to acknowledge the relatively large number of figures that have been included with permission in this book from Gray's Atlas of Anatomy 3e (ISBN: 9780323636391). We would like to express our sincere thanks to the authors of this leading anatomy atlas, Richard L. Drake, A. Wayne Vogl, Adam W. M. Mitchell, Richard Tibbets and Paul Richardson.

Hester Lacey

I would like to thank all my previous surgical mentors overs the years whose pearls of wisdom and friendship make the surgical community such a special place to be part of.

Giles Davies

Series editor's acknowledgement

We would like to express our sincere gratitude to those who have provided their support and expertise in preparing this fourth edition of the *Crash Course* series. Our junior doctor contributors' participation in crafting the manuscript has been indispensable. Their first-hand experience and current medical knowledge have infused realism and practicality into our content.

Our faculty editors deserve a special note of thanks. They have extensively validated the correctness of the information, ensuring that the content is not just accurate but also contemporaneous, credible, and aligns with the latest medical standards.

We extend our heartfelt thanks to our publisher, Elsevier. Their staff have demonstrated an unwavering commitment to quality, maintaining the high standards set since the first edition. Their insights have routinely enriched the content and process alike.

Our Commissioning Editor, Jeremy Bowes, deserves a special mention for his consistent support and guiding hand throughout the development process. His directions and advice have bettered this edition and spurred us on our quest for excellence.

We are greatly indebted to Alex Mortimer for her wisdom, practical insights and valuable guidance. A big thank you to our Content Strategists, Trinity Hutton and Cloe Holland-Borosh, who need special acknowledgement for meticulously outlining the direction and scope of the content. They've managed to mix details with a strategic plan, keeping our readers in mind.

Lastly, much gratitude is owed to our Content Product Managers, Taranpreet Kaur, Ayan Dhar, Shivani Pal and Tapajyoti Chaudhuri, who have juggled the numerous day-to-day tasks with utmost dedication and perseverance. Despite the ever-approaching deadlines, they have shown remarkable patience and steadfast determination, ensuring that each step of the book's development was accomplished seamlessly.

In conclusion, we sincerely thank each of these wonderful people for their outstanding contributions and support, without which this work wouldn't have been achieved. Their passion, commitment and collaborative effort have helped us bring this edition together.

Philip Xiu

Rapid UKMLA Index

The UKMLA Curriculum Conditions Priority levels have been based on the below:

Level 1: Conditions that a newly qualified doctor should have a good knowledge of and be able to recognise and manage.
Level 2: Conditions requiring knowledge for recognising and confirming diagnosis and planning first-line management in straightforward cases.
Level 3: Conditions where recognition of clinical presentation and describing principles of management are important.

Table 1 UKMLA Conditions and Where to Find Them

Priority List	UKMLA Conditions	Chapter	Page
3	Acid-base abnormality	Chapter 2: The lower gastrointestinal tract Chapter 4: Endocrine surgery	64, 75 106, 137, 142
1	Acne vulgaris	Chapter 9: Plastics and skin surgery	311
2	Acoustic neuroma	Chapter 8: Ear, nose and throat	262–267, 287–288, 290
3	Acute cholangitis	Chapter 1: The upper gastrointestinal tract	6–7, 16, 37, 41–43
1	Acute kidney injury	Chapter 7: Urology	213
1	Acute pancreatitis	Chapter 1: The upper gastrointestinal tract	6–10,13–14, 16–18, 31, 37, 41–49
1	Addison's disease	Chapter 4: Endocrine surgery	140–141
2	Alcoholic hepatitis	Chapter 1: The upper gastrointestinal tract	16–17
1	Allergic disorder	Chapter 8: Ear, nose and throat	269–270, 293–295
1	Anal fissure	Chapter 2: The lower gastrointestinal tract	54, 58, 62, 64–66, 70, 84–86
1	Anaphylaxis	Chapter 8: Ear, nose and throat	272
1	Aneurysms, ischaemic limb and occlusions	Chapter 6: Vascular surgery Chapter 10: Cardiothoracic surgery	180, 194–196, 198 338, 348–350
1	Aortic aneurysm	Chapter 6: Vascular surgery Chapter 10: Cardiothoracic surgery	171, 180, 194–198 338, 339, 348, 349, 352, 367
2	Aortic dissection	Chapter 6: Vascular surgery Chapter 10: Cardiothoracic surgery	182, 188, 189, 196, 198 335, 338, 339, 341, 348, 349, 351–353, 357, 358, 367
1	Aortic valve disease	Chapter 10: Cardiothoracic surgery	338, 339, 343, 345, 356–359, 368
1	Appendicitis	Chapter 2: The lower gastrointestinal tract	66–69, 88
1	Arrhythmias	Chapter 6: Vascular surgery Chapter 10: Cardiothoracic surgery	197, 200, 201 339, 341–342, 347, 355, 358

continued

Table 1 UKMLA Conditions and Where to Find Them—cont'd

continued

Table 1 UKMLA Conditions and Where to Find Them—cont'd

continued

Table 1 UKMLA Conditions and Where to Find Them—cont'd

Contents

Contents

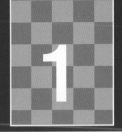

CLINICAL ANATOMY

The gastrointestinal tract (GIT) stretches from the mouth to the anus. The upper GIT includes structures from the mouth to the suspensory muscle of the duodenum, including includes the oesophagus, stomach, liver, biliary tract and pancreas.

The oesophagus is a muscular tube which carries food and liquids from the oropharynx to the gastric cardia (Fig. 1.1). The upper sphincter, at C6, prevents air entry into the GIT. The oesophagus crosses the diaphragm at T10, where the lower sphincter prevents the reflux of gastric contents and relaxes to allow passage of food into the stomach. The smooth muscle of the oesophagus transports food from the oropharynx to the stomach via peristalsis.

The stomach acts as a reservoir for ingested food (Fig. 1.2). The curvatures of the stomach attach to the greater and lesser omentum. Muscular stomach contractions churn and partially digest food before delivering it via the pyloric sphincter to the duodenum.

The liver lies in the right hypochondrium (Fig. 1.3). The liver is supplied by the right and left hepatic arteries and drained by the portal system. The falciform ligament attaches the liver to the anterior abdominal wall and divides the liver into right and left lobes. The right lobe divides further into the quadrate and the caudate lobe. The gallbladder lies on the visceral surface between the right and quadrate lobes (Fig. 1.4). The gallbladder receives bile from the liver, concentrates it and stores it before secreting it into the duodenum via the Sphincter of Oddi.

The pancreas is a retroperitoneal organ that lies posteriorly to the stomach and extends from the duodenum to the spleen (Fig. 1.5). Exocrine acinar glands release digestive enzymes into the duodenum, to aid protein digestion. The endocrine pancreatic islet cells are responsible for blood sugar regulation via secretion of insulin and glucagon.

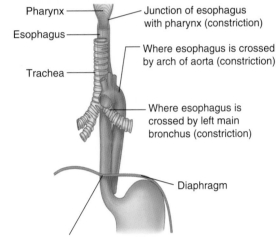

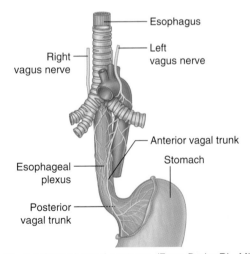

Fig. 1.1 Oesophageal anatomy. (From Drake RL, Mitchell AWM, Vogl AW. *Gray's Anatomy for Students Flash Cards,* 5th Edition. Elsevier; 2024.)

UPPER GASTROINTESTINAL PRESENTATIONS

History taking

Opening the consultation
Introduce yourself and confirm the patient's details.

Presenting complaint (PC)
Begin with an open question to identify the presenting complaint.

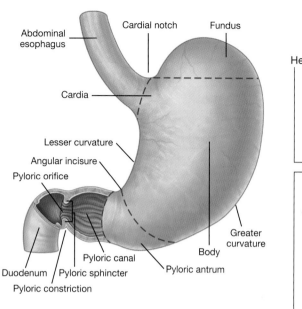

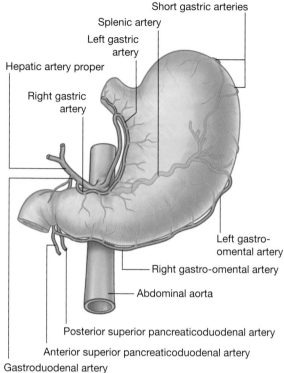

Fig. 1.2 Anatomy of the stomach. (From Vogl AW, Mitchell AWM, Drake RL. *Gray's Basic Anatomy*. Churchill Livingstone, Elsevier Inc. 2013.)

CLINICAL NOTES

- If the patient presents with pain, offer analgesia before taking the history.
- This will benefit the consultation and gain you marks for empathy in exams.

History of presenting complaint (HPC)

Explore the presenting complaint in more detail, using SOCRATES:

- Site: identify the location of the symptoms and whether this has changed over time.
- Onset: identify when the symptom started and whether it was sudden or gradual.
- Character: pain may be aching, sharp or burning in nature.
- Radiation: retroperitoneal pain radiates to the back, ureteric pain 'loin to groin' and diaphragmatic irritation may cause shoulder tip pain.
- Onset: When did the symptom start? Was it sudden or gradual?
- Character: ask the patient to describe the symptom in their own words.
- Radiation: assess whether the symptom moves anywhere else.
- Associated symptoms: screen for other symptoms of GIT pathology.

- Timing: assess whether symptoms are constant, come and go and how they have changed over time.
- Exacerbating and relieving factors: Does anything make the pain better or worse? The pain may be made worse with position or with movement, such as lying down. Food may exacerbate or relieve the pain. Identify if there are certain foods that make the pain better or worse.
- Severity – ask the patient to grade the pain on a scale of 1 to 10.

HINTS AND TIPS

The characteristics of pain can provide useful information for the diagnosis:

- Visceral pain is aching and poorly localized
- Peritoneal inflammation results in severe localized pain
- Organ rupture typically causes sudden onset, tearing pain
- Colicky pain is sharp and severe and intermittent with muscular spasms.
- Burning pain commonly relates to dyspepsia

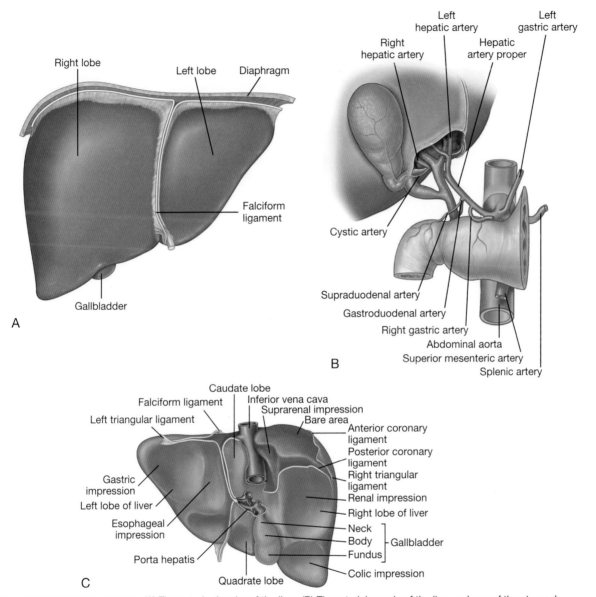

Fig. 1.3 Hepatobiliary anatomy. (A) The anterior border of the liver. (B) The arterial supply of the liver, pylorus of the stomach and gallbladder. (C) The posterior border of the liver. (From Vogl AW, Mitchell AWM, Drake RL. *Gray's Basic Anatomy*. Churchill Livingstone, Elsevier Inc. 2013.)

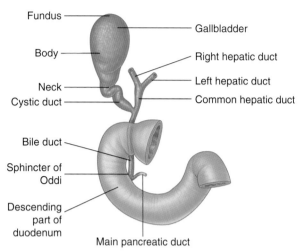

Fundus
Gallbladder
Body
Right hepatic duct
Neck
Left hepatic duct
Cystic duct
Common hepatic duct
Bile duct
Sphincter of Oddi
Descending part of duodenum
Main pancreatic duct

Fig. 1.4 The biliary tree. (From Vogl AW, Mitchell AWM, Drake RL. *Gray's Anatomy for Students An Instant Review*, 4th Edition - South Asia Edition. Elsevier; 2020.)

RED FLAG

There are several red flag features in upper GI histories that put patients at high risk for life-threatening causes:
- Severe, sudden onset pain
- Pain that wakes the patient from sleep
- Haematemesis or melaena
- Fever, jaundice, right upper quadrant pain
- Peritoneal signs – guarding and rigidity, rebound tenderness
- Haemodynamic instability
- Unintentional weight loss
- Rapidly progressive symptoms

Common presentations in upper GIT histories include:

- Acute abdominal pain: one of the most common presentations. The differential ranges from benign to life-threatening.

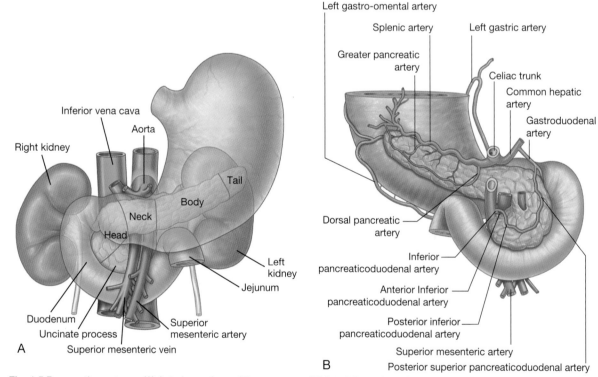

Inferior vena cava
Aorta
Right kidney
Tail
Body
Neck
Head
Left kidney
Jejunum
Duodenum
Uncinate process
Superior mesenteric artery
Superior mesenteric vein

A

Left gastro-omental artery
Splenic artery
Left gastric artery
Greater pancreatic artery
Celiac trunk
Common hepatic artery
Gastroduodenal artery
Dorsal pancreatic artery
Inferior pancreaticoduodenal artery
Anterior Inferior pancreaticoduodenal artery
Posterior inferior pancreaticoduodenal artery
Superior mesenteric artery
Posterior superior pancreaticoduodenal artery

B

Fig. 1.5 Pancreatic anatomy. (A) Anterior surface of the pancreas. (B) Arterial supply to the pancreas. (From Vogl AW, Mitchell AWM, Drake RL. *Gray's Basic Anatomy*. Churchill Livingstone, Elsevier Inc. 2013.)

- Dyspepsia: epigastric or retrosternal pain which radiates to the chest, associated with nausea, bloating, an acidic taste in the mouth and flatulence.
- Dysphagia: swallowing difficulty, which may be painful (odynophagia).
- Nausea and vomiting: very common, and often occur alongside other symptoms.
- Haematemesis, melaena and haematochezia: haematemesis describes vomit containing blood, melaena is the passage of partially digested blood in stool, and haematochezia is the passage of fresh blood per rectum respectively. All are indicators of upper gastrointestinal tract bleed (UGIB).
- Jaundice: the yellow discolouration of the skin associated with the deposition of bile pigments in the skin and sclera, indicating hepatobiliary pathology.

Systemic screen

A brief systemic screen should be performed to evaluate for associated symptoms.

HINTS AND TIPS

The mnemonic **FLAWS** can be used to screen for systemic features:
- **F** – Fever
- **L** – Lethargy
- **A** – Appetite loss
- **W** – Weight change
- **S** – Night sweats

Past medical history

Enquire about other medical conditions, past surgeries and any recent investigations or procedures that may be related to the underlying diagnosis.

Drug history

Document a complete drug history, and assess compliance, recent changes and over-the-counter medication use. It is essential to document allergy status.

CLINICAL NOTES

- A good drug history can provide invaluable diagnostic information.
- Many medications can cause nausea and vomiting.
- New prescriptions associated with symptoms may provide the diagnosis.
- Poor medication compliance may explain new or worsening symptoms of underlying disease.

Family history

Screen for conditions that run in the family and record the age of diagnosis.

Social history

Screen for risk factors in the social history

- Baseline functional status: to assess the impact of symptoms and ability to cope at home.
- Alcohol use: excess alcohol use is associated with gastric and hepatobiliary disease.
- Smoking: corrosive effects on the gastric mucosa make smoking a significant risk factor for GIT pathology. Record the number of pack years.
- Recreational drug use: intravenous drug use is associated with systemic illness and infective pathology.
- Diet and weight: obesity and high-fat diets increase the risk of GIT disease.
- Sexual history: assess for new sexual partners and unprotected sexual intercourse.

CLINICAL NOTES

- Alcoholism is often under-reported, particularly in the elderly.
- If there is evidence of problem drinking, screen for alcohol dependence using the **CAGE** mnemonic:
  - **C** – do you ever feel you need to cut down on your drinking?
  - **A** – does it annoy you when people comment on your drinking?
  - **G** – do you ever feel guilty about your drinking?
  - **E** – do you ever need an eye-opener to get you up in the morning?

HINTS AND TIPS

Sexual history, travel history, and alcohol and intravenous drug use, can help determine nonsurgical causes of jaundice.

Ideas, concerns and expectations

Eliciting the patient's ideas, concerns and expectations, to identify what they wanted to get out of the consultation, and any concerns you can address to alleviate anxiety.

Closing the consultation

Summarize the history back to the patient, answer any questions and thank them for their time.

DIFFERENTIAL DIAGNOSIS

Acute abdominal pain

The differential diagnosis of acute abdominal pain is guided by the location of the pain (Fig. 1.6).

CLINICAL NOTES

- Visceral pain can be poorly localized, and you should not discount a diagnosis based on location alone.
- An AAA can present with diffuse abdominal pain or localized pain in any abdominal area, with radiation to the flanks or groin.

Figs 1.7 and 1.8 outline the approach to the patient with acute abdominal pain.

RED FLAG

Immediately life-threatening causes of acute abdominal pain include:
- Aortic dissection
- Myocardial infarction
- Ruptured AAA
- Acute pancreatitis
- Acute cholangitis
- Acute upper GI bleeding
- Perforated peptic ulcer
- Appendicitis
- Acute mesenteric ischaemia
- Ruptured ectopic pregnancy

Investigations for acute abdominal pain

1. Bedside
   - Observations: to identify haemodynamic instability and evidence of infection.

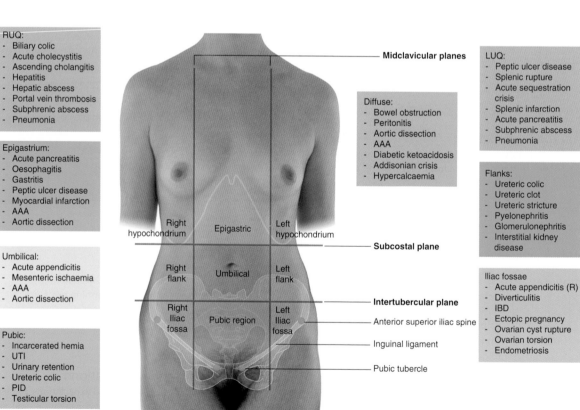

RUQ:
- Biliary colic
- Acute cholecystitis
- Ascending cholangitis
- Hepatitis
- Hepatic abscess
- Portal vein thrombosis
- Subphrenic abscess
- Pneumonia

Epigastrium:
- Acute pancreatitis
- Oesophagitis
- Gastritis
- Peptic ulcer disease
- Myocardial infarction
- AAA
- Aortic dissection

Umbilical:
- Acute appendicitis
- Mesenteric ischaemia
- AAA
- Aortic dissection

Pubic:
- Incarcerated hernia
- UTI
- Urinary retention
- Ureteric colic
- PID
- Testicular torsion

Diffuse:
- Bowel obstruction
- Peritonitis
- Aortic dissection
- AAA
- Diabetic ketoacidosis
- Addisonian crisis
- Hypercalcaemia

LUQ:
- Peptic ulcer disease
- Splenic rupture
- Acute sequestration crisis
- Splenic infarction
- Acute pancreatitis
- Subphrenic abscess
- Pneumonia

Flanks:
- Ureteric colic
- Ureteric clot
- Ureteric stricture
- Pyelonephritis
- Glomerulonephritis
- Interstitial kidney disease

Iliac fossae:
- Acute appendicitis (R)
- Diverticulitis
- IBD
- Ectopic pregnancy
- Ovarian cyst rupture
- Ovarian torsion
- Endometriosis

Midclavicular planes

Subcostal plane

Intertubercular plane

Anterior superior iliac spine

Inguinal ligament

Pubic tubercle

Right hypochondrium — Epigastric — Left hypochondrium

Right flank — Umbilical — Left flank

Right Iliac fossa — Pubic region — Left Iliac fossa

Fig. 1.6 The abdominal regions. (From Mitchell AWM, Vogl AW, Drake RL. *Gray's Anatomy for Students*, 5th Edition. Elsevier; 2024.)

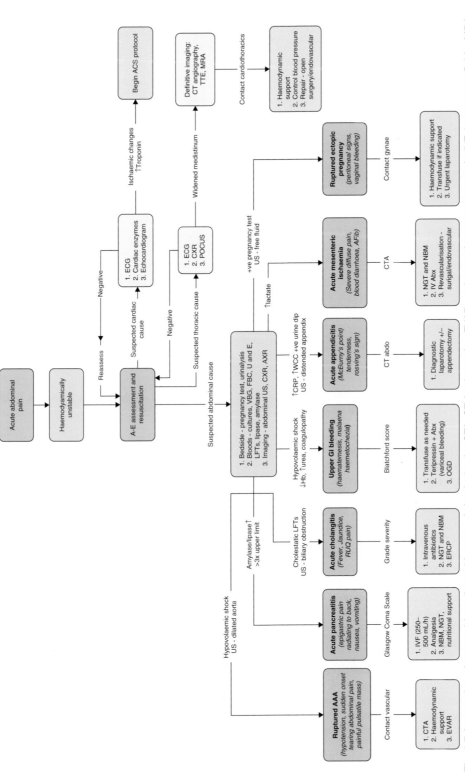

Fig. 1.7 Approach to the unstable patient with acute abdominal pain. *CTA*, CT Angiography; *CTA*, CT Angiography; *EVAR*, endovascular aneurysm repair; *IVF*, intravenous fluids; *MRA*, magnetic resonance angiography; *NGT*, nasogastric tube; *NBM*, nil by mouth; *OGD*, oesophagogastroduodenoscopy; *POCUS*, point-of-care ultrasound; *TTE*, transthoracic echocardiogram; *TVUSS*, transvaginal ultrasound.

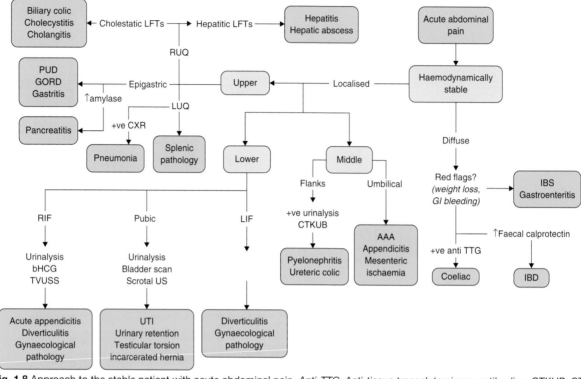

Fig. 1.8 Approach to the stable patient with acute abdominal pain. *Anti-TTG*, Anti-tissue transglutaminase antibodies; *CTKUB*, CT kidneys, ureters, bladder; *TVUSS*, transvaginal ultrasound.

- ECG: ischaemic changes indicate acute coronary syndrome (ACS) or thoracic pathology.
- Urinalysis: +ve for leukocytes, nitrites, in urinary tract infection (UTI) or pyelonephritis. Often abnormal in appendicitis.
- Pregnancy test: indicated in any female of childbearing age. +ve pregnancy test, abdominal pain and vaginal bleeding suggest ectopic pregnancy.
- Capillary blood glucose (CBG): hyperglycaemia may indicate diabetic ketoacidosis (DKA). Hypoglycaemia is associated with Addison disease.
- Stool sample: ↑ faecal calprotectin indicates inflammatory bowel disease (IBD). *Clostridium difficile* - toxin should be tested for in profuse watery diarrhoea and abdominal pain.

2. Bloods
- Blood cultures: to assess for abdominal sepsis.
- VBG: ↑ lactate indicates sepsis or mesenteric ischaemia.
- FBC: ↑WCC is associated with infection. Anaemia indicates acute or chronic blood loss.
- U&E: ↑ Urea/creatinine indicate acute kidney injury (AKI). Urea may be raised in acute UGIB.

- LFTs: ↑ALT/AST and ALP/γGT indicate hepatobiliary pathology.
- Amylase/Lipase: ↑in acute pancreatitis.
- Clotting: there may be coagulopathy in acute and chronic liver disease. May be deranged in acute UGIB.
- Bone profile: hypercalcemia can cause ureteric calculi and pancreatitis and may indicate underlying malignancy. Hypocalcaemia is a complication of pancreatitis.
- Group and Save: two samples to be sent to prepare for surgery.
- Troponin: ↑ in ACS

COMMON PITFALLS

Amylase is a useful marker for pancreatitis, however, is not specific and may be raised in other conditions including bowel obstruction, perforated peptic ulcer or DKA.

3. Imaging
    - Abdominal ultrasound (US): may show biliary or ureteral dilation, intraabdominal masses or aneurysms.
    - Chest X-ray (CXR): pneumoperitoneum indicates bowel perforation. Consolidation may be evident in lower lobe pneumonia.
    - Abdominal X-ray (AXR): dilated loops of bowel indicate obstruction. A volvulus presents with a classic 'coffee bean' sign. Thumb printing and lead pipe colon indicate IBD. Renal stones may be radiopaque.
    - Computed tomography (CT): for detailed examination of masses, aneurysms, perforations and retroperitoneal structures.
    - Magnetic resonance cholangiopancreatography (MRCP): used to visualize the biliary tree in patients unsuitable for endoscopic retrograde cholangiopancreatography (ERCP).
    - Oesophagogastroduodenoscopy (OGD): to diagnose and treat bleeding peptic ulcers or varices.
    - ERCP: to allow visualization of the biliary tree and treatment of obstruction.

COMMON PITFALLS

- Approximately 30% of acute perforations are not evident on an erect chest radiograph.
- The absence of pneumoperitoneum does not exclude the diagnosis.
- Beware of a silent perforation in the elderly and patients on corticosteroids.

Chronic abdominal pain

Chronic abdominal pain has a range of aetiologies (Fig. 1.9).

Investigations for chronic abdominal pain
1. Bedside
    - Weight: weight changes may point towards a diagnosis of peptic ulcer disease (PUD) or abdominal malignancy.
    - Stool sample: ↑faecal calprotectin in IBD.
2. Bloods
    - FBC: anaemia secondary to chronic UGIB can occur in PUD or malignancy.
    - U&E: ↑Urea/creatinine indicates AKI. Chronic diarrhoea in IBS, coeliac disease, IBD and chronic pancreatitis may result in ↓K.
    - LFTs: cholestatic picture (↑ALP/γGT) indicates biliary pathology or pancreatic cancer.

- Anti-TTG antibodies: ↑ in coeliac disease.
3. Imaging
    - Abdominal US: first line to assess biliary tree pathology, abdominal ascites or characterize abdominal masses.
    - AXR: may demonstrate bowel obstruction. A calcified pancreas or ureteric stones may be radiopaque.
    - OGD: to detect and treat PUD.
    - Colonoscopy: to detect IBD and colon cancer.

CLINICAL NOTES

Colonoscopy findings of Crohn disease include:
- Skip lesions
- Cobblestoning
- Deep ulcerations
Colonoscopy findings of ulcerative colitis include:
- Oedema
- Superficial erythema
- A 'starry sky' appearance of profuse shallow ulcers

Dyspepsia

The differential diagnosis of dyspepsia should consider the timing of dyspepsia, its relationship with food and associated abdominal pain (Fig. 1.10).

HINTS AND TIPS

Assess symptoms in relation to food (i.e., spicy foods, tomatoes, caffeine, chocolate), and position (i.e., lying flat).

Investigations for dyspepsia
1. Bedside
    - ECG: may detect ischaemic changes in underlying ACS.
    - Weight: weight changes may indicate PUD or malignancy.
    - Helicobacter pylori (H. pylori) testing: via urea breath test or stool sample, to diagnose the cause of gastro-oesophageal reflux disease (GORD) or PUD.
2. Bloods
    - FBC: anaemia suggests UGIB
    - U&Es: ↑Urea/creatinine indicates AKI which may be related to associated vomiting or diarrhoea.
    - LFTs: biliary pathology can cause dyspepsia.
    - Troponin: ↑ in ACS.

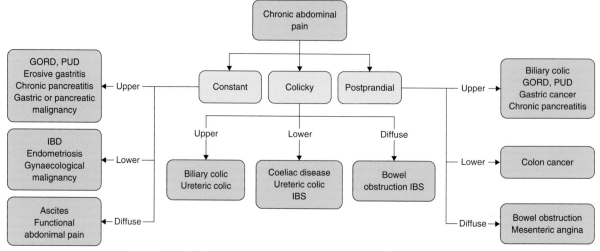

Fig. 1.9 Differential diagnosis of chronic abdominal pain. *PUD*, Peptic ulcer disease.

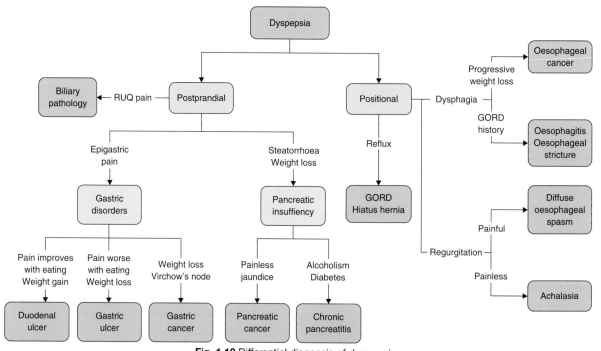

Fig. 1.10 Differential diagnosis of dyspepsia.

3. Imaging
   - Barium swallow: to detect oesophageal strictures or cancer, hiatal hernias, GORD and oesophageal motility disorders that may cause dyspepsia.
   - OGD: to detect PUD, Barrett's oesophagus or oesophageal perforation, or malignancy. CLO testing for H. pylori can be performed, which provides an immediate diagnosis.
   - Oesophageal manometry: to assess for oesophageal dysmotility.
   - Abdominal US: to detect biliary tree dilatation or gallbladder inflammation.

RED FLAG

ALARMS symptoms are red flag features of dyspepsia and should raise suspicion of underlying malignancy:
- **A**naemia
- **L**oss of weight and anorexia
- **A**ge (>50 years)
- **R**ecent onset/rapidly progressive symptoms
- **M**elaena/haematemesis (signs of UGIB)
- **S**wallowing difficulties (dysphagia)

Dysphagia

Dysphagia is a complex symptom and a red flag for serious pathology (Fig. 1.11).

CLINICAL NOTES

Associated symptoms may include:
- Effortless or painful regurgitation
- Halitosis (bad breath)
- Dyspepsia
- Breathlessness, cough or chest pain
- Fatigue and weight loss
  Progressive dysphagia will affect solid foods first, then softer foods and finally liquids.

Investigations for dysphagia
1. Bedside
   - Weight: associated weight loss indicates severe, clinically significant dysphagia.
   - Sputum sample: aspiration pneumonia from atypical organisms can develop related to dysphagia.
2. Bloods
   - FBC: anaemia indicates occult UGIB, associated with malignancy.
   - TFTs: a large goitre can compress the oesophagus and result in dysphagia.
3. Imaging
   - OGD: for direct visualization of structural abnormalities or mucosal lesions.
   - Barium swallow: to detect motility disorders and characterize structural abnormalities.
   - Oesophageal manometry: evaluates the peristaltic function of the oesophagus during swallowing, to diagnose oesophageal motility disorders.
   - CXR: lobar consolidation indicates aspiration pneumonia.

- CT head: ischaemic or haemorrhagic stroke may present with acute dysphagia and unilateral focal neurology.
- CT thorax: if external oesophageal compression is suspected.

Nausea and vomiting

Nausea is exceedingly common and can relate to systemic or gastrointestinal disease (Fig. 1.12).

CLINICAL NOTES

Determine the number and frequency of episodes, colour and contents of vomit, timing and relationship to eating, and associated appetite loss.

Nausea and vomiting can be associated with several acutely life-threatening conditions, and red flag symptoms warrant urgent investigation and management (Fig. 1.13).

RED FLAG

A triad of profuse, repeated vomiting, severe retrosternal pain and surgical emphysema are red flag features for oesophageal perforation.

Investigations for nausea and vomiting
1. Bedside
   - Observations: hypotension and tachycardia relate to hypovolaemic shock, and fever may indicate systemic infection.
   - ECG: ischaemic changes suggest ACS.
   - Urinalysis: may be abnormal in acute appendicitis. Urinary ketones suggest DKA.
   - CBG: hyperglycaemia associated with vomiting suggests DKA or hyperosmolar hyperglycaemic state (HHS).
   - Stool sample: may detect organisms in infective gastroenteritis.
   - H. pylori testing: indicated in cases of suspected GORD and PUD.
   - Pregnancy test: an important differential in females of childbearing age!
2. Bloods
   - Blood cultures: in febrile, acutely unwell patients, to identify sepsis.
   - VBG: ↑ lactate suggests sepsis, DKA or bowel ischaemia. Significant vomiting can result in hypochloraemic hypokalaemic metabolic alkalosis.

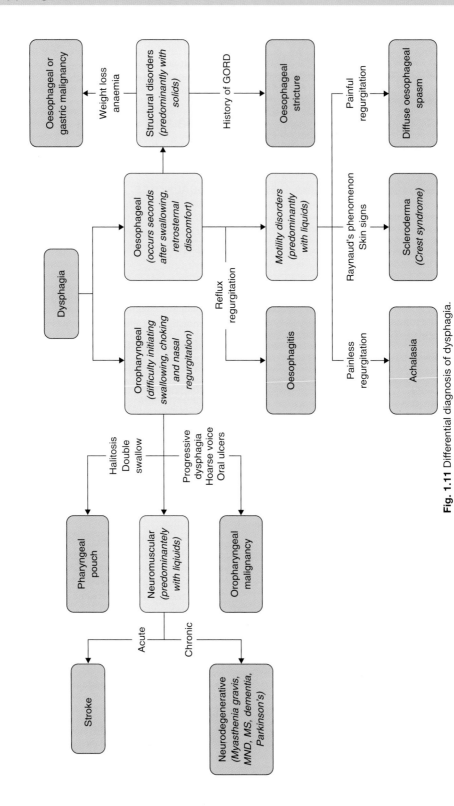

Fig. 1.11 Differential diagnosis of dysphagia.

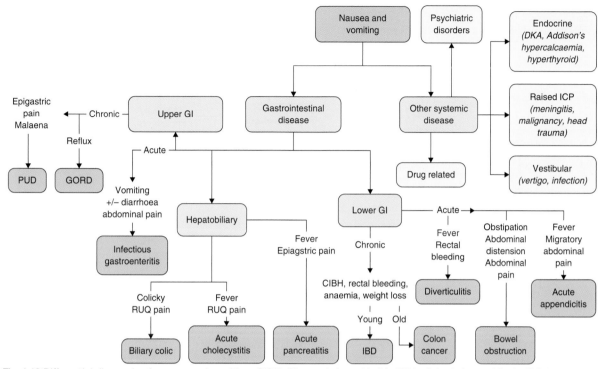

Fig. 1.12 Differential diagnosis of nausea and vomiting. *CIBH*, Change in bowel habit; *DKA*, diabetic ketoacidosis; *ICP*, intracranial pressure.

- FBC: ↑WCC indicates infection or inflammation. Anaemia may suggest associated UGIB in malignancy or PUD.
- U&Es: ↑ urea/creatinine indicates prerenal AKI in severe vomiting.
- LFTs: may be deranged in hepatobiliary pathology.
- Amylase/lipase: ↑ suggests acute pancreatitis, PUD or bowel obstruction.
- Bone profile: hypercalcemia is associated with nausea and vomiting, related to malignancy, parathyroid or renal pathology.
- TFTs: thyrotoxicosis can result in nausea and vomiting.
3. Imaging
   - AXR: may demonstrate small or large bowel obstruction.
   - OGD: indicated to diagnose and treat oesophageal and gastric pathology.
   - Abdominal US/CT: to diagnose abdominal pathology including pancreatitis, hepatobiliary pathology and appendicitis.
   - ERCP/MRCP: to diagnose and treat hepatobiliary pathology.
   - Colonoscopy: if there is suspicion of colonic malignancy or IBD.

Further imaging can be considered if intracranial pathology or systemic malignancy is suspected.

There are several treatment options for nausea. Tailoring the choice of antiemetic to the likely differential can result in rapid and effective relief of symptoms (Table 1.1).

COMMON PITFALLS

- Metoclopramide is prokinetic, and contraindicated in small bowel obstruction.
- Caution in diabetes, due to the effects of increased stomach emptying on blood sugar.
- Antidopaminergic effects mean it should be avoided in combination with antipsychotics, due to the risk of extrapyramidal side effects.

Haematemesis and melaena

Haematemesis may be bright red, indicating brisk GIT bleeding or partially digested, described as 'coffee ground' vomiting. Melaena is the passage of blood per rectum, characterized by offensive-smelling, black, tarry stool (Fig. 1.14).

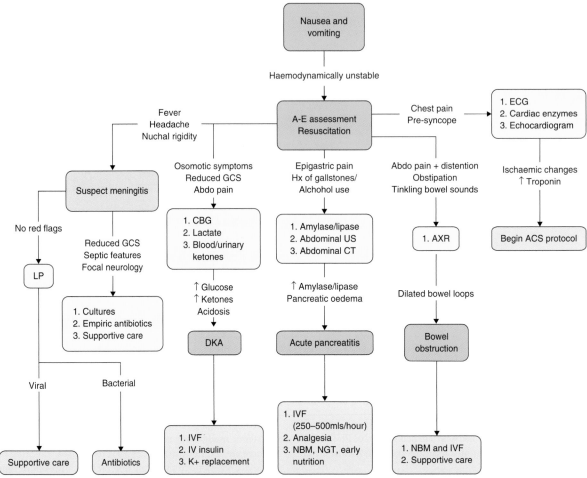

Fig. 1.13 Approach to the unstable patient with nausea and vomiting. *ACS*, Acute coronary syndrome; *CBG*, capillary blood glucose; *GCS*, Glasgow Coma Scale; *IVF*, intravenous fluids; *NGT*, nasogastric tube.

Table 1.1 Classes of antiemetics and their indications

Drug	Class	Indications	Side-effects
Metoclopramide	Dopamine receptor antagonist	Gastroparesis – aids gastric emptying	GI upset Reduced seizure threshold EPS/NMS
Prochlorperazine		Vestibular nausea	
Domperidone		Nausea and vomiting in Parkinson disease	GI upset Hyperprolactinaemia
Ondansetron	5-HT3 antagonist	Chemotherapy-induced nausea, postoperative nausea and vomiting	QT interval prolongation Serotonin syndrome
Cyclizine	H1 antagonist	Vestibular nausea	Sedating Anticholinergic effects
Dexamethasone	Glucocorticoid	Chemotherapy-induced nausea, postoperative nausea and vomiting	Cushing syndrome Hyperglycaemia

EPS, Extrapyramidal side effects; NMS, neuroleptic malignant syndrome.

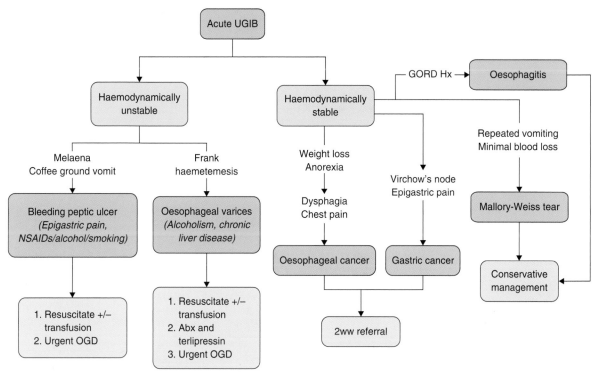

Fig. 1.14 Approach to the patient with acute UGIB. *OGD*, Oesophagogastroduodenoscopy.

CLINICAL NOTES

- The Blatchford score should be used to risk stratify prior to endoscopy.
- The Rockall score is used to determine the risk of rebleeding after endoscopy, and suitability for early discharge.

RED FLAG

- An acute UGIB is a surgical emergency.
- Urgent assessment and resuscitation is required with treatment initiated to prevent further blood loss.
- In stable patients with UGIB or new anaemia, be suspicious for underlying malignancy.

Investigations for UGIB

1. Bedside
   - Observations: acute blood loss will present with tachycardia and hypotension.
   - ECG: to exclude cardiac causes of epigastric/chest pain, tachycardia and hypotension.

2. Bloods
   - FBC and clotting: anaemia and coagulopathy occur with severe bleeds.
   - U&Es: ↑urea relates to partial digestion of blood proteins. Significant blood loss can cause AKI.
   - LFTs: liver disease can increase the risk of varices and coagulopathy.
   - G&S and CXM: two separate group and save samples should be sent to prepare for transfer to theatre. In acute bleeds, cross-matching up to six units of blood is appropriate.

3. Imaging
   - OGD: the gold standard diagnostic and therapeutic intervention for acute UGIB. Diagnostic biopsies can be done for malignancy, and haemostasis can be achieved using cautery, banding or clipping in variceal bleeding or bleeding peptic ulcers.

Jaundice

The approach to the patient with jaundice should be guided by the pattern of abnormality on liver function tests, which can help establish whether pathology is prehepatic, hepatic or posthepatic (Fig. 1.15).

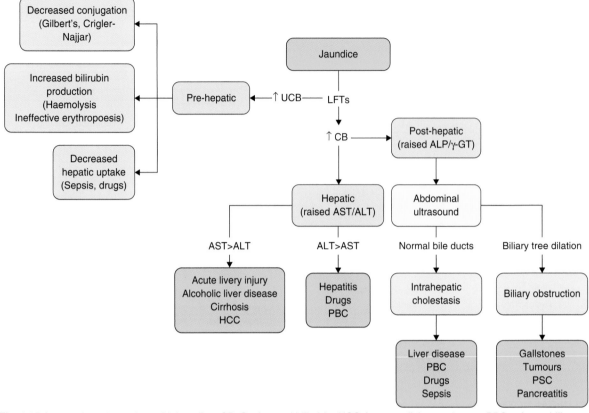

Fig. 1.15 Approach to the patient with jaundice. *CB*, Conjugated bilirubin; *HCC*, hepatocellular carcinoma; *PBC*, primary biliary cirrhosis; *PSC*, primary sclerosing cholangitis; *UCB*, unconjugated bilirubin.

CLINICAL NOTES

- Jaundice may be insidious or acute in onset.
- Associated symptoms including RUQ pain, pyrexia, pruritus, dark urine, pale stools and flu-like symptoms guide the likely diagnosis.

Investigations for jaundice

1. Bedside
   - Observations: acute pancreatitis or cholangitis can cause sepsis, presenting with pyrexia, hypotension and tachycardia.
   - Urinalysis: ↑urinary bilirubin suggests conjugated bilirubinaemia in hepatic or posthepatic pathology. Haemoglobinuria may be present in prehepatic jaundice.
   - Pregnancy test: cholestasis of pregnancy can cause jaundice.

2. Bloods
   - Blood cultures: indicated in suspected intra-abdominal sepsis.
   - VBG: ↑ lactate suggests sepsis.
   - FBC: anaemia may indicate acute haemolysis or bleeding. ↑ WCC indicates infection.
   - LFTs: ↑bilirubin is diagnostic of jaundice. ↑ AST/ALT suggests a hepatic cause, and ALP/γ-GT a cholestatic cause (Table 1.2).
   - Clotting screen: coagulopathy can relate to liver.
   - Albumin: hypoalbuminemia indicates acute or chronic liver disease.
   - Amylase/lipase: ↑ in acute pancreatitis, which can cause jaundice or result from biliary tree obstruction.
   - Hepatitis serology: to screen for viral hepatitis.
   - Autoimmune screen: to assess for antismooth muscle, antimitochondrial and antinuclear antibodies, implicated in autoimmune hepatitis, primary biliary cirrhosis (PBC) and primary sclerosing cholangitis (PSC), respectively.

Table 1.2 Investigation findings for jaundice

Test	Prehepatic jaundice	Hepatic jaundice	Posthepatic jaundice
Unconjugated bilirubin	↑↑	↑	Normal
Conjugated bilirubin	Normal	↑	↑↑
AST/ALT	Normal	↑ ↑↑ in alcoholic hepatitis (AST/ALT >2)	Normal
ALP	Normal	↑	↑↑
γ-GT	Normal	↑ ↑↑ in alcoholic hepatitis	↑↑
Urinary bilirubin	Normal	↑	↑↑
Urinary urobilinogen	↑↑	Normal of ↑	↓
Urine colour	Normal Dark in haemoglobinuria	Normal or dark	Dark
Stool colour	Dark	Normal, dark or pale	Pale

- Tumour markers: CA 19-9 can be raised in pancreatic cancer or cholangiocarcinoma, which cause painless jaundice.
3. Imaging
   - Abdominal US: to diagnose biliary tree pathology, liver parenchymal disease or abdominal masses.
   - ERCP: diagnostic and therapeutic in biliary pathology, with stone removal or stent placement in strictures or external compression.
   - MRCP: to diagnose biliary pathology in patients unsuitable for ERCP.
   - Abdominal CT: for detailed assessment of intra-abdominal masses.
   - Liver biopsy: for detailed assessment of liver disease in alcoholic liver disease (ALD), cirrhosis and hepatocellular carcinoma (HCC).

THE ABDOMINAL EXAM

Gather appropriate equipment and prepare for the examination.

HINTS AND TIPS

The acronym **WIPER** can be used to prepare for an examination:
- **W**ash your hands
- **I**ntroduce yourself
- **P**atient details
- **E**xplain the procedure and **E**xpose appropriately
- **R**eposition patient

General inspection

Inspect from the end of the bed, to assess for clues as to the underlying pathology:

- Pain: there may be obvious pain. Ensure they are comfortable and offer analgesia where possible.
- Pallor: may suggest anaemia relating to acute or chronic blood loss or malnutrition.
- Dehydration: demonstrated by reduced skin turgor, and dry mucous membranes.
- Jaundice: yellow pigmentation to the skin or sclera suggests hepatobiliary or pancreatic pathology.
- Cachexia: pathological muscle wasting, suspicious of malignancy.
- Restlessness/agitation: commonly seen in gastrointestinal or ureteric colic.
- Still: peritonitic patients will be still, with movement exacerbating the pain.
- Sitting forward: may suggest retroperitoneal pathology.
- Equipment: mobility aids, medications and medical devices including feeding tubes, stoma bags or surgical drains can offer hints as to the underlying diagnosis.

Observations

- Temperature: pyrexia indicates acute infection. In significant shock, relating to blood loss, peritonitis or pancreatitis, patients may be hypothermic.
- Respiratory rate: rapid, shallow breathing may indicate sepsis or peritonitis.
- Blood pressure: hypotension can relate to haemorrhage, shock or interstitial fluid losses in peritonitis.
- Pulse: tachycardia can relate to hypotension or sepsis.

- SpO$_2$%: hypoxia can occur in severe pancreatitis, liver failure or sepsis.

Peripheral examination

Hands and arms
Clinical signs in the hands can suggest underlying abdominal pathology.

- Radial pulse: assess the rate and rhythm.
- Clubbing: loss of the angle between the nail and the nail bed can relate to IBD, coeliac disease or cirrhosis.
- Koilonychia: spooning of the nails associated with anaemia and malabsorption.
- Leukonychia: whitening of the nail bed associated with hypoalbuminemia in chronic liver disease (CLD).
- Palmar erythema: related to elevated oestrogen levels in pregnancy or CLD.
- Dupuytren's contracture: thickening of the palmar fascia seen in alcoholism, diabetes and CLD.
- Asterixis: flapping tremor seen in CLD due to hyperammonaemia.
- Bruising/excoriations: bruising in the arm and excoriations may suggest clotting abnormalities and pruritis in CLD or cholestasis. Needle track marks may indicate IVDU.
- Acanthosis nigricans: darkening of the axillary skin associated with insulin resistance and gastric cancer. Axillary hair loss can indicate anaemia and malnutrition.

Face and neck
Examine the face, neck and chest for further signs of abdominal pathology

- Conjunctival pallor: suggests anaemia, and scleral icterus underlying cholestasis.
- Angular stomatitis: irritation of the corners of the mouth that can occur with iron deficiency anaemia, malabsorption or GI malignancy.
- Glossitis: smooth enlargement of the tongue associated with malabsorption.
- Aphthous ulcers: signs of nutritional deficiencies or Crohn disease.
- Cervical lymphadenopathy: associated with malignancy. Trosier's sign is an enlarged Virchow's node in the left supraclavicular fossa, associated with gastric cancer.
- Spider naevi: >5 spider naevi is associated with CLD.
- Gynaecomastia: can result from impaired oestrogen metabolism in CLD.

CLINICAL NOTES

Stigmata of chronic liver disease are related to the underlying metabolic disturbance:

- Impaired bilirubin metabolism – jaundice, pruritis
- Portal hypertension – hepatomegaly, splenomegaly, ascites, caput medusa and peripheral oedema
- Elevated oestrogen – gynecomastia, spider naevi, palmar erythema
- Elevated ammonia – hepatic encephalopathy, asterixis
- Hypoalbuminemia – leukonychia, peripheral oedema
- Coagulopathy – bleeding and bruising

Examination of the abdomen

Inspection
Inspect the abdomen carefully for:

- Scars: may indicate previous operations, increasing the risk of adhesions and bowel obstruction.
- Distention: relating to the 6 Fs – fat, fluids, flatus, faeces, fetus or fulminant masses.
- Hernias: irreducible or strangulated hernias can cause pain and small bowel obstruction.
- Pulsatility: prominent abdominal pulsations may suggest abdominal aortic aneurysm.
- Movement: the still patient with shallow breathing indicates peritonitis.
- Bruising: Cullen's (umbilical) and Grey Turner's (flank) bruising are associated with haemorrhagic pancreatitis.
- Caput medusae: distended paraumbilical veins associated with portal hypertension.
- Stomas: colostomies are flush to the skin and contain solid stool. Ileostomies and urostomies are spouted. Ileostomies contain liquid stool and urostomies contain urine.

COMMON PITFALLS

- Location should not be relied upon to determine the type of stoma.
- Inspecting the contents and for the presence of a spout are more reliable methods of determining stoma type.

Palpation

Position the patient lying flat. Lightly palpate the nine abdominal regions, assessing for clinical signs of abdominal pathology. Examine areas of pain last.

- Tenderness: monitor the patient's facial expressions. Pain may indicate local pathology in the associated abdominal region.
- Rebound tenderness: sharp abdominal pain upon release of pressure on the abdomen. A sign of peritonitis.
- Guarding: involuntary muscle spasm indicating underlying peritoneal irritation.
- Rovsing's sign: palpation of the left iliac fossa causing pain in the right iliac fossa, associated with appendicitis.
- Masses: large or superficial masses such as hernias may be palpable.

Deep palpation follows light palpation. Characterize any masses identified:

- Location: which abdominal quadrant.
- Size and shape.
- Consistency: smooth, irregular, hard or soft.
- Mobility: free or tethered to underlying structures.
- Pulsatility: a pulsatile mass suggests an aneurysm.

Palpation of the abdominal organs:

- Liver: assess for hepatomegaly by systematically palpating from the right iliac fossa to the right upper quadrant, feeling for a liver edge when palpating on deep inspiration.
- Gallbladder: biliary pathology can cause gallbladder enlargement. Assess for Murphy's sign by palpating the gallbladder, and asking the patient to take a deep breath in. Sudden cessation of breathing with inspiration suggests gallbladder inflammation.
- Spleen: assess for splenomegaly by systematically palpating from the right iliac fossa to the right upper quadrant, feeling for the splenic notch on deep inspiration.
- Kidneys: ballot the kidneys by placing one hand behind the flank on the patient's back and one hand just below the costal margin on the same side. Push your hands together to assess for enlargement of the lower pole of the kidney as the patient breathes in.
- Aorta: palpate the aorta just above the umbilicus. The aorta should feel pulsatile, but not expansile. An expansile aorta suggests an AAA.
- Bladder: palpate the suprapubic area to assess for urinary obstruction or retention.

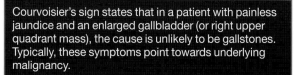

RED FLAG

Courvoisier's sign states that in a patient with painless jaundice and an enlarged gallbladder (or right upper quadrant mass), the cause is unlikely to be gallstones. Typically, these symptoms point towards underlying malignancy.

Percussion

Hepatomegaly, splenomegaly and a distended bladder will have a dull percussion note.

Shifting dullness

Ascites can be detected by identifying shifting dullness:

- Percuss the abdomen from the umbilicus to the flank.
- If an area with a dull percussion note is reached, this suggests abdominal fluid.
- Locate the area of dullness and ask the patient to turn to the opposite side.
- If the same area now has a resonant percussion note, this indicates fluid has shifted with the effects of gravity, suggesting free fluid in the abdomen.

Auscultation

Auscultate for bowel sounds:

- Hyperactive: increased intestinal activity, such as diarrhoea.
- Absent: obstruction or generalized ileus in peritonitis.
- Tinkling: bowel obstruction.

Auscultate the aorta and iliac arteries to detect bruits, associated with aneurysms and vascular disease.

Completing the examination

Wash your hands, thank the patient for their time and summarize your findings.

Further tests include:

- Digital rectal examination: to diagnose faecal impaction or assess for rectal bleeding.
- External genitalia: to assess for genitourinary pathology related to abdominal symptoms.
- Hernial orifices: a complete hernia exam is indicated if there is evidence of hernias.

OESOPHAGEAL DISORDERS

Gastro-oesophageal reflux disease

GORD is a chronic condition where reflux of the stomach contents into the oesophagus results in irritation to the oesophageal mucosa. It is common, affecting up to 20% of the population each year. It results from inappropriate relaxation of the lower oesophageal sphincter (LES), increased intragastric pressure, or anatomical abnormalities. Risk factors include smoking, caffeine and alcohol consumption, obesity, pregnancy and drugs that reduce the LES pressure, including CCBs, anticholinergics, benzodiazepines and nitrates. There is a wide differential diagnosis of the underlying aetiology, including oesophageal, gastric and biliary disorders (Fig 1.16).

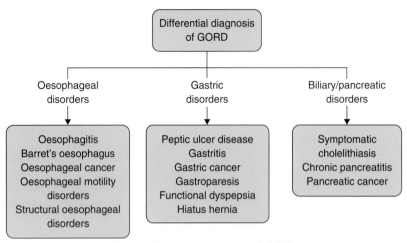

Fig. 1.16 Differential diagnosis of GORD.

Symptoms and signs

Symptoms include:

- Dyspepsia (heartburn)
- Regurgitation of acid into the mouth
- Epigastric pain
- Nausea +/– vomiting
- Halitosis
- Belching, bloating, excessive flatus (flatulent dyspepsia)
- Dysphagia

Symptoms are typically exacerbated by lying down after eating or heavy, spicy or fatty foods.

RED FLAG

Red flags in GORD histories that warrant a 2-week referral include ALARMS:

- A – Aged over 55
- L – Loss of appetite and weight
- A – Anaemia
- R – Recent onset or rapidly progressive symptoms
- M – Melaena or haematemesis
- S – Swallowing difficulties (dysphagia and odynophagia)

Investigations

Relevant investigations include:

- H. pylori testing: H. pylori is a gram-negative aerobic bacterium that lives in the stomach, and erodes the mucosal lining of the stomach, exposing the epithelium to the stomach acid, resulting in gastritis and ulcers. Testing can be done using a stool test or urea breath test.
- Barium swallow: to diagnose structural lesions including strictures or malignancy.
- OGD: for patients with red flag features, to diagnose oesophagitis, ulcers or malignancy, and take tissue biopsies for histology.

Management

Management involves testing and treating for H. pylori, and acid-reducing therapies (Fig. 1.17, Table 1.3).

Surgical options for refractory symptoms include:

- Fundoplication: the proximal stomach is wrapped around the LES, increasing sphincter pressure and preventing reflux.
- Dilation and stenting: to treat fibrotic or compressive strictures.

Complications

Complications related to the chronic irritation and inflammation of the oesophageal mucosa:

- Oesophagitis: inflammation, ulceration and bleeding of the oesophageal mucosa.
- Stricture: healed oesophagitis can develop into a fibrotic stricture, resulting in dysphagia (Fig. 1.18).
- Barrett's oesophagus: premalignant metaplasia of the oesophageal epithelium from squamous to columnar epithelium, which may progress to dysplasia and malignant change.

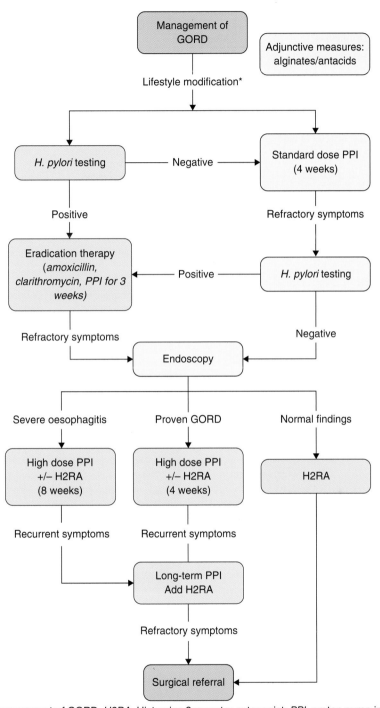

Fig. 1.17 Approach to management of GORD. *H2RA*, Histamine 2 receptor antagonist; *PPI*, proton pump inhibitor. *Lifestyle changes include weight loss for overweight people; smoking cessation for tobacco smokers; head-of-bed-elevation; and avoidance of late-night eating if nocturnal symptoms are present.

Table 1.3 Different acid-reducing therapies

Medication	Drug class	Mechanism	Side effects
Omeprazole Lansoprazole Pantoprazole	Proton-pump inhibitor	Bind to and inhibit the hydrogen-potassium ATPase pump that resides on parietal cell, blocking gastric acid secretion	Short term – GI upset Long term – nutritional deficiencies, hyponatremia hypocalcaemia, osteoporosis, chronic kidney disease, *Clostridium difficile* infections.
Famotidine	H2-receptor antagonist	Bind to histamine H2 receptors located on gastric parietal cells, competitively inhibiting histamine binding and decreasing gastric acid secretion	Headache, dizziness, constipation, diarrhoea
Sodium alginate	Alginate	Forms a protective layer that floats on top of the stomach contents of your stomach, preventing reflux into the oesophagus	GI upset
Calcium carbonate, magnesium carbonate (Rennie's)	Antacid	Neutralize stomach acids	GI upset
Metoclopramide	D2 receptor antagonists	Increases lower oesophageal tone to reduce reflux of stomach contents, increases stomach emptying and reduces intragastric pressure	GI upset Reduced seizure threshold Extrapyramidal side effects Neuroleptic malignant syndrome

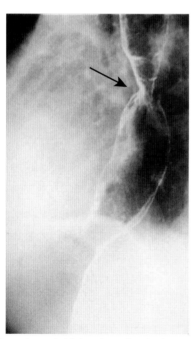

Fig. 1.18 Oesophageal stricture (*arrow*) on barium swallow. Narrowing of the oesophagus at the gastroesophageal junction, indicating oesophageal stricture. (From East CA, Dhillon RS. *Ear, Nose and Throat and Head and Neck Surgery: An Illustrated Colour Text,* 4th Edition. Elsevier; 2012.)

RED FLAG

- Oesophageal perforation can occur spontaneously, due to violent vomiting, or as a complication of stricture dilation, particularly in underlying malignancy. Symptoms include:
  - Sudden onset chest and abdominal pain
  - Circulatory collapse
  - Pyrexia
  - Surgical emphysema in the supraclavicular region
- Perforation can lead to mediastinitis, which has a high mortality rate. Urgent surgical repair is indicated, or chest drain and antibiotic therapy if the patient is unfit for surgery.

Oesophageal adenocarcinoma

Oesophageal adenocarcinoma results from the dysplastic transformation of Barrett's oesophagus. Relevant risk factors include long-standing, poorly controlled GORD, male sex, obesity, smoking and older age. Patients with Barrett's oesophagus should have regular surveillance endoscopies to identify and treat high-grade dysplasia with endoscopic ablation or surgical resection, to prevent development of malignancy (Fig. 1.19).

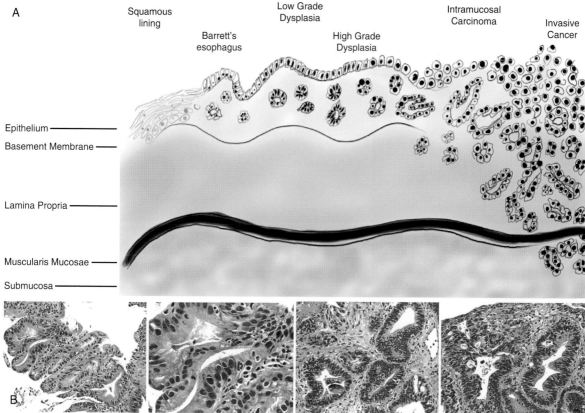

Fig. 1.19 Dysplastic progression of Barrett's oesophagus to oesophageal adenocarcinoma. (A) Histological progression from normal squamous lining to Barrett's oesophagus to dysplasia and then oesophageal adenocarcinoma. (B) Histologic progression of Barrett's oesophagus from no dysplasia to low-grade dysplasia, high-grade dysplasia and oesophageal adenocarcinoma. (From A. Konda VJA, et al. *Quality in Barrett's Esophagus: Diagnosis and Management.* Elsevier; 2022. B. Salemme M, et al. *Intestinal metaplasia in Barrett's oesophagus: An essential factor to predict the risk of dysplasia and cancer development.* Volume 48, Issue 2, February 2016, Pages 144–147.)

Symptoms and signs
Oesophageal adenocarcinoma is often asymptomatic initially. When symptoms develop, they include:

- Progressive dysphagia
- Chest pain
- Dyspepsia
- UGIB (haematemesis or melaena)
- Iron deficiency anaemia
- Weight loss
- Hoarseness and persistent cough

Investigations
Endoscopy and biopsy allow direct visualization of the tumour and histological diagnosis.

A barium swallow can be used prior to endoscopy to identify tumour position, size and related structural abnormalities of the oesophagus (Fig. 1.20).

Management
Management options include:

- Localized disease: oesophagectomy with neoadjuvant chemoradiotherapy.
- Advanced disease: palliative treatment, including stenting, chemoradiation, brachytherapy or endoscopic laser therapy.

Most patients present late, with advanced disease and are suitable for palliation only. The prognosis is very poor, with overall 5-year survival of only 4%.

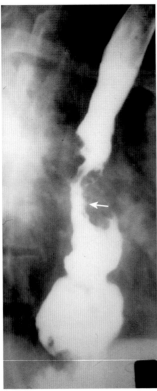

Fig. 1.20 Oesophageal adenocarcinoma. Barium swallowing demonstrating the classical 'apple core lesion' of stenosis and proximal dilation. (From Kontoyannis A, Sweetland H. *Crash Course: Surgery*. 3rd Edition. Elsevier; 2008.)

Oesophageal motility disorders

Oesophageal motility disorders include both hypomobility disorders and hypermobility disorders (Table 1.4, Fig. 1.21):

- Achalasia
- Diffuse oesophageal spasm
- Pharyngeal pouch

CLINICAL NOTES

- Regurgitation of the stomach contents in achalasia, DES and pharyngeal pouch can all result in aspiration pneumonia.
- Recurrent aspiration pneumonia should raise suspicion of underlying oesophageal dysmotility.

CLINICAL NOTES

Endoscopy should be avoided in pharyngeal pouch due to the risk of perforating the pouch.

Table 1.4 Oesophageal motility disorders

Disorder	Aetiology	Clinical features	Investigation	Management
Achalasia	Degeneration of the myenteric nerve plexus, failure of LES relaxation	Dysphagia to solids and liquid Effortless regurgitation when lying flat Weight loss Retrosternal pain	*Barium swallow* – dilated distal oesophagus *Oesophageal manometry* – failure of LES relaxation	*Medical* – botox injections, nitrates, CCBs *Surgical* – dilation or myotomy
DES	Idiopathic oesophageal hypermotility	Intermittent dysphagia to liquids Exacerbated by very hot/cold foods Retrosternal chest pain Acid reflux Hoarseness or recurrent cough	*Barium swallow* – corkscrew oesophagus *Oesophageal manometry* – premature contractions and hypermobility	*Conservative* – lifestyle modifications *Medical* – nitrates, CCBs, PDE5 inhibitors, botox injections *Surgical* – dilation and myotomy
Pharyngeal pouch	Impaired relaxation of the cricopharyngeus and pharyngeal herniation	Dysphagia Neck swelling Halitosis 'Double swallow'	A barium swallow will delineate the lesion	Excision Endoscopic stapling

CCBs, *Calcium channel blockers*; DES, *diffuse oesophageal spasm*; LES, *lower oesopha–geal sphincter*.

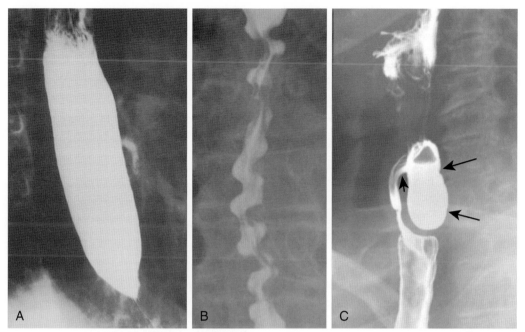

Fig. 1.21 Barium swallow findings in oesophageal motility disorders. (A) Barium swallow demonstrating 'bird's beak' appearance of the oesophagus in achalasia. (B) Corkscrew oesophagus in diffuse oesophageal spasm. (C) Pharyngeal pouch at the cricopharyngeus. (From (A) Dawit L, et al. *Medicine Morning Report Subspecialties: Beyond the Pearls*. Elsevier; 2023. (B, C) Goldman L, Schafer AI. *Goldman-Cecil Medicine*. 26th Edition. Elsevier; 2020.)

GASTRIC DISORDERS

Gastritis

Gastritis is the inflammation of the gastric mucosa, which can cause erosive lesions in the mucous lining, progressing to ulceration, bleeding and perforation. Risk factors include H. pylori infection, NSAIDs, aspirin or steroids use, alcohol and smoking, or systemic critical illness. There is an increased risk of gastric cancer in chronic gastritis.

Symptoms and signs
Typical features include:

- Dyspepsia
- Epigastric pain
- Haematemesis or melaena

Management
Management involves:

- Lifestyle changes: cessation of irritants (i.e., NSAIDs, alcohol, smoking), weight loss
- Acid-reducing therapies: PPIs, H2RAs

- H. pylori testing: and eradication therapy given if detected (amoxicillin, clarithromycin and high-dose PPIs)
- OGD: to diagnose and treat complications including erosions or ulcerations and take biopsies if there is evidence of malignancy

RED FLAG

Symptoms of gastritis alongside unintentional weight loss and progressive dysphagia are red flag features for upper GI malignancy, and warrant urgent investigation.

Peptic ulcer disease

Peptic ulcer disease (PUD) describes the presence of ulcerations within the GIT, commonly occurring in the stomach or the first section of the duodenum. PUD results from breakdown in mucosal defence mechanisms, because of increased or inappropriate acid or proteolytic enzyme secretion. The strongest risk factor for PUD is H. pylori infection. Other risk factors include NSAID/corticosteroid use, alcohol, smoking and critical illness.

Symptoms and signs

The typical features of PUD relate to the likely location of the ulcer (Table 1.5).

Investigations

Investigations include

- H. pylori testing: and eradication if present can be done in primary care for patients without red flag features.

- OGD: indicated urgently for patients with red flag features, or those who test negative for H. pylori (Fig. 1.22). Bleeding ulcers can be cauterized, and biopsies can be taken to identify malignancy. CLO testing for H. pylori provides an immediate diagnosis

Management

Management of PUD involves H. pylori eradication and management of complications (Fig. 1.23).

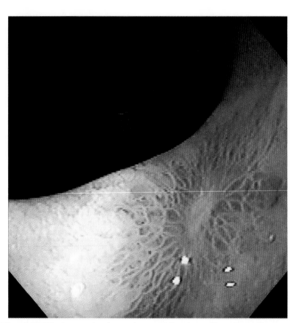

Fig. 1.22 Endoscopic view of a gastric ulcer. (Courtesy Feras Alissa, MD, Pittsburgh, PA; and Cary Sauer, MD, Atlanta, GA.)

Table 1.5 Gastric versus duodenal ulcers

	Gastric ulcer	Duodenal ulcer
Incidence	15% of ulcers 1:1 male to female Ages 50–60	80% of ulcers 2:1 male to female Ages 20–50
Aetiology	H. pylori infection (25%–50%) NSAID use	H. pylori infection (40%–70%) Zollinger-Ellison syndrome
Symptoms	Epigastric pain worse after eating Weight loss Haematemesis/vomiting Early satiety Dyspepsia	Epigastric pain relieved by eating Weight gain Nocturnal pain Radiation of pain to the back Melaena Bloating
Complications	Bleeding Perforation Gastric carcinoma	Bleeding Perforation Gastric outlet obstruction

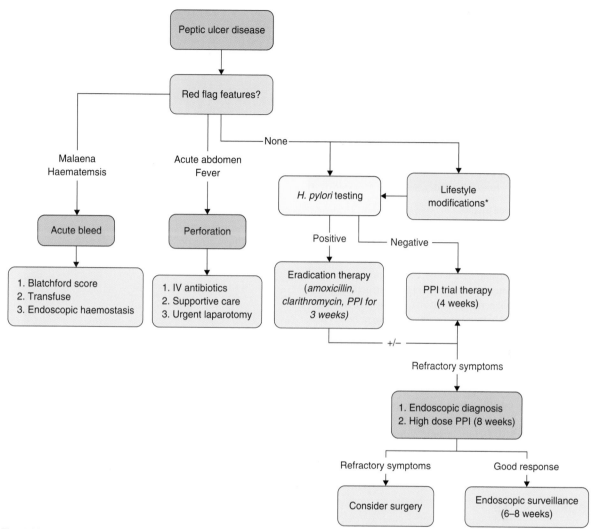

Fig. 1.23 Approach to patients with peptic ulcer disease. *Lifestyle modification includes stopping NSAIDs or other medications that trigger symptoms, reducing alcohol, tobacco and caffeine intake and modifying stress levels where possible.

CLINICAL NOTES

Patients treated for PUD need repeat endoscopy within 6–8 weeks to ensure resolution.

Complications

RED FLAG

An acutely bleeding ulcer presents with UGIB and should be managed with haemodynamic support and endoscopic cautery.

Further complications include:

- Malignant transformation: more common with gastric ulcers.
- Gastric outlet obstruction: chronic ulceration can result in scarring and fibrosis, presenting with progressive vomiting of undigested food and weight loss. Surgical management involves gastroenterostomy to bypass the obstruction.
- Fistula formation: penetration of an ulcer through the GIT wall into adjacent organs such as the pancreas or biliary tree. Can result in intraabdominal sepsis.
- Iron deficiency anaemia: as the result of chronically UGIB.

Gastric cancer

Gastric cancer is the third most common gastrointestinal cancer in the United Kingdom. It tends to present late and has a poor prognosis. Risk factors include chronic H. pylori infection, PUD and genetic conditions that increase the risk of GIT malignancy including HNPCC. Other risk factors include obesity, smoking, EBV infection and diets high in nitrates and salts.

CLINICAL NOTES

The stomach is the commonest site of primary extranodal lymphoma, from the mucosa associated lymphoid tissue (MALT). Risk factors include H. pylori infection.

Symptoms and signs

Gastric cancer is often asymptomatic in the early stages. When symptoms develop, they include ALARMS features of upper GIT malignancy:

- Anaemia
- Loss of weight and anorexia
- Age (>50 years)
- Recent onset/rapidly progressive symptoms
- Melaena/haematemesis
- Swallowing difficulties (dysphagia)

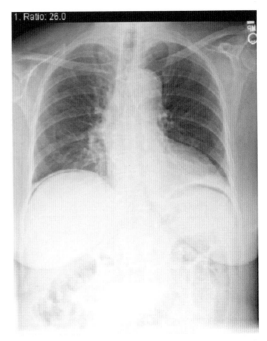

Fig. 1.24 Pneumoperitoneum on erect chest X-ray indicating gastrointestinal perforation. Air is evident under the right hemidiaphragm. (From Brakenridge S, et al. *Textbook of Critical Care,* 8th Edition. Elsevier; 2024.)

Other features include:

- Abdominal pain
- Palpable abdominal mass
- Early satiety
- Nausea and vomiting
- Constitutional features of malignancy

Investigations

Diagnosis is made via OGD and biopsy for histology analysis. Staging imaging includes CXR, abdominal US and CT Chest Abdomen and Pelvis.

CLINICAL NOTES

CEA and CA19-9 are nonspecific serologic biomarkers for abdominal malignancy and may be raised in gastric cancer.

Management

Management should follow an MDT approach, based on the realistic goals of treatment, considering the extent and location of disease, and patient's wishes. The mainstay of treatment for localized disease is surgical resection with radical lymph node dissection, with neoadjuvant and adjuvant chemotherapy (Fig. 1.25).

- Total gastrectomy: suitable for cancer in the proximal or middle of the stomach.
- Subtotal gastrectomy: for cancer confined to the distal or proximal stomach.
- Oesophagectomy: for adenocarcinomas of the oesophagogastric junction.

Most patients present with late-stage disease. Unresectable or metastatic tumours should be managed with palliation, focusing on symptoms control and improving quality of life.

- Pain management: adequate analgesia with opiates.
- Surgery: gastroenterostomy or stenting for gastric outlet obstruction.
- Nutritional support: enteral nutrition is preferred, including nasogastric, nasojejunal, gastrostomy or jejunostomy.
- Management of complications: endoscopic management of UGIB and therapeutic paracentesis for ascites.

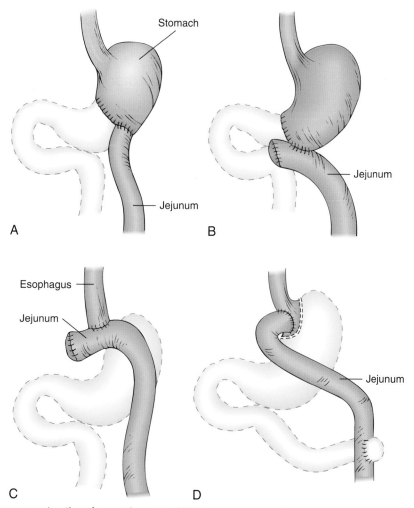

Fig. 1.25 Surgical management options for gastric cancer. (A) Total gastrectomy; (B) subtotal gastrectomy; (C) reconstructive procedures, including Roux-en-Y bypass (anastomosis of the small intestine to the oesophagus) ensure ongoing functioning of the GIT. (From Grodner M, et al. *Nutritional Foundations and Clinical Applications*. 8th Edition. Elsevier; 2023.)

Complications

Complications include:

- Metastatic spread: regional spread to adjacent organs, lymphatic spread via the thoracic duct, or haematogenous spread via the portal system, to the liver and the lungs.
- Gastric outlet obstruction: presenting with postprandial vomiting, early satiety, weight loss, a palpable abdominal mass and abdominal distension.

HINTS AND TIPS

Metastasis most commonly affects the Bone, Brain, Liver and Lung (BBLL). Locally progressive disease may present with symptoms of invasion into adjacent organs:

- Jaundice
- Pancreatic insufficiency – steatorrhoea and hyperglycaemia
- Ascites
- Hepatomegaly
- Rectal bleeding
- Chest pain

Postgastrectomy complications include:

- Malabsorption: due to reduced gastric digestion of food.
- Small intestinal bacterial overgrowth syndrome: in the bypassed intestinal segment, presenting with diarrhoea or steatorrhoea, weight loss and nutritional deficiencies.

- Dumping syndrome: a bypassed pyloric sphincter can result in rapid emptying of stomach contents into the small intestine, increasing intestinal motility and resulting in nausea, vomiting, diarrhoea and abdominal pain after eating.
- Malignancy: developing in the gastric remnant.

HEPATOBILIARY DISORDERS

The liver plays an essential role in many body systems, including the coagulation system, immune system and gastrointestinal system (Fig. 1.26).

Jaundice

Jaundice occurs due to disruption of bilirubin metabolism, and can relate to prehepatic, hepatic or posthepatic (Fig. 1.27, Table 1.6). Jaundice is clinically visible when serum bilirubin rises above 30 mmol/L.

Hepatic disorders

Liver injury

Damage to the liver can be acute, chronic or acute on chronic (Fig. 1.28, Table 1.7).

Investigations

Investigations for a suspected liver injury include a full liver panel:

- LFTs
- Clotting screen
- Hepatitis serology

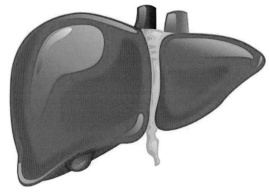

Metabolism
Drugs/toxins
Alcohol
Ammonia -> urea
Hormones
Fatty acids

Protein synthesis
Clotting factors
Albumin
Immunoglobulins
Acute phase proteins

Blood sugar regulation
Glycolysis
Glycogenesis
Glycogenolysis
Gluconeogenesis

Lipid synthesis
Cholesterol
Triglycerides

Bile synthesis
Bilirubin conjugation
Bile acid production
Bile secretion

Micronutrient storage
Copper
Zinc
Magnesium
Iron
Vitamins ADEK, B_{12}

Immunological
Pathogen detection and clearance
Induction of immune tolerance
Storage of immune cells

Fig. 1.26 Functions of the liver.

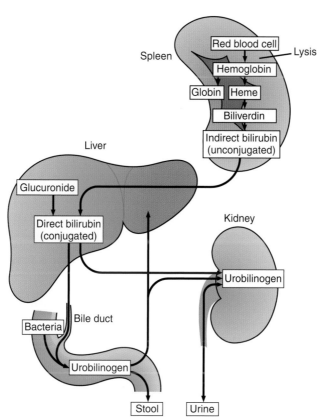

Fig. 1.27 Bilirubin metabolism. Unconjugated bilirubin (UCB) is a breakdown product of heme metabolism and travels bound to albumin in the serum. UCB is conjugated in the liver and excreted into the biliary tract, where it forms part of bile. Conjugated bilirubin is broken down in the small intestine to stercobilin, which makes stool brown, and urobilinogen, which makes urine yellow. (From MacDonald SA. *Pagana's Canadian Manual of Diagnostic and Laboratory Tests*, 3rd Edition. Elsevier; 2024.)

Table 1.6 Causes of jaundice

	Prehepatic	Hepatic	Posthepatic
Pathophysiology	↑ Haemolysis • Haemolytic anaemia • Haemolytic transfusion reactionsIneffective erythropoiesis Thalassemia Pernicious anaemiaIncreased bilirubin production • Massive blood transfusionImpaired hepatic uptake of bilirubin • ↓ hepatic blood flow • Medications	↓ Bilirubin conjugation • Gilbert syndrome • Crigler-Najjar syndromeHepatocellular injury • ALI/CLDIntrahepatic cholestasis • PBC • Intrahepatic cholestasis of pregnancy	Extrahepatic cholestasis • Malignancy • Gallstone-related disease • PSC • Pancreatitis
Symptoms	Jaundice, malaise, pallor +/- fever, SOB, petechiae	Jaundice, fever, malaise, RUQ pain Ascites Hepatosplenomegaly	Jaundice, dark urine, pale stools, pruritus* +/- RUQ pain, mass, nausea and vomiting
Ix	↑UCB	↑UCB and ↑CB (mixed) ↑AST/ALT, γ-GT	↑CB ↑ALP/γ-GT

ALI, *Acute liver injury;* CB, *conjugated bilirubin;* CLD, *chronic liver disease;* PSC, *primary sclerosing cholangitis;* UCB, *unconjugated bilirubin.*
Pruritus occurs due to the precipitation of excess bile salts into the skin.

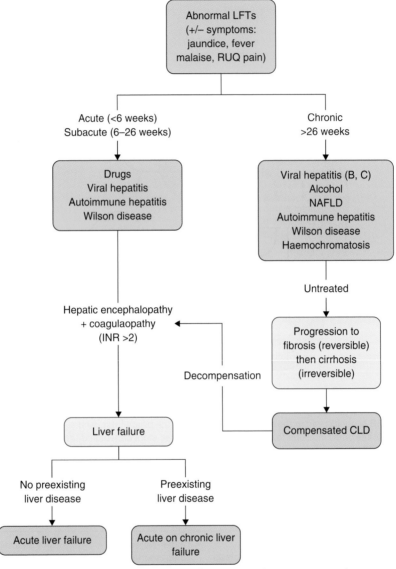

Fig. 1.28 Classification of liver injury. *CLD*, Chronic liver disease. *Decompensation occurs secondary to precipitants, including viruses, drugs, alcohol, ischaemia, surgery or sepsis.

- Antibody screen – antinuclear, antismooth muscle, liver kidney microsomal and antimitochondrial antibodies
- Serum A1AT levels
- Serum copper and ceruloplasmin
- Serum ferritin

A liver US should then be performed to investigate for parenchymal disease.

Portal hypertension

Portal hypertension describes a pathologic increase in portal venous pressure above 15 mmHg that develops as the result of obstructed portal venous blood flow. This can occur as the result of hepatobiliary or systemic pathology. The most common cause is cirrhosis (Table 1.8).

Table 1.7 Types of liver damage

	ALF	CLD	ACLF
Definition	Rapidly progressive (<26 weeks) severe liver injury, with abnormal liver enzymes, coagulopathy and encephalopathy No preexisting liver disease	Progressive deterioration in liver function over 6 months	**Acute decompensation of CLD,** with multiorgan failure Presence of severe liver injury, including abnormal liver enzymes, coagulopathy and encephalopathy
Aetiology	Hepatotoxic medications (paracetamol overdose most common) Viral hepatitis Wilson disease Malignant infiltration	Alcohol Chronic hepatitis Chronic medication abuse PBC/PSC Haemochromatosis Wilson disease	Hepatotoxic medications Alcohol Hepatitis Ischaemia Surgery Sepsis
Symptoms	Hepatic encephalopathy Jaundice Ascites	Fatigue Malaise Anorexia/weight loss Pruritus jaundice Hepatosplenomegaly	Hepatic encephalopathy Variceal bleeding Jaundice Ascites
Investigations	↑↑ALT/AST ↑↑ Ammonia ↓↓Platelets ↓CBG ↑Urea and creatinine ↑ PT/INR	Liver panel Abdominal CT	↑↑ALT/AST ↑↑ Ammonia ↓↓Platelets ↓CBG ↑Urea and creatinine ↑ PT/INR
Management	Urgent resuscitation Urgent liver transplant *N*-acetylcysteine (in paracetamol overdose)	Abstinence Nutritional support Low salt diet Spironolactone Propranolol	Haemodynamic resuscitation Respiratory support Lactulose* Control ICP Early referral for liver transplant
Complications	Death Coagulopathy Multiorgan failure	Ascites, SBP Hepatic encephalopathy Portal hypertension Coagulopathy + bleeding Peripheral oedema HCC	Death Hepatorenal syndrome** Coagulopathy Multiorgan failure Death

ACLF, Acute on chronic liver failure; ALF, acute liver failure; CBG, capillary blood glucose; CLD, chronic liver disease; PSC, primary sclerosing cholangitis.
*Lactulose increases GIT clearance of ammonia.
**Hepatorenal syndrome is an acute deterioration in kidney function in patients with advanced liver disease. It is reversible with rapid effective treatment of liver disease.

Table 1.8 Causes of portal hypertension

Prehepatic	Intrahepatic	Posthepatic
Portal vein thrombosis Splenic vein thrombosis SVC occlusion	Cirrhosis Primary biliary cirrhosis Hepatic metastases Schistosomiasis Polycystic liver disease	Budd–Chiari syndrome Right-sided heart failure Constrictive pericarditis

Symptoms and signs

Clinical features include:

- Symptoms of CLD: jaundice, encephalopathy, nausea and anorexia, malaise

- Stigmata of chronic liver disease
- Portosystemic anastomosis: paraumbilical, oesophageal, gastric, retroperitoneal or anorectal, with associated complications including varices and UGIB (Figs 1.29–1.30)
- Fluid retention – splenomegaly, ascites and peripheral oedema

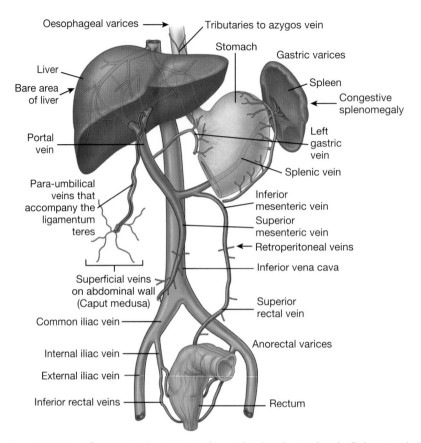

Oesophageal varices ⟶
Tributaries to azygos vein
Stomach
Gastric varices
Liver
Bare area of liver
Spleen
⟵ Congestive splenomegaly
Portal vein
Left gastric vein
Splenic vein
Para-umbilical veins that accompany the ligamentum teres
Inferior mesenteric vein
Superior mesenteric vein
⟵ Retroperitoneal veins
Inferior vena cava
Superficial veins on abdominal wall (Caput medusa)
Superior rectal vein
Common iliac vein
Anorectal varices
Internal iliac vein
External iliac vein
Inferior rectal veins
Rectum

Fig. 1.29 Portosystemic anastomoses. Portosystemic anastomosis can develop due to chronically increased portal pressure and the diversion of blood from the high-pressure portal system. (From Mitchell AWM, Drake R, Drake RL. *Gray's Basic Anatomy*. Churchill Livingstone, Elsevier Inc. 2013.)

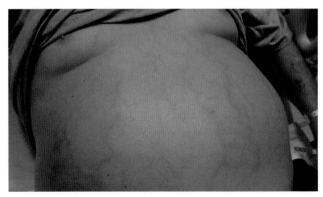

Fig. 1.30 Caput medusae. Dilated superficial veins over the anterior abdominal wall indicating paraumbilical varices. (From Dennis M, et al. Symptome verstehen - Interpretation klinischer Zeichen. Elsevier Urban-Fischer Germany; 2019.)

Investigation

Diagnosis can typically be made from clinical features alone. Further investigation including abdominal US/CT can be done if there is diagnostic uncertainty, or acute portal hypertension, which may relate to reversible causes including portal vein thrombosis.

Management

Management includes medical therapy, to reduce portal pressures, or surgical intervention to divert blood flow and reduce portal pressure:

- Medical: Nonselective beta-blockers (propranolol), which induce splanchnic vasoconstriction, reducing portal blood pressures and anastomotic blood flow
- Surgical: Transjugular intrahepatic portosystemic shunts (TIPS), used where there are persistent or refractory complications including bleeding, ascites, thromboses or hepatorenal syndrome (Fig. 1.31)

Hepatocellular carcinoma

Hepatocellular carcinoma (HCC) is the commonest primary liver malignancy. It typically occurs in those with underlying liver disease, including cirrhosis or chronic hepatitis.

HINTS AND TIPS

- Metastatic tumours are the commonest type of liver tumour. The most common origin of metastases include:
  - Breast
  - Colon
  - Stomach
  - Pancreas
  - Lung
  - Prostate
- They have a poor prognosis, hence typically are managed with palliation

CLINICAL NOTES

- Benign liver tumours including adenoma, haemangioma and focal nodular hyperplasia are rare.
- Risk factors include excess oestrogen exposure.
- They are largely asymptomatic and often found incidentally.
- Conservative management is typical, unless lesions are large, or symptomatic.
- There is a small risk of malignant transformation.

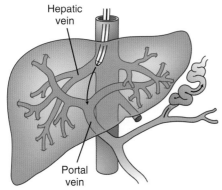
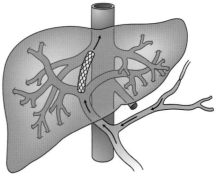

Fig. 1.31 Transjugular intrahepatic portosystemic shunt. A needle catheter is inserted through the internal jugular vein, through the liver, and into the portal vein as it enters the liver, allowing blood to drain from the portal vein directly into the systemic circulation, reducing the high-pressure portal circulation (From Townsend C, Beauchamp RD, Evers BM, Mattox K, eds. *Sabiston Textbook of Surgery: The Biological Basis of Modern Surgical Practice*. 21st Edition. Elsevier; 2022.)

Symptoms and signs

HCC typically presents late. Nonspecific features may include:

- Abdominal pain
- Weight loss and anorexia
- Stigmata of CLD, including ascites and jaundice

Investigations

Screening for HCC should take place every 6 months for those with cirrhosis or chronic hepatitis infections, and includes:

- Serum α-fetoprotein (AFP) levels
- Abdominal US

Diagnosis should be confirmed with CT and liver biopsy if screening is suggestive of HCC (Fig. 1.32).

Management

Management of all malignancies should follow an MDT approach and consider the patient's functional status and wishes, and the likely outcomes of treatment. As HCC typically presents late, the prognosis is generally poor.

- Curative treatment: for tumours detected early, including resection or radiofrequency ablation, +/– liver transplant where available.
- Palliative treatment: for advanced tumours, including noncurative regional chemo/radioembolization, or systemic chemotherapy.

Biliary disorders

Gallstones and biliary colic

Gallstones (cholelithiasis) are abnormal collections in the gallbladder that develop as the result of chronic cholestasis and cholesterol precipitation from bile. Pigmented gallstones occur secondary to imbalances in metabolites of bilirubin as the result of haemolysis or infection. Predisposing factors include obesity, the metabolic syndrome, malabsorptive disease and oestrogen exposure.

HINTS AND TIPS

Risk factors for gallstones include the **6 F's**:
- Fat
- Fair
- Female
- Fertile
- Forty
- Family history

Symptoms and signs

Most gallstones are asymptomatic and may be picked up incidentally on abdominal imaging. Intermittent obstruction of the cystic duct by gallstones results in biliary colic:

- Postprandial severe RUQ pain
- Radiating to the epigastrium, shoulder and back

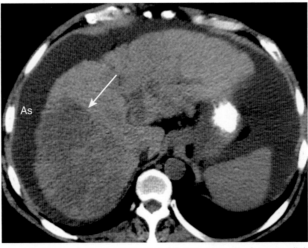

Fig. 1.32 Hepatocellular carcinoma. Contrast-enhanced abdominal CT demonstrating hepatocellular carcinoma *(arrow)*. (From Herring W, Summerton SL. *Learning Radiology: Recognizing the Basics,* 5th Edition. Elsevier; 2024.)

- Nausea, vomiting
- Flatulent dyspepsia
- Pain typically resolves within several hours after eating.

Investigations

Symptomatic gallstones should be investigated with an abdominal US (Fig. 1.33).

> **HINTS AND TIPS**
>
> - Over 90% of gallstones are not calcified and so do not show up on a plain abdominal radiograph (Fig. 1.34).
> - Pure cholesterol stones are radiolucent.

> **CLINICAL NOTES**
>
> - FBC and LFTs are typically normal in uncomplicated cholelithiasis, even in symptomatic gallstones.
> - Derangements in FBC and LFTs indicate underlying infection and biliary obstruction.

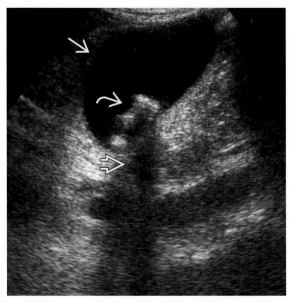

Fig. 1.33 Ultrasound findings of multiple gallstones within the gallbladder with posterior acoustic shadowing. (From Zaheer A, Raman SP. *Diagnostic Imaging: Gastrointestinal,* 4th Edition. Elsevier; 2022.)

Management

A conservative approach is indicated for asymptomatic gallstones. For biliary colic, management includes:

- Conservative: weight loss and reduced fat intake.
- Medical: analgesia, antispasmodics and antiemetics, with bile dissolution therapy (Ursodeoxycholic acid) used in those unsuitable for surgery.
- Surgical: Elective laparoscopic cholecystectomy for symptomatic cholelithiasis, or asymptomatic cases at increased risk of complications. Extracorporeal shock wave lithotripsy (ESWL) can be used to fragment stones and encourage passage into the duodenum.

Complications

Complications include:

- Cholecystitis: inflammation of the gallbladder due to cholestasis.
- Choledocholithiasis: the presence of gallstones within the common bile duct (CBD) (Fig. 1.35).
- Obstructive jaundice: obstruction to biliary flow, which can occur as the result of choledocholithiasis, presenting with pruritus, pale stools and dark urine.
- Cholangitis: infection of the CBD, typically due to choledocholithiasis.
- Gallstone pancreatitis: pancreatic inflammation due to obstruction of the pancreatic duct.
- Enteric fistula: an abnormal connection between the biliary tree and the GIT. Can result in gallstone ileus with passage of large stones into the duodenum.
- Cholangiocarcinoma: carcinoma of the gallbladder associated with chronic inflammation and cholelithiasis.

> **RED FLAG**
>
> - Complications of gallstones including cholecystitis, cholangitis and pancreatitis are surgical emergencies due to the risk of abdominal sepsis. Emergency management involves management of sepsis:
>   - Fluids, oxygen and empirical antibiotics
>   - Lactate, urine output and blood cultures
> - Further management includes supportive care and urgent stone removal by ERCP or cholecystectomy.

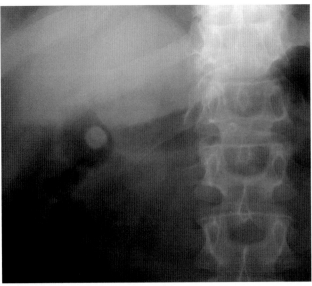

Fig. 1.34 Calcified gallstones on abdominal X-ray. Approximately 10%–20% of gallstones are radiopaque and visible on an abdominal radiograph. (From Horton-Szar D, Kelly BE, Bickle I. *Crash Course: Imaging*. Elsevier; 2007.)

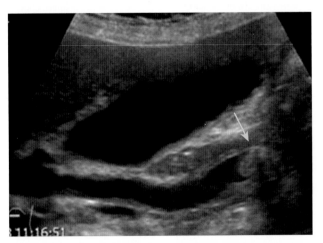

Fig. 1.35 Abdominal US of the common bile duct. Dilated common bile duct, with filling defect, suggestive of calculus. (From Hagen-Ansert, SL. *From Textbook of Diagnostic Sonography*, 9th Edition. Elsevier; 2023.)

CLINICAL NOTES

Cholangiocarcinoma is rare and has a poor prognosis. Symptoms include:

- Fatigue, fever, weight loss
- Jaundice, dark urine, pale stools, pruritus
- A palpable, nontender mass in the RUQ (Courvoisier's sign)

Acute cholecystitis

Acute cholecystitis describes the acute inflammation of the gallbladder, typically occurring following gallstone obstruction of the cystic duct. Bacterial infection can be superimposed, typically with gram-negative organisms including Escherichia coli, Klebsiella and Enterobacter. It is a surgical emergency, due to the risk of abdominal sepsis.

Symptoms and signs

Key features include:

- RUQ pain
- Positive Murphy's sign
- Fever
- Nausea and vomiting

Investigations

The diagnosis is based on the following criteria:

- Local inflammation: RUQ pain and Murphy's sign.
- Systemic inflammation: fever or raised inflammatory markers.
- Imaging findings: gallbladder inflammation on abdominal US (Fig. 1.36).

Management

The initial management of acute cholecystitis should follow an A–E approach (Fig. 1.37).

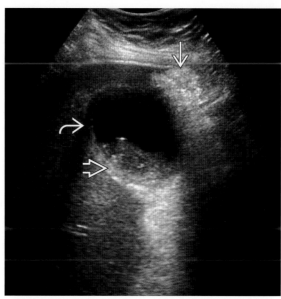

Fig. 1.36 Abdominal US findings in cholecystitis. Gallstones are evident in the gallbladder, with associated wall thickening, oedema distention and mural air. If US is inconclusive, abdominal CT or MRI can be considered. (From Bhatt S, Wasnik AP, Lane BF, Wong-You-Cheong J, Morgan TA, Kamaya A. *Diagnostic Ultrasound: Abdomen & Pelvis,* 2nd Edition. Elsevier; 2022.)

Surgical management includes:

- Cholecystectomy: the definitive treatment. Associated choledocholithiasis should be treated with stone extraction pre- or postoperatively.
- Percutaneous cholecystostomy: temporizing gallbladder drainage for unstable patients. Elective cholecystectomy can be arranged when the patient is stable enough for surgery.

Complications

Complications include:

- Gangrenous cholecystitis: ischaemic necrosis that can develop in severe cholecystitis.

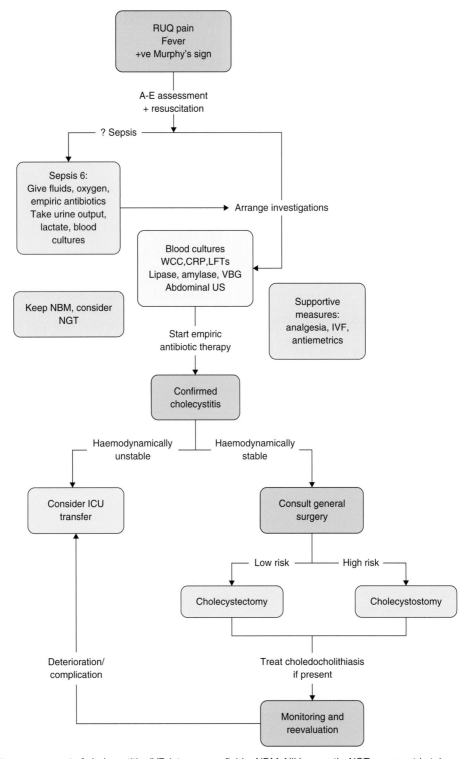

Fig. 1.37 Acute management of cholecystitis. *IVF*, intravenous fluids; *NBM*, Nil by mouth; *NGT*, nasogastric tube.

- Gallbladder perforation: ischaemic necrosis can result in perforation, which presents with generalized peritonitis and a focal defect in the gallbladder wall on imaging. Urgent laparotomy and cholecystectomy are required.
- Cholecystoenteric fistula: an abnormal connection between the lumen of the gallbladder and the adjacent bowel, risking development of gallstone ileus.
- Gallbladder empyema: pus-filled distention of the gallbladder. Percutaneous drainage is done before elective cholecystectomy, 6 weeks after symptom resolution.
- Chronic cholecystitis: chronic low-grade inflammation of the gallbladder secondary to recurrent acute cholecystitis. Symptoms are like acute cholecystitis, but milder, and often self-limiting. Management includes low-fat diets and elective cholecystectomy (Fig. 1.38).

HINTS AND TIPS

Chronic cholecystitis can result in gallbladder calcification and risks cholangiocarcinoma (Fig. 1.39). Elective cholecystectomy is required.

Ascending cholangitis

Ascending cholangitis is the acute inflammation of the biliary tree, which can develop secondary to CBD obstruction and biliary stasis, as the result of stones or strictures. Infection may also be introduced during ERCP. It is a surgical emergency, due to the risk of abdominal sepsis.

Symptoms and signs

The key symptoms include Charcot's triad:

- RUQ pain
- Fever
- Jaundice

  Other features include signs of sepsis:

- Hypotension and tachycardia
- Confusion and mental status changes
- Nausea and vomiting

HINTS AND TIPS

- Elderly patients may present atypically, with absence of pain and jaundice.
- Acute hepatitis or pancreatitis, may also present with fever, jaundice and RUQ pain, and should be considered in the differential diagnosis.

Investigations

Diagnosis is based on the following criteria:

- Systemic signs of inflammation: fever, ↑CRP, ↑WCC
- Evidence of cholestasis: jaundice, or cholestatic LFTs including ↑ALP and GGT↑
- Imaging: dilated CBD and periductal inflammation, +/− choledocholithiasis on abdominal imaging (Fig. 1.40)

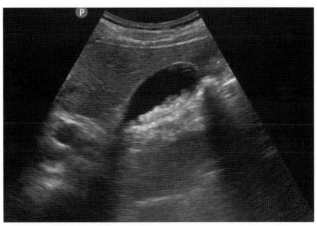

Fig. 1.38 Patient with chronic cholecystitis, with an oedematous thick-walled gallbladder with multiple small stones. (From Hagen-Ansert SL. *Textbook of Diagnostic Sonography,* 9th Edition. Elsevier; 2023.)

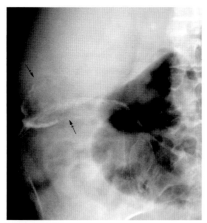

Fig. 1.39 Porcelain gallbladder. Calcification of the walls of the gallbladder. There is a strong association with malignancy. (From Horton-Szar D, Kelly BE, Bickle I. *Crash Course: Imaging*. Elsevier; 2007.)

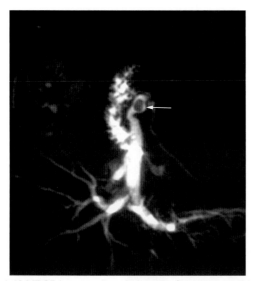

Fig. 1.40 MRCP in ascending cholangitis. Stones are visible as filling defects within the bile ducts. (From Horton-Szar D, Kelly BE, Bickle I. *Crash Course: Imaging*. Elsevier; 2007.)

Further blood tests include:

- Blood cultures/VBG: to diagnose intraabdominal sepsis
- Coagulation screen: coagulopathy may develop in severe cholangitis

Management

The management of ascending cholangitis involves an A–E approach with urgent haemodynamic support and management of sepsis (Fig. 1.41).

Definitive management includes:

- ERCP with sphincterotomy: to drain the gallbladder and treat choledocholithiasis (Fig. 1.42).
- Interval cholecystectomy: performed following the resolution of the acute episode.
- Biliary stenting: for biliary strictures or external compression relating to underlying malignancy.

Complications

Complications include:

- Sepsis: and subsequent hypovolaemic shock, multiorgan dysfunction and death.
- Biliary strictures: developing following the acute episode, predisposing to further episodes and cholangitis and cholangiocarcinoma.

PANCREATIC DISORDERS

Acute pancreatitis

Acute pancreatitis is the inflammation of the pancreas. Gallstones and alcohol use account for 95% of cases. Risk factors include obesity, high-fat diets, smoking, diabetes and cystic fibrosis, which predispose to acute episodes following exposure to triggers. Acinar cell injury as the result of alcohol or obstructed enzyme flow results in autodigestion of the pancreatic tissue by proteolytic enzymes, leading to massive release of inflammatory cells and cytokines, resulting in pancreatic inflammation and a widespread systemic inflammatory response. Pancreatitis is a surgical emergency and can develop into a severe life-threatening illness.

HINTS AND TIPS

The causes of pancreatitis can be remembered by the mnemonic I GET SMASHED:

- **I**diopathic
- **G**allstones
- **E**TOH excess
- **T**rauma
- **S**teroids
- **M**umps
- **A**utoimmune
- **S**corpion stings
- **H**ypertriglyceridemia/hypercalcaemia
- **E**RCP
- **D**rugs (azathioprine, furosemide, tetracyclines and sodium valproate)

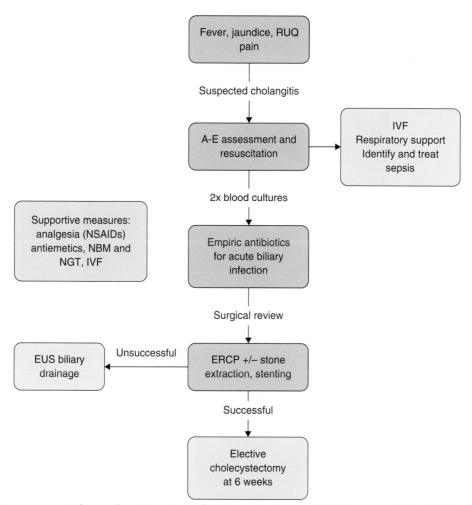

Fig. 1.41 Acute management of ascending cholangitis. *EUS*, Endoscopic ultrasound; *IVF*, Intravenous fluids; *NGT*, nasogastric tube.

Symptoms and signs

The key symptoms include:

- Severe epigastric pain radiating to the back
- Nausea and vomiting
- Fever

HINTS AND TIPS

- Pain in pancreatitis has several characteristic features:
  - Severe constant pain
  - Radiating to the back, or right or left hypochondrium
  - Worse after meals and when lying flat
  - Improves leaning forward
- Diffuse tenderness and guarding suggest acute peritonitis.

Other features include:

- Jaundice: in biliary pancreatitis, indicating cholestasis
- Abdominal distention/ascites: in necrotizing pancreatitis
- Chest pain/dyspnoea: indicating the development of pulmonary complications
- Abdominal bruising: retroperitoneal haemorrhage can occur in severe pancreatitis (Fig. 1.43)
- Shock: tachycardia, hypotension and oliguria

Investigations

The diagnosis of pancreatitis is based on:

- Typical clinical features
- ↑ Pancreatic enzymes: lipase or amylase > 3× the upper limit of normal
- Imaging demonstrating pancreatic inflammation

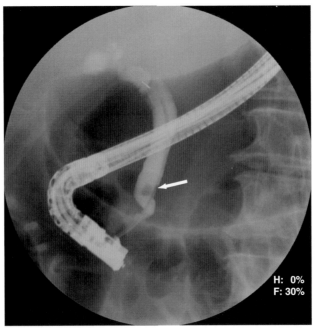

Fig. 1.42 Endoscopic retrograde cholangiopancreatography. Intraoperative cholangiogram demonstrating bile duct stone during ERCP. (From Townsend CM, et al. *Sabiston Textbook of Surgery*. 21st Edition. St Louis, Elsevier; 2022.)

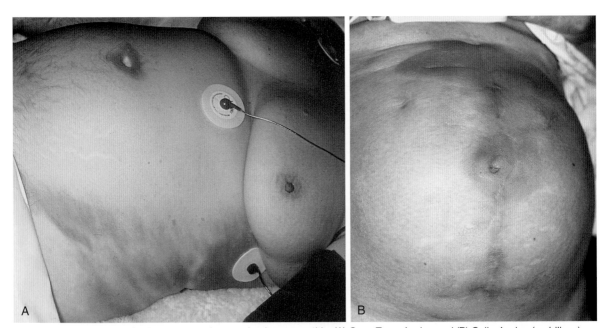

Fig. 1.43 Abdominal exam findings in acute haemorrhagic pancreatitis. (A) Grey–Turner's sign and (B) Cullen's sign (umbilicus). (From Jarnagin WR. *Blumgart's Surgery of the Liver, Biliary Tract and Pancreas*. 5th Edition. Saunders; 2012.)

Pancreatic imaging involves:

- Abdominal US: to identify gallstones, pancreatic oedema, peripancreatic fluid and pancreatic pseudocysts, or walled-off necrosis.
- CT abdomen: may demonstrate pancreatic oedema, peripancreatic fat stranding and necrotic complications (Fig. 1.44).
- ERCP: to diagnose and treat gallstone pancreatitis.

Management

Management should follow an A–E approach with appropriate stabilization and resuscitation (Fig. 1.45).

Long-term management includes:

- Abstinence from alcohol: support includes medical detox or anti-craving medications, social support and psychological therapies
- Surgical debridement: for necrotizing pancreatitis
- Cholecystectomy: if gallstones are the underlying aetiology

Complications

The complications of acute pancreatitis can be severe and life-threatening:

- Hypovolemic shock: release of inflammatory mediators leads to increased vascular permeability, third spacing of intravascular fluid, hypotension and tachycardia.
- Necrotizing pancreatitis: hypotension and decreased organ perfusion lead to necrosis of pancreatic tissue.
- Sepsis: superimposed infection of a necrotic pancreas can lead to septicaemia and multiorgan failure. Renal failure is a common complication of pancreatic sepsis.
- Hypocalcaemia: increased lipase release from the pancreas leads to release of free fatty acids, which bind serum calcium, leading to hypocalcaemia, which has neurological, musculoskeletal and cardiovascular complications.
- Respiratory: pneumonia, respiratory failure and ARDS due to a systemic inflammation. Respiratory complications are a sensitive indicator of severity and mortality risk.
- Chronic pancreatitis: irreversible damage to the structure and function of the pancreas that occurs following repeated episodes of acute pancreatitis.

Chronic pancreatitis

Recurrent episodes of acute pancreatitis can cause progressive and irreversible damage to the pancreas, impairing its exocrine and endocrine functions and triggering the development of chronic pancreatitis. Long-term heavy use of alcohol is the most common cause, however, ductal obstruction secondary to strictures or gallstones can also predispose to development. Smoking is a significant risk factor.

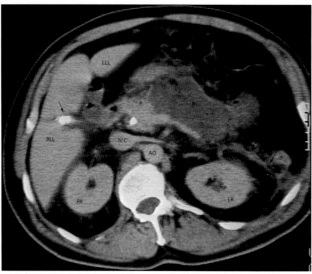

Fig. 1.44 CT abdomen demonstrating pancreatitis. *P,* Normal pancreatic head. *Necrotic and inflamed pancreatic body and tail, *arrow,* gallstone within the gallbladder. (From Horton-Szar D, Kelly BE, Bickle I. *Crash Course: Imaging.* Elsevier; 2007.)

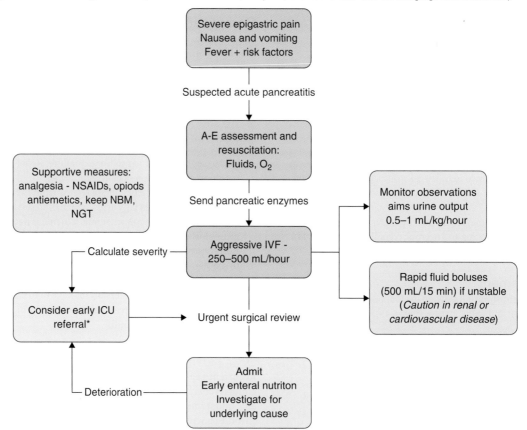

Fig. 1.45 Management of acute pancreatitis. ICU referral is typically indicated if there is concurrent organ dysfunction/failure, evidence of sepsis, ongoing significant fluid requirements, or in older age or high-risk groups. The Glasgow-Imrie criteria is a useful marker of severity. Scores over 3 are typically referred to ICU. *NBM,* Nil by mouth; *NGT,* nasogastric tube

Symptoms and signs

Symptoms include:

- Chronic, constant, severe, epigastric pain, that radiates to the back, and relieved bending forward.
- Postprandial pain.
- Nausea and vomiting.
- Features of pancreatic exocrine and endocrine insufficiency (Table 1.9).

HINTS AND TIPS

In the late stages of chronic pancreatitis, pain may be absent.

Investigations

The diagnosis of chronic pancreatitis is based on:

- Typical clinical features and risk factors.
- Tests of pancreatic function – faecal elastase is a marker of exocrine insufficiency.
- Typical imaging findings.

HINTS AND TIPS

Pancreatic enzymes including amylase and lipase may normal in chronic pancreatitis, even in acute exacerbations, and should not be relied upon for diagnosis.

Imaging in chronic pancreatitis involves:

- Abdominal US: pancreatic calcification, ductal strictures and dilation, and gallstones.
- Abdominal X-ray: pancreatic calcification may be radiopaque, which is highly specific for chronic pancreatitis (Fig. 1.46).

Table 1.9 Features of pancreatic exocrine and endocrine insufficiency in chronic pancreatitis

Exocrine symptoms	Endocrine symptoms
Steatorrhoea	Polyuria and polydipsia
Cramping abdominal pain	Hyperglycaemia
Bloating	Fatigue
Fat-soluble vitamin deficiencies (ADEK)	Weight loss
Malabsorption	
Weight loss	

- Abdominal CT: demonstrating pancreatic duct dilation and calcification. A 'chain of lakes' appearance of the pancreatic duct is typical. Malignancy can also be excluded (Fig. 1.47).

Management

Management involves preventing progression and management of chronic pain.

- Analgesia: following the WHO analgesia ladder, begin with nonopioid oral analgesics (paracetamol/NSAIDs). Opioid analgesia should be avoided where possible, due to issues with tolerance and addiction. Adjuvant options include tricyclic antidepressants, selective serotonin reuptake inhibitors, serotonin and norepinephrine reuptake inhibitors and gabapentin.
- Abstinence: from both alcohol and smoking is essential. Alcohol abstinence therapies and nicotine replacement therapies can be offered.
- Management of comorbidities: key to reducing morbidity and mortality.
- Pancreatic enzyme replacement (Creon): taken with meals to reduce symptoms of malabsorption and vitamin deficiencies.

CLINICAL NOTES

- Beware of prescribing tricyclic antidepressants in those with previous substance abuse.
- These medications are commonly abused and are very dangerous in overdose.

Surgical management includes partial or total pancreatic resection:

- Pancreaticoduodenectomy (Whipple procedure).
- Distal pancreatectomy.
- Total pancreatectomy – the only known cure, limited to patients with severe unretractable pain, where all other measures have failed.

Complications

- Recurrent acute pancreatitis: chronic pancreatitis predisposes patients to acute pancreatitis.
- Vitamin ADEK deficiency: pancreatic exocrine insufficiency can lead to fat-soluble vitamin deficiency, and complications including weight loss, malnutrition and osteoporosis.
- Pancreatogenic diabetes: endocrine pancreatic insufficiency leads to insulin-dependant diabetes mellitus.

- Pancreatic pseudocysts: encapsulated collections of pancreatic fluid that present with a painless abdominal mass and pressure effects on surrounding organs.
- Pancreatic ascites: secondary to ductal disruption or rupture of a pseudocyst, presenting with abdominal distention and pain, dyspnoea and peripheral oedema.
- Pancreatic cancer: chronic pancreatitis is a key risk factor for the development of pancreatic cancer, particularly in patients with longstanding disease.

Table 1.10 outlines the differences between acute and chronic pancreatitis.

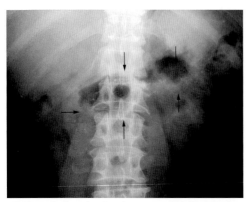

Fig. 1.46 X-ray findings in chronic pancreatitis. Speckled calcifications are visible in the upper abdomen. The location is consistent with the head and body of the pancreas. (From Horton-Szar D, Kelly BE, Bickle I. *Crash Course: Imaging*. Elsevier; 2007.)

Pancreatic cancer

Pancreatic cancer is the fifth most common cause of cancer-related deaths in the United Kingdom. The prognosis is poor, due to the late onset of symptoms and diagnosis. Most cancers arise from the pancreatic head and are exocrine tumours, with 95% ductal adenocarcinomas. Risk factors include smoking, chronic pancreatitis, alcohol excess, obesity and type 2 diabetes.

CLINICAL NOTES

- An insulinoma is an insulin-secreting endocrine tumour of the pancreas. They are associated with multiple endocrine neoplasia.
- Symptoms include recurrent hypoglycaemic episodes.
- They are typically benign and solitary, and respond well to surgical resection.

HINTS AND TIPS

- Occupational exposure to dyes is a commonly examined risk factor for pancreatic cancer.
- Screen for occupational risk factors in any history suspicious of malignancy.

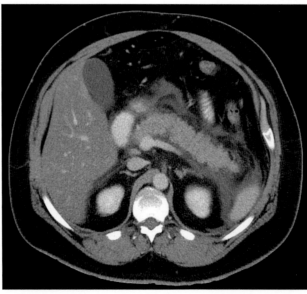

Fig. 1.47 CT abdomen and pelvis in a patient with acute pancreatitis showing pancreatic enlargement, edema and peripancreatic fluid. The patient had recurrent alcoholic pancreatitis. (From Omar AM. *USMLE Step 2 CK Plus*. Elsevier; 2023.)

Table 1.10 Acute versus chronic pancreatitis

	Acute	Chronic
Description	Acute inflammation, reversible damage	Progressive inflammation, irreversible damage Impaired exocrine and endocrine functions
Aetiology (most common)	Acute alcohol excess Gallstones	Chronic alcohol excess Ductal obstruction Smoking
Disease course	Sudden onset	Recurrent, progressive, relapsing-remitting
Symptoms	Severe epigastric pain Radiating to the back, relieves sitting forward, worse after eating Nausea and vomiting Fever	Chronic constant epigastric pain Radiating to the back, relieves sitting forward, worse after eating Abdominal cramping, bloating, Diarrhoea/steatorrhoea Flatulence Nausea
Investigations	↑ Lipase/amylase ↓ Calcium Abdominal US – oedema, fluids, necrosis, pseudocysts Abdominal CT – oedema, fat stranding	Lipase/amylase often normal ↓ faecal elastase Abdominal US – oedema, calcifications Abdominal CT – duct dilation, stenosis, calcifications – chain of lakes
Management	Aggressive fluid resuscitation Early enteral feeding Oxygen +/- ERCP/cholecystectomy	Pain management Abstinence Enzyme replacement Surgery for intractable pain
Complications	Pseudocysts, abscess, fistula Shock, sepsis ARDS, pleural effusion Hypocalcaemia Multiorgan failure, death	Chronic pain Opiate addiction Exocrine insufficiency – malnutrition, malabsorption Endocrine insufficiency – diabetes Pseudocysts, abscesses Pancreatic cancer
Prognosis	30% mortality in organ failure	Dependant on adherence to abstinence and comorbidities

Symptoms and signs

Early disease is typically asymptomatic. Symptoms develop late, and include:

- Courvoisier's sign: painless jaundice and abdominal mass.
- Pancreatic exocrine insufficiency: malabsorption and steatorrhea.
- Pancreatic endocrine insufficiency: impaired glucose tolerance.
- Constitutional symptoms: fever, lethargy, appetite and weight loss, night sweats.
- Hypercoagulability: pancreatic cancer is associated with superficial migratory thrombophlebitis (Trousseau syndrome), predisposing to VTE.

RED FLAG

Painless jaundice in an older adult with a history of smoking or alcohol abuse is highly suspicious of pancreatic cancer. Courvoisier's law states that a painless, palpable gallbladder and jaundice is unlikely to represent gallstones. In these cases, symptoms are more likely to relate to biliary or pancreatic malignancy.

CLINICAL NOTES

New diabetes and associated osmotic symptoms may be an early diagnostic clue for pancreatic cancer.

Investigations

Suspected pancreatic cancer should be investigated with abdominal imaging:

- Abdominal US: the initial imaging modality.
- Abdominal CT with contrast: if there is high clinical suspicion for malignancy, to evaluate local spread and determine resectability.
- Endoscopic US: to confirm the diagnosis and take tissue samples for histology.
- CTCAP: for staging and assessment of metastasis (Fig. 1.48).

> **CLINICAL NOTES**
>
> The 'double-duct' sign on CT, with dilation of the CBD and pancreatic duct suggests tumour related biliary tree obstruction.

> **CLINICAL NOTES**
>
> CA 19-9 is a tumour marker used to evaluate progression and treatment response. It is not recommended for diagnostic or screening purposes.

Management

Management of all malignancies involves an MDT approach, considering the realistic goals of treatment and patient wishes. Tumours detected early may be resectable, however, most present late and are inoperable. Treatment is therefore palliative and revolves around supportive care and the management of complications.

Palliative management includes:

- Chemoradiotherapy: to shrink the tumour and reduce symptoms. May allow for surgical resection if the response is dramatic.
- Pain management: severe pain is common and should be managed using the WHO pain ladder, with early specialist support. Refractory pain can be treated with coeliac ganglion nerve block or splanchnicectomy.
- Nutritional support: enteral nutrition, with pancreatic enzyme replacement as needed.

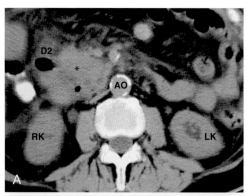

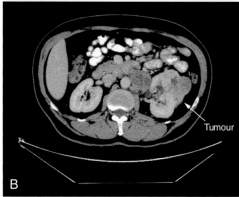

Fig. 1.48 Pancreatic cancer. (A) *Demonstrates the enlarged pancreatic head and gland atrophy. (B) Demonstrates metastatic disease in the left kidney and left para-aortic lymphadenopathy (*). *AO,* Aorta; *D2,* the second part of duodenum; *LK,* left kidney; *RK,* right kidney. (From Horton-Szar D, Kelly BE, Bickle I. *Crash Course: Imaging.* Elsevier; 2007.)

Patients should be followed up frequently to monitor the response to treatment and assess for complications.

Complications

Complications include:

- Metastases: to local structures including the liver, lymphatics, duodenum, stomach, colon and lungs.
- Biliary obstruction: managing with ERCP and stenting.
- Gastric outlet obstruction: managed with endoscopic stenting.
- Malignant ascites: managed with intermittent paracentesis or spironolactone.

Chapter Summary

- A ruptured AAA can present with diffuse abdominal pain or pain localized to any abdominal region, and should always be considered in the differential diagnosis.
- Melaena and haematemesis are always red flags. Melaena is more commonly associated with bleeding peptic ulcers and haematemesis with ruptured oesophageal varices.
- Patients with dyspepsia should be screened for ALARM features, which are associated with underlying oesophageal or gastric malignancy.
- H. pylori is the most significant risk factor for GORD, gastritis and PUD, and should be tested for and eradicated as the first step in management.
- Risk factors for gallstones are the 6 Fs – fat, fair, female, fertile, forty, family history.
- You can differentiate between cholecystitis and cholangitis by the presence of jaundice, which is part of Charcot's triad of ascending cholangitis.
- The first step in the assessment of jaundice should be LFTs, which can differentiate between prehepatic, hepatic and posthepatic causes.
- Severe epigastric pain radiating to the back, vomiting and fever, is likely to represent acute pancreatitis. The most common causes are gallstones and alcohol.
- Pancreatitis is acutely life-threatening, and aggressive fluid resuscitation is the most important step in the management.
- Courvoisier's sign states that jaundice and a palpable gallbladder are likely to represent underlying malignancy of the pancreas and gallbladder.

Continued

● Chapter Summary—cont'd

UKMLA Conditions

Acute cholangitis
Acute pancreatitis
Adverse drug effects
Alcoholic hepatitis
Anaemia
Appendicitis
Change in bowel habit
Change in stool colour
Cholecystitis
Cirrhosis
Diabetic ketoacidosis
Diarrhoea
Gallstones and biliary colic
Gastric cancer
Gastro-oesophageal reflux disease
Gastrointestinal perforation
Intestinal ischaemia
Hepatitis
Hyperemesis
Inflammatory bowel disease
Irritable bowel syndrome
Liver failure
Malabsorption
Malnutrition
Mesenteric adenitis
Metastatic disease
Oesophageal cancer
Pancreatic cancer
Peptic ulcer disease and gastritis
Peritonitis
Sepsis
Shock
Speech and language problems
Viral gastroenteritis
Vitamin B_{12} and/or folate deficiency
Vomiting

UKMLA Presentations

Abdominal distension
Abdominal mass
Acute abdominal pain
Ascites
Bleeding from upper GI tract
Change in bowel habit
Change in stool colour
Chronic abdominal pain
Decreased appetite
Diabetic ketoacidosis
Diarrhoea
Fever
Food intolerance
Jaundice
Massive haemorrhage
Melaena
Nausea
Night sweats
Organomegaly
Pruritus
Sepsis
Shock
Speech and language problems
Swallowing problems
Vomiting
Weight gain/weight loss

The lower gastrointestinal tract 2

CLINICAL ANATOMY

The lower gastrointestinal tract (GIT) extends from the suspensory muscle of the duodenum to the anus. The small intestine extends from the stomach pylorus to the ileocecal valve. It is divided into the duodenum, jejunum, and ileum. The jejunum and the upper ileum digest and absorb fats, carbohydrates, and proteins. Bile salts and vitamin B_{12} are absorbed from the terminal ileum (Fig. 2.1).

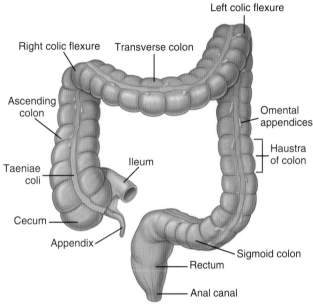

Fig. 2.2 The large intestine. (From Vogl AW, Mitchell AWM, Drake RL. *Gray's Basic Anatomy.* Churchill Livingstone, Elsevier Inc. 2013.)

The large intestine (colon) begins at the caecum and terminates at the anal canal. Absorption of fluids and salts in the colon produces solid stool for excretion (Fig. 2.2).

The greater and lesser omentum are folds of peritoneum that surround the intestines and connect to abdominal organs. The omentum stores fat and contributes to immune regulation and limit the spread of intraabdominal infection. The mesentery is formed from a double fold of peritoneum, and contains vasculature, lymphatics and nerves that supply the intestine, and attaches the intestines to the posterior abdominal wall (Fig. 2.3).

The superior mesenteric artery branches from the abdominal aorta at L2 to supply the ascending and transverse colon. The inferior mesenteric artery branches from the aorta at L3 to supply the terminal transverse, descending and sigmoid colon, rectum, and anal canal (Fig. 2.4).

The enteric nervous system consists of the myenteric and submucosal plexus in the gut wall, and regulates gastrointestinal secretions, blood flow and peristalsis (Fig. 2.5).

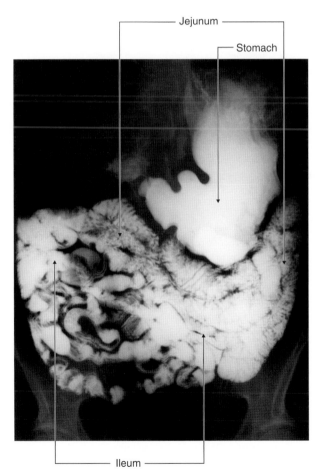

Fig. 2.1 The small intestine. Barium swallow delineating the small intestine. (From Vogl AW, Drake RL, Mitchell AWM. *Gray's Anatomy for Students,* 5th Edition. Elsevier; 2024.)

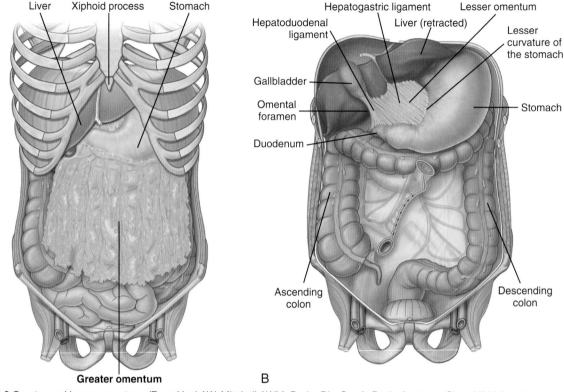

Fig. 2.3 Greater and lesser omentum. (From Vogl AW, Mitchell AWM, Drake RL. *Gray's Basic Anatomy.* Churchill Livingstone, Elsevier Inc. 2013.)

LOWER GI PRESENTATIONS

History taking

Opening the consultation
Introduce yourself and confirm the patient's details.

Presenting complaint (PC)
Begin with an open question to identify the presenting complaint.

History of presenting complaint (HPC)
Explore the presenting complaint in more detail, using SOCRATES. Common symptoms of lower GI pathology include:

- Abdominal pain: sharp localized pain suggests peritoneal inflammation.

- Change in bowel habit (CIBH): constipation may relate to diet or obstructive pathology. Diarrhoea may relate to inflammation or infection. There may be associated blood, mucous, and colicky abdominal pain.
- Abdominal distention: typically relating to bowel obstruction, ascites, or irritable bowel syndrome (IBS). There may be associated pain, nausea or vomiting, or change in bowel habit.
- Abdominal mass: may be firm, soft, tender, or painless. May be related to malignancy or organomegaly.
- Rectal bleeding: fresh red blood separate from the stool is suggestive of anorectal disease. Melaena is suggestive of bleeding higher in the GIT.
- Anorectal pain: severe pain on defecation suggests anal fissure. Associated swelling suggests prolapse or haemorrhoids. There may be bleeding or itch.
- Weight loss: may relate relating to malabsorptive or malignant disease.

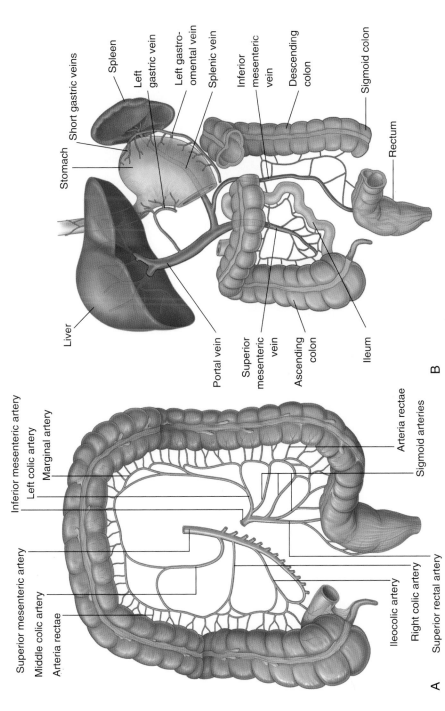

Fig. 2.4 Vascular supply to intestines. (From Vogl AW, Mitchell AWM, Drake RL. *Gray's Basic Anatomy*. Churchill Livingstone, Elsevier Inc. 2013.)

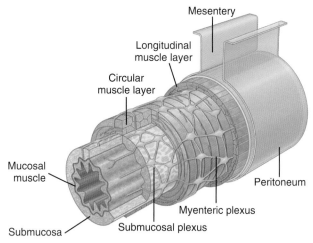

Fig. 2.5 The enteric nervous system. (From Vogl AW, Mitchell AWM, Drake RL. *Gray's Basic Anatomy.* Churchill Livingstone, Elsevier Inc. 2013.)

RED FLAG

Red flags in lower GI history include:

- Obstipation: complete constipation with no passing of flatus. Indicates bowel obstruction.
- Rectal bleeding: significant rectal bleeding is a red flag for colitis or malignancy.
- Anaemia: new unexplained anaemia in an older adult is suggestive of blood loss from the GIT, which may be related to cancer.
- Weight loss: unintentional weight loss is a red flag for malignancy or inflammatory bowel disease (IBD).
- Tenesmus: the sensation of incomplete emptying of the rectum. It is usually associated with a rectal mass or IBD.

Systemic screen

Perform a brief systemic screen to evaluate for associated symptoms and constitutional features. A brief menstrual history should be obtained in females.

HINTS AND TIPS

Organomegaly, ascites, or bowel obstruction may suggest malignancy, associated with constitutional features (FLAWS):

- F – Fever
- L – Lethargy
- A – Anorexia
- W – Weight loss
- N – Night sweats

Past medical history

Screen for associated past medical conditions, surgeries, investigations and procedures.

Drug history

A complete drug history should be obtained, assessing compliance, recent changes or side effects, over-the-counter use and allergies.

HINTS AND TIPS

- Many drugs can cause gastrointestinal upset.
- Recent antibiotic use associated with profuse watery diarrhoea suggests C. difficile infection.

Family history

Hereditary conditions may increase the risk of IBD or intestinal malignancy. Screen for young relatives with a history of colorectal cancer (CRC).

Social history

Obtain a complete social history:

- Functional status: to assess independence, support needs and impact of symptoms.
- Smoking: smoking is a risk factor for Crohn's disease and malignancy.
- Alcohol: may be associated with liver pathology or GIT bleeding.
- Diet and weight: processed diets high in red meat and fat increase the risk of colorectal malignancy.
- Foreign travel: may be related to infective pathology.

Ideas, concerns and expectations

Eliciting the patient's ideas, concerns and expectations, to identify what they want to get out of the consultation, and any concerns you can address to alleviate anxiety.

Closing the consultation

Summarize the history back to the patient, answer any questions and thank them for their time.

DIFFERENTIAL DIAGNOSES

Change in bowel habit

The differential diagnoses of a CIBH relates to the nature of symptoms (Fig. 2.6).

CLINICAL NOTES

- Perform a thorough fluid status assessment.
- Significant diarrhoea risks dehydration.
- Constipation may be precipitated or worsened by fluid losses.
- Bowel obstruction is associated with intraabdominal fluid losses.

RED FLAG

- In acute diarrhoea, consider sepsis.
- Fever and haemodynamic instability may be present.
- Urgent admission and treatment with IV antibiotics is essential.

Investigations for CIBH

1. Bedside
   - Observations: assess for pyrexia and identify haemodynamic instability.
   - Stool MC&S: to diagnose infective gastroenteritis. C. difficile toxin testing can be performed, and parasitic causes excluded.
   - Faecal calprotectin: ↑ in IBD.
   - Faecal elastase: ↑ in pancreatic insufficiency.
2. Bloods
   - FBC: ↑WCC is associated with infection or inflammation. Microcytic anaemia is associated with chronic blood loss. Macrocytic anaemia suggests malabsorption.
   - CRP/ESR: non-specific markers of inflammation, significantly increased in IBD.
   - U&E: significant diarrhoea can result in acute kidney injury (AKI) and electrolyte abnormalities.
   - Bone profile: hypercalcaemia is associated with constipation.
   - TFT: hyperthyroidism may cause diarrhoea, and hypothyroidism constipation.
   - CEA: a tumour marker increased in CRC.
3. Imaging
   - Abdominal X-ray (AXR): to identify acute complications of diarrhoea including ileus or toxic megacolon or diagnose bowel obstruction or faecal impaction.
   - CT colonography: for detailed assessment of intraluminal obstruction, strictures or masses.
   - Rigid sigmoidoscopy: to visualize the rectum and lower sigmoid. Neoplastic lesions or inflammatory changes in this area can be biopsied.
   - Flexible sigmoidoscopy/colonoscopy: to visualize the colon to the splenic flexure, and caecum in colonoscopy. Biopsies can be taken, or polyps removed.
   - Barium enema: for visualizing colonic mucosa. Suitable where strictures or severe diverticular disease prevent colonoscopy.

Laxative options to manage constipation should consider lifestyle factors and treatment course (Table 2.1).

CLINICAL NOTES

- Laxatives are avoided in intestinal obstruction or ileus, due to the risk of perforation with stimulant laxatives or faecal impaction with bulk forming laxatives.
- Loperamide may be considered short-term for mild-to-moderate diarrhoea, but should be avoided in infective diarrhoea or IBD, due to the risk of toxic megacolon.

Abdominal mass and distension

The differential diagnoses of abdominal mass or distension includes benign and malignant lesions of the GIT (Fig. 2.7).

HINTS AND TIPS

Causes of abdominal distension include the **6 F's**:

- Fat
- Fluid
- Flatus
- Faeces
- Foetus
- Fulminant mass

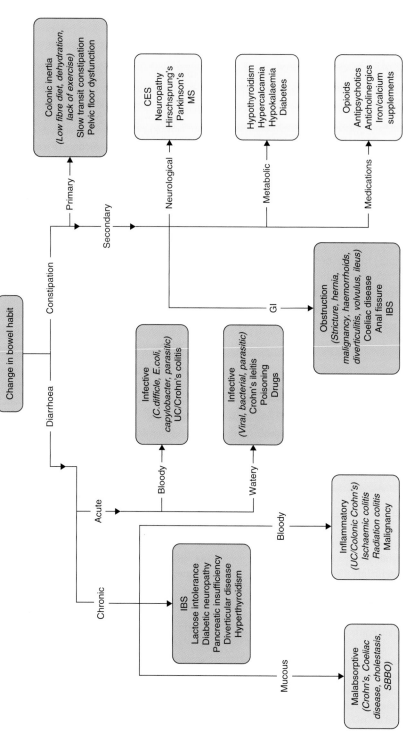

Fig. 2.6 Differential diagnosis of change in bowel habit. *CES*, Cauda equina syndrome; *IBS*, inflammatory bowel syndrome; *MS*, multiple sclerosis; *SBBO*, small bowel bacterial overgrowth; *UC*, ulcerative colitis.

Table 2.1 Laxatives

Classification	Mechanism	Example	Indication
Stimulant	Stimulates myenteric plexus, increased peristalsis,	Senna, bisacodyl	Short-term relief of acute constipation Decreased bowel motility
Osmotic	Attract water into intestinal lumen	Lactulose, Movicol	Chronic constipation
Stool softener	Promotes fat and water mixture to stool	Docusate sodium	Chronic constipation
Bulk-forming	Distends stool, promotes stool water retention	Fybogel, ispaghula husk	Low dietary fibre intake

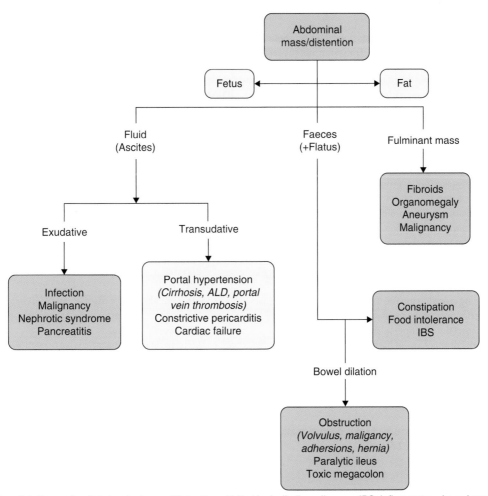

Fig. 2.7 Differential diagnosis of abdominal mass/distention. *ALD*, Alcoholic liver disease; *IBS*, inflammatory bowel syndrome.

Investigations for abdominal mass and distension

1. Bedside
   - Urinalysis: may show haematuria in renal tumours, or severe UTI.
   - Pregnancy test: indicated in any female of childbearing age.
   - Ascitic tap: ascitic fluid can be sent for MC&S to differentiate between transudative and exudative causes and look for malignant cells.
2. Bloods
   - FBC: ↑ WCC is associated with inflammatory pathology.
   - U&E: to assess for AKI, chronic kidney disease (CKD) or electrolyte derangement.
   - LFTs: hypoalbuminemia suggests poor liver synthetic function and may cause ascites. Transaminitis suggests hepatic pathology.
   - Tumour markers: ↑ CEA is associated with CRC, CA-125, with ovarian malignancy, and bHCG and AFP with ovarian or testicular teratoma.
3. Imaging
   - Abdominal US: to assess for ascites, organomegaly, masses and cysts.
   - AXR: distended loops of bowel suggest obstruction or pseudo-obstruction. A 'ground-glass' appearance suggests ascites.
   - CXR: pneumoperitoneum indicates perforation, associated with obstruction.
   - Intravenous urogram: to assess kidney anatomy and function in renal masses.
   - CT abdomen: for detailed assessment of abdominal viscera.
   - Barium enema: for imaging caecal masses and visualizing colonic mucosa. Can differentiate large bowel obstruction from pseudo-obstruction.
   - Small bowel fluoroscopy: to characterize small bowel functional or mechanical pathology.
   - Ultrasound-guided biopsy: to provide a histological diagnosis of a mass

Malnutrition

The causes of malnutrition include chronic disease, malabsorption, and lifestyle factors (Fig. 2.8).

CLINICAL NOTES

- Surgical patients are at high risk for perioperative malnutrition.
- Malnutrition increases the risk of infection and delayed wound healing.
- BMI and MUST scores should be calculated pre-operatively and monitored during the postoperative period.
- Nutritional support should be given as required, with enteral nutrition preferred.
- Total parenteral nutrition (TPN) is considered if bowel function is poor postoperatively.

Investigations for malnutrition

1. Bedside
   - Weight: weight should be measured to assess and monitor nutritional status.
   - CBG: severe malnourishment will manifest with hypoglycaemia.
   - ECG: cardiac muscle wasting risks arrhythmias.
   - Faecal elastase: elevation suggests pancreatic insufficiency, which can result in malabsorption and malnutrition.
   - Faecal calprotectin: elevated in IBD. Crohn's disease is associated with malnutrition due to small bowel disease.
2. Bloods
   - FBC: malabsorptive disease can result in anaemia.
   - U&Es: may demonstrate electrolyte abnormalities or AKI in dehydration.
   - LFTs: hypoalbuminaemia is associated with malnutrition.
   - TFTs: hyperthyroidism can result in malnutrition due to chronic diarrhoea.
   - Bone profile: hypophosphatemia and hypocalcaemia may indicate malnutrition.
   - B_{12}/folate: malabsorption of vitamin B results from ileal disease.

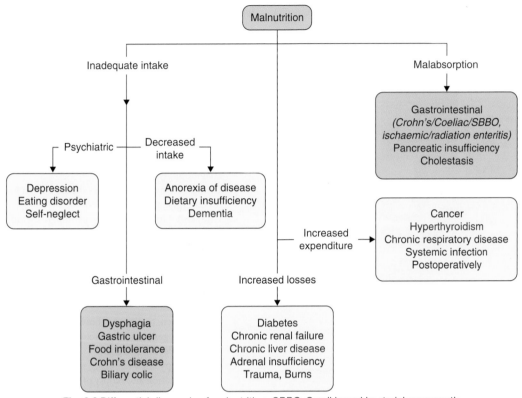

Fig. 2.8 Differential diagnosis of malnutrition. *SBBO,* Small bowel bacterial overgrowth.

3. Imaging
   - AXR: may demonstrate lead pipe colon or thumbprinting in IBD.
   - CTTAP: full body imaging may be performed if there is suspicion for malignancy.

DIFFERENTIALS

- Short gut syndrome results from resection of large stretches of intestine.
- Crohn's disease, radiation enteritis or mesenteric infarction are common causes.
- Resection to <1 m results in significant malabsorption and nutrient and vitamin deficiencies.
- TPN is necessary.

Management of malnutrition involves adequate nutritional support and identification of the underlying cause. Feeding options include:

- Supplements: specific nutrient replacement or provision of nutrient-dense food or drink.
- Enteral nutrition: nasogastric or nasojejunal tubes, or long-term, percutaneous routes gastrostomy or jejunostomy.

- Parenteral nutrition: delivery of complete nutritional requirements through central venous access. Used when enteral nutrition is not possible (Fig. 2.9).

RED FLAG

- Refeeding syndrome is a life-threatening condition resulting from rapid reintroduction of nutrition in chronic malnutrition.
- Massive insulin release results in acute hypophosphatemia, hypokalaemia and hypomagnesaemia.
- Features include arrhythmias, seizures and rhabdomyolysis.
- To avoid refeeding syndrome, food should be reintroduced slowly, and electrolytes monitored and replaced where required.

Lower GI bleeding

The differential diagnosis of lower GI bleeding (LGIB) includes inflammatory, infective, and malignant pathology. The appearance of the blood passed can help identify the location of GIT bleeding (Figs 2.10–2.11).

The approach to a patient with an LGIB involves resuscitation and urgent haemostasis (Fig. 2.12).

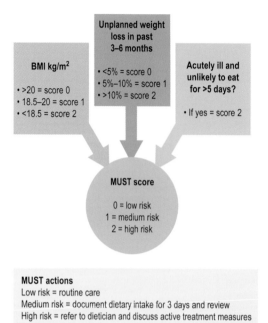

Fig. 2.9 Must score. The must score should be calculated to assess risk and need for nutritional support. (The 'Malnutrition Universal Screening Tool' ('MUST') is reproduced here with the kind permission of BAPEN (British Association for Parenteral and Enteral Nutrition). For further information on 'MUST' see www.bapen.org.uk.)

Investigations for LGIB

1. Bedside
   - Stool MC&S: severe diarrhoea associated with rectal bleeding suggests parasitic infection.
   - Faecal calprotectin: ↑ in IBD. Ulcerative colitis (UC) presents with LGIB.
2. Bloods
   - FBC: normocytic anaemia suggests acute blood loss, and microcytic anaemia suggests chronic bleeds.
   - U&Es: severe volume loss can result in AKI.
   - Clotting screen: severe bleeding will manifest with coagulopathy.
   - Group and save: two samples should be sent to prepare for emergency surgery and crossmatch for transfusion.
   - CRP/ESR: ↑ in inflammatory pathology including IBD.
   - Autoimmune screen: LGIB may relate to autoimmune pathology.
   - CEA: ↑ suggests CRC.
3. Imaging
   - CT angiography: to localize the bleeding site and attempt haemostasis.
   - CT abdomen: to diagnose bowel ischemia or fistula.
   - Oesophagogastroduodenoscopy (OGD): to exclude upper GI bleeding (UGIB).
   - Colonoscopy: for visualizing angiodysplasia, and characterization and biopsy of intestinal masses.
   - Proctoscopy: to assess for anorectal lesions. Sclerotherapy or banding can be applied directly if haemorrhoids are identified.

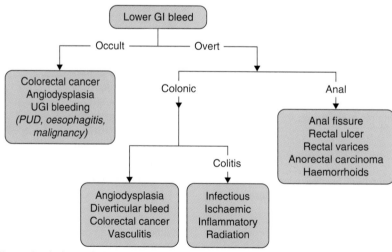

Fig. 2.10 Differential diagnosis of a lower GI bleed. Occult bleeding may be diagnosed on a FIT test or suspected due to unexplained iron deficiency anaemia.

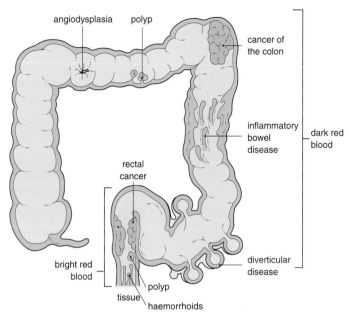

Fig. 2.11 Causes of lower GI bleeding. (From Kontoyannis A, Sweetland H. *Crash Course: Surgery*, 3rd Edition. Elsevier; 2008.)

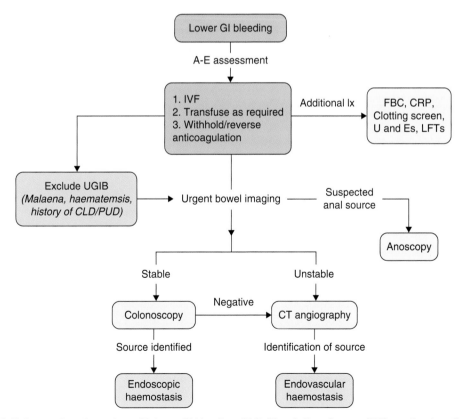

Fig. 2.12 Approach to the patient with lower GI bleeding. *CLD,* Chronic liver disease; *PUD,* peptic ulcer disease.

63

HINTS AND TIPS

In rectal bleeding managed conservatively, close haemoglobin monitoring is required to evaluate the need for transfusion.

CLINICAL NOTES

- Angiodysplasia is a vascular abnormality common in the elderly which can cause spontaneous severe rectal bleeding.
- Dilated tortuous vessels and 'cherry red' areas are seen on colonoscopy.

Anorectal pain

The differential diagnosis of anorectal pain includes infective and traumatic pathology (Fig. 2.13).

Investigations for anorectal pain

1. Bedside
   - FIT testing: to evaluate for occult LGIB.
   - CBG: hyperglycaemia and diabetes are associated with anorectal abscesses.
   - Fluid MC&S: anorectal fluid should be cultured to identify pathogens and guide antibiotic therapy.

2. Bloods
   - FBC: to evaluate for anaemia relating to blood loss. ↑WCC suggests an abscess.
   - U&Es: severe abscess infection can result in metabolic acidosis and AKI.
   - HIV testing: advised in all those with anal carcinoma if status is unknown.

3. Imaging
   - Pelvic CT: to assess for primary anal tumours and evaluate local spread.
   - Proctoscopy: direct inspection of the anal cavity to identify fistula or masses.
   - Anorectal US: to evaluate for sphincter pathology and anorectal malignancy.
   - Anorectal manometry: elevated sphincter pressures are associated with sphincter spasm in anal fissure.
   - Anoscopy and biopsy: to visualize an anorectal mass and obtain tissue samples for histology.

DIFFERENTIAL

- A perianal haematoma results from rupture of a perianal capillary.
- Symptoms include irreducible painless anal swelling.
- The majority resolve spontaneously within a few days.
- If non-resolving, evacuation under anaesthesia can be performed.

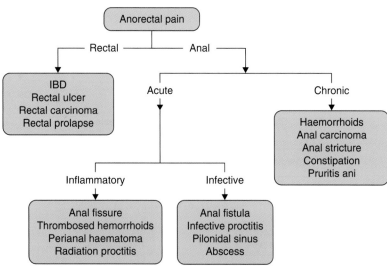

Fig. 2.13 Differential diagnosis of anorectal pain. *IBD*, Inflammatory bowel disease.

DIGITAL RECTAL EXAM

Rectal examination

A digital rectal examination (DRE) is essential to assess rectal symptoms or CIBH. Equipment required includes lubricant, paper towels and appropriate personal protective equipment (PEE).

General inspection

End-of-the-bed assessment can indicate underlying pathology:

- Weight loss: cachexia is severe muscle wasting associated with malignancy.
- Pallor: associated with anaemia, which may be related to chronic GIT bleeding.
- Lymphadenopathy: generalized, tender lymphadenopathy is associated with systemic immunosuppression including HIV infection.
- Skin rashes: rashes may be present in systemic inflammatory disorders or immunosuppression. Both increase the risk of anorectal abscesses and malignancy.
- Red eye: both painful and painless red eye can represent extraintestinal manifestations of IBD, which can present with anorectal symptoms.

Inspection

Separate the buttocks and inspect the perianal skin:

- Skin tags: small perianal skin tags are common and are associated with fissures.
- Haemorrhoids: external haemorrhoids may be visible as swellings near the anal verge.
- Fissure: tears in the anal canal are commonly located posteriorly and suggest chronic constipation. They are extremely painful.
- Fistula: anal fistulae are associated with IBD, anal abscesses and diverticular disease. There will be local erythema inflammation and anal discharge.
- Excoriations: suggest pruritis ani associated with anal pathology.
- Swelling: abscess may be visible with reddened, indurated overlying skin. Pilonidal abscesses lie in the natal cleft, with midline pitting representing infected hair follicles.
- Bleeding: visible anal bleeding may relate to haemorrhoids or anal malignancy.
- Rectal prolapse: ask the patient to cough. Appearance of a concentric mass suggests prolapse, or blue vascular lesions internal haemorrhoids.

Palpation

Lubricate the examining finger and insert gently into the anal canal.

- Rectum: rotate your finger 360 degrees to assess the rectal wall. Assess the size, location and texture of masses, and for hard stool in the rectum.
- Prostate: palpate the prostate anteriorly and assess size, lobar symmetry and consistency. A midline sulcus should be palpable. Asymmetry suggests malignancy.

- Anal tone: assess anal tone by asking the patient to contract on your finger. Reduced tone suggests spinal cord lesions, IBD or rectal trauma. High sphincter tone suggests anorectal spasm.
- Canal irregularities: fissures may be palpable as indurated lesions on the anal verge.

HINTS AND TIPS

Goodsall's rule states that anterior fistula communicate directly into the anal canal, and posterior fistula communicate in the midline.

RED FLAG

- Cauda equina syndrome results from compression of the cauda equina in the spinal cord.
- Symptoms include lower limb paralysis, lower back pain, saddle anaesthesia and loss of sphincter control.
- Reduced anal sphincter tone and faecal incontinence may be evident on DRE.
- Urgent lumbosacral MRI should be performed.

Withdraw your finger and inspect for blood or mucous on the glove.

- Melaena: dark, foul, tarry stool suggestive of UGIB
- Fresh red blood: associated with LGIB and IBD
- Mucous: associated with malabsorptive conditions

HINTS AND TIPS

- Crohn's disease presents with anal fistulae, fissures and abscesses.
- UC is associated with profuse bloody diarrhoea.

Completing the examination

Provide the patient with paper towels to clean themselves and offer them privacy to get dressed. Dispose of PPE, wash your hands and summarize your findings.

Further investigations include:

- OGD/coloscopy: to investigate any evidence of LGIB.
- Proctoscopy/sigmoidoscopy: for assessment of anorectal masses, and treatment of haemorrhoids.

INTESTINAL DISORDERS

Peritonitis

Peritonitis is the acute inflammation of the peritoneum. Secondary peritonitis relates to bacterial translocation from an intraabdominal source, typically appendicitis, diverticulitis, pancreatitis or organ perforation. Spontaneous bacterial peritonitis (SBP) describes bacterial infection of ascitic fluid without an identified intraabdominal source. It is common in patients with chronic liver disease (CLD).

Symptoms and signs

Symptoms include:

- Abdominal pain: severe and generalized.
- Peritonism: abdominal rigidity, rebound tenderness, guarding.
- Gastrointestinal upset: nausea, vomiting, CIBH, paralytic ileus.
- Haemodynamic instability: fever, tachycardia and hypotension.
- Altered mental status: associated with systemic infection or hepatic encephalopathy.

HINTS AND TIPS

- SBP may be asymptomatic.
- Have a high index of suspicion in patients with known ascites.

Investigations

Investigations include:

- FBC/CRP: systemic inflammation presents with ↑WBC/CRP.
- U&Es: AKI can relate to sepsis or hepatorenal syndrome.
- LFTs: deranged acutely in intraabdominal sepsis or relating to CLD.
- Clotting screen: CLD can manifest with coagulopathy.
- Blood cultures: two sets should be taken before antibiotics are given.
- Abdominal US: will show peritoneal inflammation and free fluid in the abdomen.
- Diagnostic paracentesis: peritoneal fluid should be sampled and sent for analysis (Fig. 2.14).

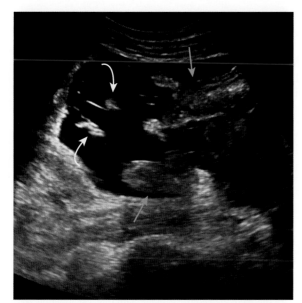

Fig. 2.14 Abdominal US in peritonitis. US demonstrating peritonitis relating to bowel perforation. Complex ascites with fibrous septa (*white arrows*) surrounds the bowel (*blue arrows*), with evident peritoneal thickening and bowel displacement. (From Kamaya A, Wong-You-Cheong J. *Diagnostic Ultrasound: Abdomen & Pelvis,* 2nd Edition. Elsevier; 2022.)

DIFFERENTIALS

- Neutrophilia ≥250/mm³ is diagnostic of peritonitis.
- In secondary peritonitis, the aetiological organisms are identified on fluid culture.
- Multiple organisms suggest perforation.
- In SBP, culture is often negative, but gram-negative species may be found.

Management

Management includes:

- Antibiotics: empirical broad-spectrum antibiotics, tailored to culture results.
- Supportive measures: IV fluids, analgesia and antipyretics, withhold nephrotoxic drugs.

Additional management of SBP involves:

- IV albumin: to reduce the risk of hepatorenal syndrome
- Repeat paracentesis: after 48 hours, to assess the response to antibiotics.
- Secondary prophylaxis: in patients with recurrent SBP, typically ciprofloxacin.

CLINICAL NOTES

Identification of the underlying cause and definitive management in secondary peritonitis is essential to prevent overwhelming sepsis and death

---

The prognosis relates to the speed of identification and administration of antibiotic therapy. Peritonitis carries a high risk of sepsis, acute organ failure and death.

Appendicitis

Appendicitis is the acute inflammation of the appendix. Appendix obstruction by infective lymphoid tissue hyperplasia or a fecalith results in local inflammation, bacterial translocation, and if severe, ischaemia, perforation and peritonitis. Appendicitis is very common, particularly in children.

Symptoms and signs

Characteristic symptoms include:

- Abdominal pain: periumbilical pain that migrates to the RIF (Fig. 2.15).
- Anorexia: associated with nausea and vomiting.
- Fever: low-grade fever is common. High temperature suggest perforation.
- Diarrhoea/constipation: due to inflammation or paralytic ileus.

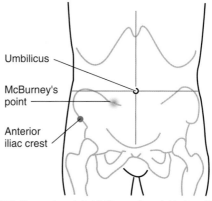

Fig. 2.15 McBurney's point. McBurney's point is two-thirds of the way from the right anterior superior iliac crest to the umbilicus. The pain migrates to this point within 12 to 24 hours of presentation. (From Ignatavicius DD, Workman ML, Rebar CR. *Medical-Surgical Nursing: Concepts for Interprofessional Collaborative Care,* 9th Edition. Elsevier; 2018.)

Typical examination features include:

- RIF tenderness: localized tenderness at McBurney's point.
- Peritonism: guarding, rigidity, and rebound tenderness in the RIF.
- Rovsing's sign: RIF pain on palpation of LIF.
- Psoas sign: RIF pain on passive extension of the right hip when lying on the left side.

HINTS AND TIPS

- Inflammation irritates the appendiceal visceral peritoneum, producing pain referred to the T10 dermatome (the umbilicus).
- Progressive inflammation irritates the parietal peritoneum, resulting in sharp localized pain over the appendix in the RIF.

Investigations

Investigations include:

- Urinalysis: may be positive, with mild leucocytosis and haematuria.
- FBC/CRP: ↑ WBC and CRP indicate inflammation.
- U&Es: vomiting and diarrhoea can result in AKI and electrolyte abnormalities.
- b-HCG: essential to exclude ectopic pregnancy in females of childbearing age.

Appendicitis is a clinical diagnosis. Imaging can be performed if the diagnosis is in doubt (Fig. 2.16).

Management

The approach to appendicitis includes resuscitation, risk stratification, and urgent surgical consult (Fig. 2.17).

CLINICAL NOTES

Laparoscopic appendectomy within 24 hours is the gold standard management.

Complications

Complications include:

- Appendiceal mass: collection of inflammatory appendiceal tissue. Managed conservatively, with interval appendectomy when acute inflammation has resolved.
- Appendiceal abscess: localized pus and necrotic appendiceal tissue, resulting from perforation, presenting with sepsis and severe RIF pain. Managed with percutaneous drainage and interval appendectomy.
- Gangrenous appendicitis: appendiceal necrosis. Requires emergency appendectomy.
- Perforation: appendiceal rupture, resulting in peritonitis. Requires emergency appendectomy.

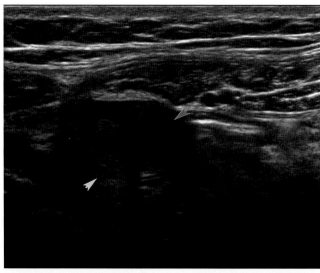

Fig. 2.16 Abdominal US in acute appendicitis. US findings include appendiceal dilation, wall thickening, and the target sign (concentric rings of hyperechogenicity) within the appendix. (From Dighe MK, Grajo JR, Lee LK. *Abdominal Imaging: Case Review Series.* Elsevier; 2022.)

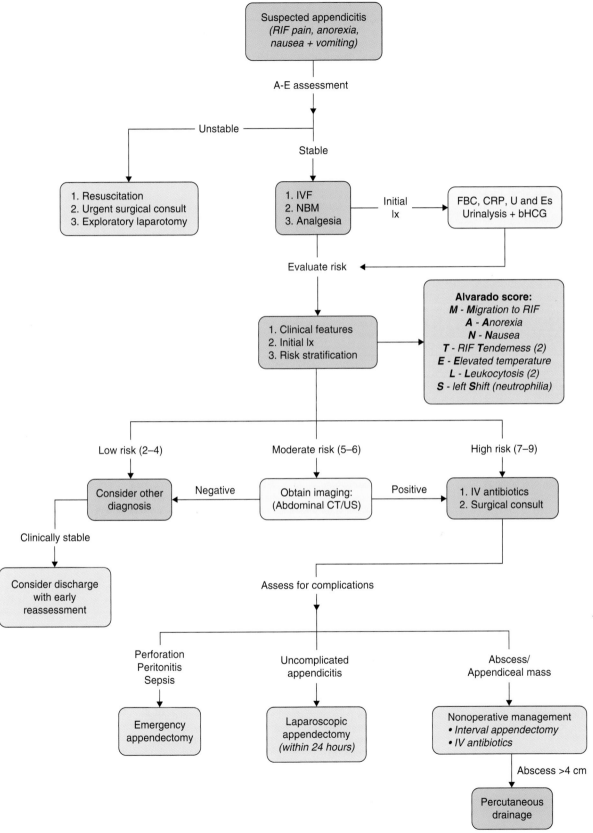

Fig. 2.17 Approach to the patient with acute appendicitis. *NBM,* Nil by mouth.

The prognosis is good, in uncomplicated cases. The mortality rate is approximately 1% in those progressing to perforation and peritonitis

Inflammatory bowel disease

IBD describes the autoimmune inflammation of the GIT. IBD is differentiated into UC and Crohn's disease, based on colonoscopy findings and clinical features. Risk factors include family history and inheritance of the HLA-B27 antigen (Table 2.2, Figs 2.18–2.20).

Table 2.2 Inflammatory bowel disease

	Crohn's	UC
Site affected	Mouth to anus (predominantly terminal ileum and colon)	Begins in rectum Ascends through colon → caecum
Symptoms	Chronic diarrhoea (+/– blood, in colitis) Abdominal pain, palpable mass Malabsorption, anaemia, weight loss	Chronic bloody diarrhoea Abdominal pain Faecal urgency, tenesmus
Investigations	↑ Faecal calprotectin ↑ CRP/ESR	↑ Faecal calprotectin ↑ CRP/ESR pANCA
Colonoscopy findings	Transmural inflammation Skip lesions Mucosal ulceration, cobblestoning Fissures, strictures, fistula	Mucosal/submucosal inflammation, oedema, friable with easy bleeding Surface erosions/ulcerations Crypt abscesses
Extraintestinal manifestations	Fatigue, low-grade fever Enteropathic arthritis Anterior uveitis, episcleritis Clubbing Erythema nodosum Pyoderma gangrenosum	Fatigue, low-grade fever Ankylosing spondylitis Anterior uveitis, episcleritis Primary sclerosis cholangitis Erythema nodosum Pyoderma gangrenosum
Treatment	Induce remission: • Corticosteroids • TNF inhibitors (infliximab) Maintain remission: • Azathioprine • Methotrexate • Sulphasalazine (5-ASA)	Induce remission: • Corticosteroids • Mesalamine (5-ASA) Maintain remission: • Mesalamine • Azathioprine (if remission achieved with steroids)
Complications	Colorectal cancer Fistula – anal, enterovaginal/vesical Perianal abscesses, ulcers Bile acid malabsorption Malnutrition, anaemia, osteoporosis Stenosis, strictures, obstruction Perforation, peritonitis	Colorectal cancer Toxic megacolon Fulminant colitis Acute/chronic GI bleeding Amyloidosis Stenosis, strictures, obstruction Perforation, peritonitis

ASA, *aminosalicylates;* pANCA, *perinuclear anti-neutrophil cytoplasmic antibodies;* TNF, *tumour necrosis factor.*

Inflammatory bowel disease (IBD)

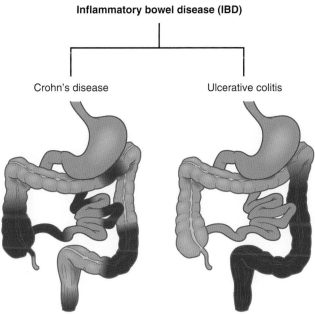

Crohn's disease   Ulcerative colitis

Fig. 2.18 Distribution of inflammatory bowel disease. Areas of inflammation in IBD. Crohn's is associated with skip lesions affecting the entire GIT. Inflammation in UC ascends proximally from the rectum to the colon. (From Harding MM. *Lewis's Medical-Surgical Nursing: Assessment and Management of Clinical Problems,* 12th Edition. Elsevier; 2023.)

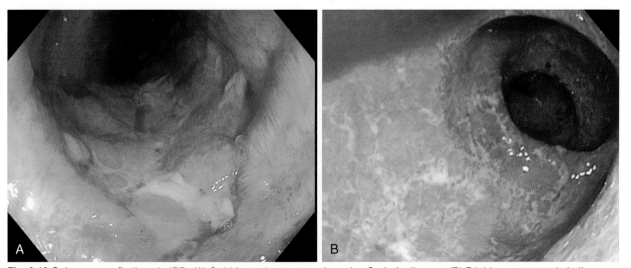

Fig. 2.19 Colonoscopy findings in IBD. (A) Cobblestoning mucosa in active Crohn's disease. (B) Friable mucosa and shallow ulcerations in UC, often described as a 'starry sky'. (From A. Chandrasekhara V, et al. *Clinical Gastrointestinal Endoscopy,* 3rd Edition. Elsevier; 2019. B. McIntire SC, Garrison J, et al. *Zitelli and Davis' Atlas of Pediatric Physical Diagnosis,* 8th Edition. Elsevier; 2023.)

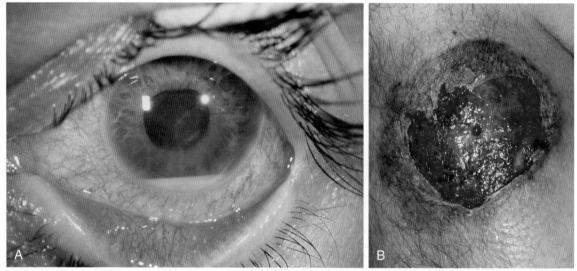

Fig. 2.20 Extraintestinal manifestation of IBD. (A) Anterior uveitis, with hyperaemia and hypopyon in the anterior chamber. (B) Pyoderma gangrenosum with a violaceous, irregular ulcer. (From A. Duker JS, Read RW, Yanoff M. *Ophthalmology,* 6th Edition. Elsevier; 2023. B. Kellerman RD, Lee EM, Wu DJ, Rajpara AN, Heidelbaugh JJ, Rakel DP. *Conn's Current Therapy 2023.* Elsevier; 2023.)

CLINICAL NOTES

- Faecal calprotectin, CRP and ESR are used to monitor disease activity.
- Endoscopic monitoring is required in the active treatment phase, but once remission has been achieved, is not routinely recommended.

RED FLAG

- Toxic megacolon presents with profuse diarrhoea, rectal bleeding, haemodynamic instability, and a distended and tender abdomen with absent bowel sounds.
- It is an indication for emergency surgery.

Acute management

IBD can present with acute flares, either as the initial presentation or as a relapse of known disease. Fulminant Crohn's disease presents with high fever, nausea, and vomiting, associated with intestinal obstruction, peritonitis, and intraabdominal abscesses. An acute flare of UC presents with fulminant colitis, with unremitting, frequent bloody diarrhoea, associated with complications including toxic megacolon (acute colonic dilation, ulcerations, and perforation). Both can result in sepsis, hypotension, multiorgan failure and death without urgent resuscitation and induction of remission (Figs 2.21–2.22).

Surgical management

Surgery is typically indicated for complications or refractory disease.

- UC: surgery can be curative and reduces the risk of colorectal cancer. Proctocolectomy with ileal pouch-anal anastomosis (J pouch) is used, to preserve continence.
- Crohn's disease: including disease resection with anastomosis or stoma formation, abscess drainage or stricturoplasty. Can induce temporary remission, but not curative. Short bowel syndrome may develop following several operations (Fig. 2.23).

Prognosis relates to the response to treatment and maintenance of remission.

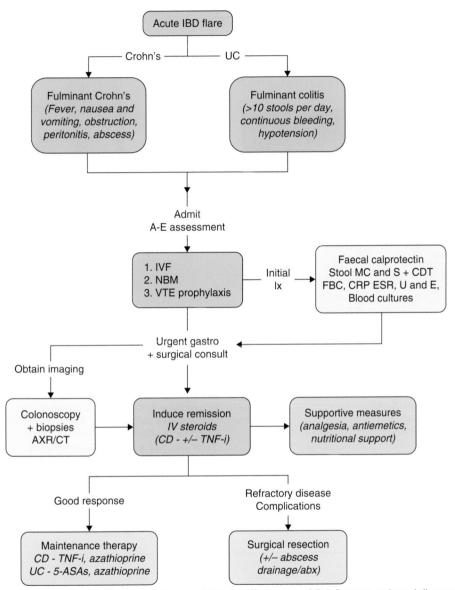

Fig. 2.21 Acute management of IBD. (*CD*, Crohn's disease; *CDT*, *C. difficile* toxin; *IBD*, inflammatory bowel disease; *NBM*, Nil by mouth; *TNF-i*, TNF inhibitor; *UC*, ulcerative colitis.)

Bowel obstruction

Bowel obstruction describes functional or mechanical obstruction to passage of bowel contents through the bowel. Mechanical obstruction can be classified as small bowel obstruction (SBO), or large bowel obstruction (LBO), depending on the location of the pathology. Functional obstruction (paralytic ileus) relates to ineffective or absent peristalsis (Table 2.3).

CLINICAL NOTES

- A closed loop bowel obstruction forms between multiple obstructing sites, for example distal colonic malignancy with a competent ileocecal valve.
- Emergency surgery is required due to the risk of rapid bowel necrosis and perforation.

Symptoms and signs

Symptoms include:

- Abdominal pain: colicky pain with progressive abdominal distension.
- Nausea and vomiting: initially bilious, progressing to feculent.

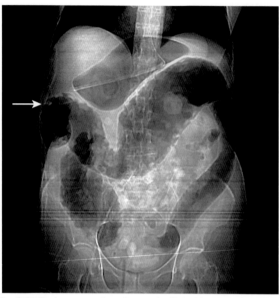

Fig. 2.22 Toxic megacolon. A grossly dilated transverse colon, indicating toxic megacolon. Wall thickening, loss of the haustral folds and 'lead-pipe' appearance of the colon is indicative of severe colitis. (From Zaheer A, Fananapazir G, Raman SP, Foster BR. *ExpertDDX: Abdomen and Pelvis,* 3rd Edition. Elsevier; 2023.)

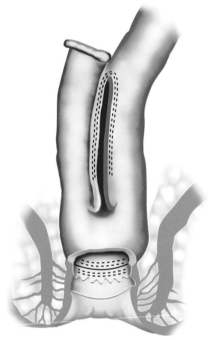

Fig. 2.23 J-pouch formation. Proctocolectomy with ileal pouch-anal anastomosis (J pouch), with resection of the entire colon, sparing of the anal sphincters, and creation of an artificial rectum using loops of small intestine. Pouchitis is a common postoperative complication. (From Araghizadeh F, Brandt LJ, Friedman LS, Feldman M, Feldman. *Sleisenger and Fordtran's Gastrointestinal and Liver Disease: Pathophysiology, Diagnosis, Management,* 10th Edition. Elsevier; 2016.)

Table 2.3 Aetiology of bowel obstruction

SBO	LBO	Paralytic ileus
Adhesions (postoperative, infective)	**Malignancy**	**Recent surgery**
Incarcerated hernias	Diverticulitis	Critical illness
Strictures	Volvulus	Atherosclerosis
Meckel's diverticulum	Adhesions	Medications - opioids, anticholinergics,
Gallstone ileus	Strictures	antiparkinson agents
Foreign body	Faecal impaction	Abdominal infection
	Foreign body	

- Constipation: in severe cases, obstipation (no passage of stool or flatus).
- Absent/decreased bowel sounds: initially hyperactive ('tinkling'), then reduced.
- Peritonism: abdominal guarding, rigidity and rebound tenderness suggest peritonitis.

Partial obstruction is possible, presenting with subacute symptoms.

DIFFERENTIALS

- A volvulus is the twisting of a bowel loop around the mesentery.
- It typically affects the sigmoid colon.
- There is a high risk of bowel necrosis and perforation.
- Risk factors include age and chronic constipation.
- Symptoms include abdominal pain, obstipation, and gross abdominal distension.
- Abdominal imaging may demonstrate the typical 'coffee-bean' sign.
- Endoscopic compression can be attempted, but if refractory, bowel resection is required.

Investigations

Investigations include:

- VBG: metabolic acidosis and ↑lactate suggest bowel ischaemia. A hypochloraemic, hypokalaemic metabolic alkalosis can occur following significant vomiting.
- FBC/CRP: ↑WBC/CRP relates to systemic inflammation and ischaemia.
- U&E: AKI and electrolyte abnormalities can result from third-spacing of fluid of vomiting.
- Abdominal imaging: CT/AXR will demonstrate bowel dilation.
- CXR: pneumoperitoneum (free air under the diaphragm) suggests perforation (Figs 2.24–2.25).

CLINICAL NOTES

In paralytic ileus, imaging demonstrate small and large diffuse bowel dilation, no obstructing lesion, and absent peristalsis.

HINTS AND TIPS

- The 3, 6, 9 rule can be used to assess for bowel dilation:
  - Small bowel >3 cm
  - Large bowel >6 cm
  - Caecum >9 cm
- Dilated bowel loops will be central in SBO and peripheral in LBO.

Management

Acute bowel obstruction is a medical emergency. Urgent resuscitation and bowel decompression are essential to prevent necrosis, perforation, and peritonitis (Fig. 2.26).

CLINICAL NOTES

- Following NG tube placement, adequate gastric aspirate (pH <5.5) should be obtained to confirm the location in the stomach.
- If adequate aspirate cannot be obtained, a chest X-ray must be ordered to confirm placement.

The prognosis relates to the speed of decompression. There is a high risk of recurrence. Frequent recurrences with failure of conservative management are an indication for surgery.

Intestinal ischaemia

Bowel ischaemia includes acute mesenteric ischaemia (AMI), chronic mesenteric ischaemia (CMI), or ischaemic colitis. Acute ischaemia typically relates to acute hypoperfusion, including severe systemic infection, hypotension, surgery, or occlusive thromboembolic disease. Atherosclerosis can result in chronic ischaemia and may precipitate acute ischaemia (Table 4.4, Figs 2.27–2.28).

HINTS AND TIPS

The classic triad of AMI includes:

- Acute abdominal pain
- Bloody diarrhoea
- Atrial fibrillation

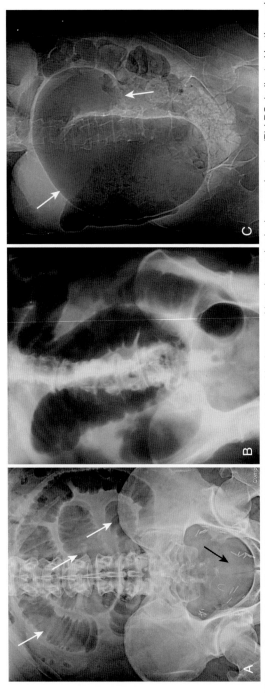

Fig. 2.24 Bowel obstruction. (A) SBO. The small bowel can be recognized by its central location and valvulae conniventes. (B) LBO, indicated by the peripheral location and presence of haustra. (C) Sigmoid volvulus, with the characteristic 'coffee-bean' sign. (From A, C. Herring CW. *Learning Radiology: Recognizing the Basics*, 5th Edition. Elsevier; 2024. B. Walls RM, Thomas N, Wu AW. *Rosen's Emergency Medicine: Concepts and Clinical Practice 2-Volume Set*, 10th Edition. Elsevier; 2023.)

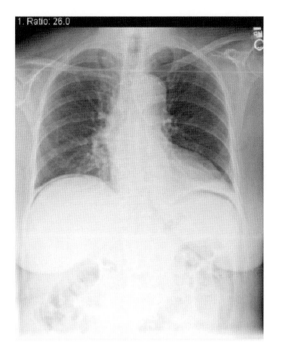

Fig. 2.25 Pneumoperitoneum. Free air under the diaphragm is suggestive of bowel perforation. (From Vincent J-L, et al. *Textbook of Critical Care,* 8th Edition. Elsevier; 2024.)

DIFFERENTIALS

- Radiation enteritis results from bowel ischemia and fibrosis following radiotherapy
- Symptoms include chronic abdominal pain, diarrhoea, and rectal bleeding.
- There is a risk of haemorrhage, perforation and obstruction.

Complications

Complications include:

- Gangrenous colitis: peritonism and fever suggest bowel necrosis and gangrene.
- Peritonitis: perforation can result in acute peritonitis, sepsis and multiorgan failure.
- Hypovolaemic shock: relating to severe diarrhoea and haemorrhage.

RED FLAG

Indications for emergency surgery include perforation, peritonitis, sepsis, massive haemorrhage and gangrenous colitis.

Prognosis relates to the speed of revascularization. The mortality of untreated ischaemia is close to 100%.

Diverticular disease

Diverticulosis describes the development of outpouchings of the colonic wall known as diverticula. Increased intraluminal pressure (typically related to constipation) and age-related intestinal wall weakness result in wall herniation, typically affecting the sigmoid colon. It is very common. Risk factors include low-fibre diets, obesity, lack of exercise, age and smoking.

Symptoms and signs

Diverticulosis is commonly asymptomatic. If symptoms develop, they include:

- Abdominal pain: intermittent colicky abdominal discomfort.
- Change in bowel habit: alternating diarrhoea and constipation.
- Diverticular complications: acute bleeding, infection, bowel obstruction and perforation.

Investigations

Asymptomatic diverticulosis may be diagnosed incidentally on abdominal imaging. Symptomatic or complicated diverticulosis is an indication for colonoscopy (Fig. 2.29).

Management

Management of diverticulosis involves preventing progression, with high-fibre diet, weight loss, increased exercise and smoking cessation, and management of complications.

Complications of diverticulosis include:

- Diverticular bleed: the most common cause of LGIB in adults, resulting in painless haematochezia. Typically resolves spontaneously. In significant bleeding, endoscopic haemostasis is required.
- Acute diverticulitis: acute diverticular inflammation, presenting with pyrexia, left lower quadrant pain, and a palpable mass, relating to pericolic inflammation.

Complications of diverticulitis include:

- Perforation: diverticulitis may proceed to perforation and generalized peritonitis.
- Pericolic abscess: perforation of diverticula can result in local abscess formation.
- Fistula formation: in acute diverticulitis, adherence of the colon to intraabdominal organs can result in vesicocolic, colovaginal or coloenteric fistula.
- Diverticular bleeding: inflammation can precipitate episodes of bleeding.

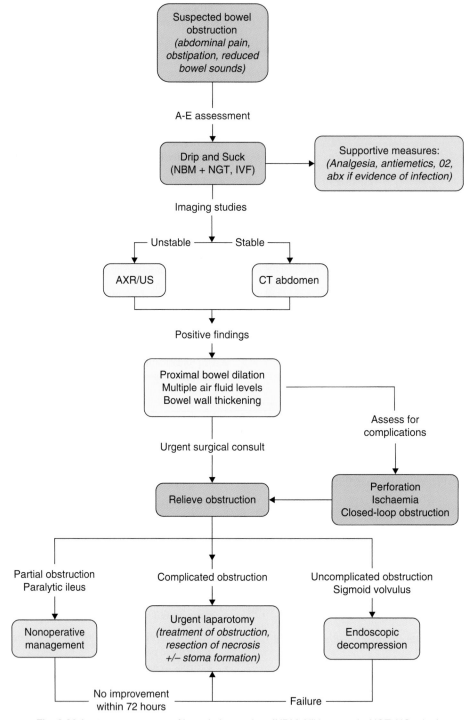

Fig. 2.26 Acute management of bowel obstruction. (*NBM*, Nil by mouth; *NGT*, NG tube.)

Table 2.4 Bowel ischaemia

	AMI	CMI	Ischaemic colitis
Aetiology	Thromboembolism (commonly due to AF) Acute hypoperfusion	Progressive atherosclerotic occlusion	Acute hypoperfusion +/− background atherosclerotic disease
Location	SMA, SMV	SMA, SMV	Watershed areas
Clinical features	Severe periumbilical pain Diarrhoea +/− blood Peritonism, sepsis	Postprandial pain Food aversion Abdominal bruit	Sudden abdominal pain Bloody diarrhoea Faecal urgency
Ix	CTA – embolism, thrombosis or dissection ↑lactate, WBC, CK, LDH	Duplex US – mesenteric stenosis Anaemia, ↓albumin	AXR/CTA – bowel wall thickening, thumbprinting ↑lactate, WBC, CK, LDH
Mx	Abx, IVF, NBM Lifelong anticoagulation Revascularization (endoscopic/surgical) Resection of necrosis	Low-fat diet, small meals Reduce vascular risk Endovascular angioplasty and stenting	Mild – supportive, bowel rest, nutritional support Severe – antibiotics and surgical resection +/− stoma formation

AF, Atrial fibrillation; CTA, CT angiography; SMA, superior mesenteric artery; SMV, superior mesenteric vein.

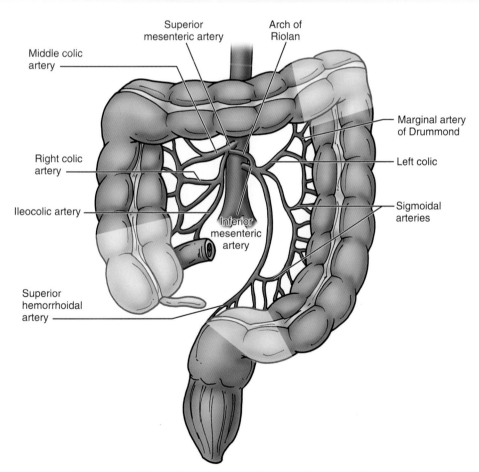

Fig. 2.27 Watershed areas of the colon, at high risk for ischaemic colitis. (From Cameron AM. *Current Surgical Therapy,* 13th Edition. Elsevier; 2020.)

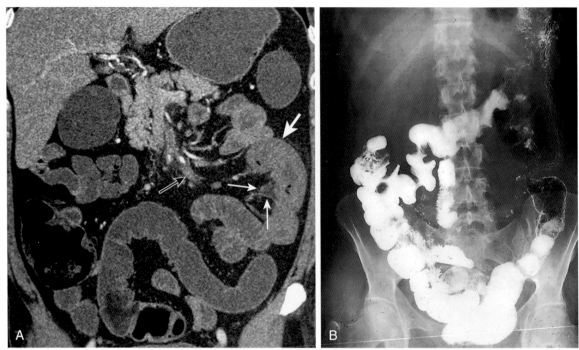

Fig. 2.28 Imaging findings in bowel ischaemia. (A) AMI relating to embolic occlusion of SMA. *Black arrow* – embolic occlusion of jejunal SMA branches, manifesting as mural thickening, oedema and hypoperfusion (*white arrows*). (B) Ischaemic colitis on X-ray, with evident mucosal oedema and 'thumb printing'. (From A. Adam A, Gourtsoyiannis N, Daskalogiannaki M. *Grainger & Allison's Diagnostic Radiology: A Textbook of Medical Imaging,* 5th Edition. Edinburgh: Churchill Livingstone, 2008. B. Garden OJ. *Principles and Practice of Surgery: Adapted International Edition,* 6th Edition. Churchill Livingstone, Elsevier; 2012.)

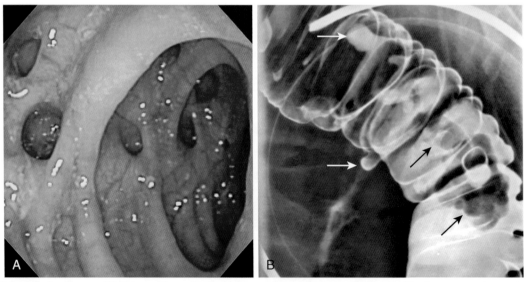

Fig. 2.29 Diverticular disease. (A) Outpouchings of colonic mucosa on colonoscopy. (B) Contrast barium enema demonstrating numerous diverticula. (From A. Feldman M, Friedman LS, Brandt LJ. *Sleisenger y Fordtran. Enfermedades digestivas y hepáticas: Fisiopatología, diagnóstico y tratamiento,* 11.ª Edición. Elsevier; 2022. B. Zaheer A, Raman SP. *Diagnostic Imaging: Gastrointestinal,* 4th Edition. Elsevier; 2022.)

- Bowel obstruction: repeated episodes of diverticulitis can result in thickening, fibrosis, and hypertrophy of the bowel wall, resulting in strictures, stenosis and bowel obstruction (Fig. 2.30).

The management of acute diverticulitis relates to Hinchey classification (Table 2.5).

The prognosis is good. Most complications resolve with conservative measures. Patients with recurrent acute complications or chronic fistula/stricture formation typically have elective colectomy, following the resolution of acute symptoms.

Colorectal carcinoma

Colorectal carcinoma (CRC) is one of the most common malignancies. CRC typically manifests due to malignant transformation of a colonic polyp. Other risk factors include older age, smoking, obesity, diets low in fibre and high in processed meat, IBD, and genetic disorders.

CLINICAL NOTES

- Polyps are typically asymptomatic.
- They are common in older adults and genetic conditions, including familial adenomatous polyposis (FAP), and hereditary nonpolyposis colorectal cancer (HNPCC).
- Polyps are typically diagnosed during colonoscopy for unexplained occult GI bleeding or anaemia.
- Visualized polyps are typically removed, due to the risk of malignant transformation, particularly with adenomas.

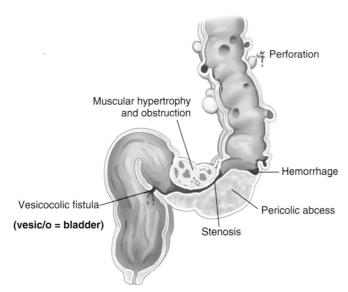

Fig. 2.30 Complications of diverticulitis. (From Shiland BJ, Zenith. *Medical Assistant: Digestive System, Nutrition, Financial Management and First AidR—Module C,* 2nd Edition. Elsevier; 2015.)

Table 2.5 Modified Hinchey classification of diverticulitis

Stage	Clinical features	Management
0	Mild diverticulitis	Uncomplicated diverticulitis: Conservative Oral antibiotics
Ia	Localized pericolic inflammation	
Ib	Local pericolic abscess	Complicated diverticulitis: Admission, IV antibiotics Percutaneous abscess drainage
II	Distant (pelvic/retroperitoneal) abscess	
III	Perforation, generalized purulent peritonitis	Emergency surgery IV antibiotics Complete bowel rest
IV	Perforation, generalized faecal peritonitis	

The lower gastrointestinal Tract

Symptoms and signs

CRC is often asymptomatic in the early stages. When symptoms develop, they include:

- Abdominal pain: mild, nonspecific abdominal discomfort or colicky pain.
- Constitutional features: fever, lethargy, appetite and weight loss, night sweats.
- Change in bowel habit: constipation or diarrhoea can occur.
- GI bleeding: melaena, haematochezia or occult bleeding (manifesting as iron-deficient anaemia) can occur, relating to the location of pathology.

RED FLAG

- New, unexplained anaemia, weight loss or GI bleeding in older adults should raise suspicion for CRC.
- Urgent colonoscopy is required.

CLINICAL NOTES

DRE may reveal melaena or a palpable lesion in rectal cancer.

Investigations

Investigations include:

- FBC: demonstrating microcytic, hypochromic anaemia.
- CEA: ↑ CRC, and monitored as a prognostic marker and to assess treatment response.
- Colonoscopy: the gold standard diagnostic test. Typical findings include an ulcerated mass, which should be biopsied for histological diagnosis.
- CTTAP: for staging and detection of local and distant metastatic disease (Fig. 2.31).

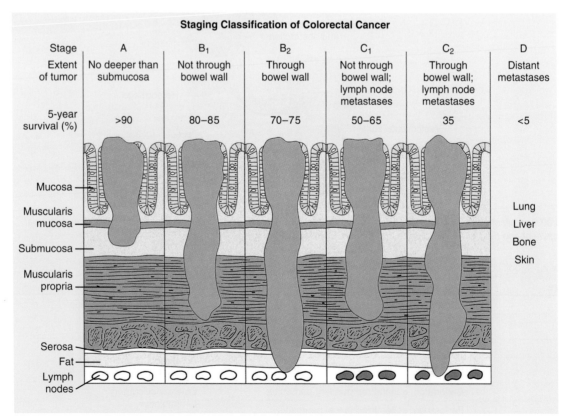

Fig. 2.31 TNM staging of CC. (From Skarin AT, Shaffer K, Wieczorek T. *Atlas of Diagnostic Oncology*, 4th Edition. Elsevier; 2010.)

82

CLINICAL NOTES

- CRC screening is offered every 2 years to those 60-75, involving a FIT test.
- Those with a positive test are invited for colonoscopy.

Management

Management should take an MDT approach, depending on the location and staging of the tumour, patient performance status, and realistic goals of treatment

- Curative treatment: offered for most patients. Resection of primary tumour, with neoadjuvant radiochemotherapy and regional lymph node dissection.

- Resection of metastasis: liver or lung metastasis may be resectable, and significantly improve cervical.
- Palliative surgery: including tumour resection or intestinal bypass, to relieve symptoms of obstructive CRC in those with unresectable metastatic disease.

The surgical approach used relates to the location of pathology (Fig. 2.32, Table 2.6).

Complications

Complications include:

- Bowel obstruction: large lesions may obstruct the bowel lumen and result in obstruction.
- Metastatic disease: liver, lung, and peritoneal metastases (peritoneal carcinomatosis) are common and may be the initial presentation of disease.

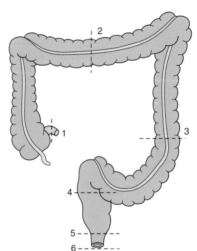

1–2: right hemicolectomy
2–4: left hemicolectomy
3–4: sigmoid colectomy
2–5: low anterior resection
3–4: resection of sigmoid colon with colostomy and closure of rectal stump (Hartmann's procedure)
3–6: abdominoperineal resection (sigmoid colon is brought out as a colostomy and anus and rectum are excised)

Fig. 2.32 Colonic surgery. (From Kontoyannis A., Sweetland H. *Crash Course: Surgery*, 3rd Edition. Elsevier; 2008.)

Table 2.6 Surgical resection of CRC

Procedure	Resection	Location of tumour
Right hemicolectomy	Distal ileum → proximal one-third transverse colon	Caecum/ascending colon
Extended right hemicolectomy	Right hemicolectomy + transverse colon	Transverse colon/hepatic flexure
Left hemicolectomy	Distal 1/3 of transverse → sigmoid colon	Descending colon
Sigmoid colectomy	Sigmoid colon	Sigmoid colon
Subtotal colectomy	Majority of colon	Multifocal lesion +/– underlying colonic disease
Anterior resection	Sigmoid colon and rectum	Rectosigmoid, upper rectum
Abdominoperineal	Anus, rectum + part of sigmoid Formation of colostomy	Distal two-third rectum

Following surgery, patients should be followed up with 6 monthly clinical assessments and CEA levels. Surveillance colonoscopy is advised at 1 year, and subsequent 3 to 5 yearly intervals, to assess for recurrence. The prognosis for localized disease is good following successful resection. For those with distant metastasis, 5-year survival is between 10% and 20%.

ANORECTAL DISORDERS

Haemorrhoids

A haemorrhoid is a dilated venous plexus with the anal canal. Increased intraabdominal pressure typically relating to chronic constipation or pregnancy, results in venous congestion. Internal haemorrhoids arise above the dentate line, and external haemorrhoids below (Fig. 2.33).

Symptoms and signs

Symptoms include:

- Bright red painless rectal bleeding following defecation
- Perianal mass secondary to haemorrhoid prolapse
- Mucous/feculent anal discharge, with associated pruritis

Internal haemorrhoids can be graded depending on the extent of prolapse (Fig. 2.34).

External haemorrhoids or grade IV internal haemorrhoids can become thrombosed, presenting with severe perianal pan, pain on defecation and tender perianal mass shiftenter(Fig. 2.35).

Investigations

Investigations include:

- DRE: to evaluate for prolapse or thrombosis.
- Anoscopy: to exclude anal fissure or anorectal carcinoma.

Management

Management of symptomatic haemorrhoids includes:

- Lifestyle modification: treatment of constipation, including increasing dietary fibre, increasing water intake and avoidance of straining.
- Topical medications: topical creams containing local anaesthetics with mild steroid can be bought over the counter to reduce pain and inflammation.

If conservative measures fail, interventional procedures include:

- Rubber band ligation

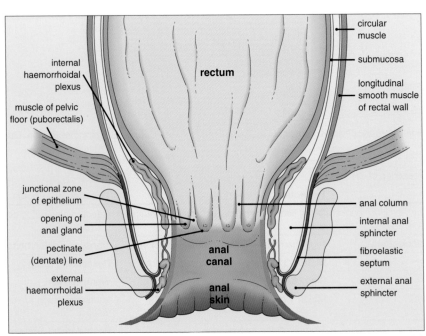

Fig. 2.33 Internal and external haemorrhoid plexi. The dentate line divides the anal canal into an upper two-thirds, that embryologically arises from endoderm, and a lower third, which arises from the ectoderm. (From Lowe JS, Anderson SI, Anderson PG. *Stevens & Lowe's Human Histology,* 5th Edition. Elsevier; 2020.)

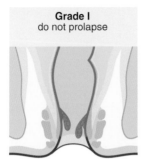
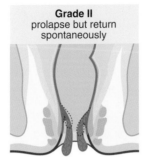
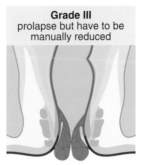

Grade I
do not prolapse

Grade II
prolapse but return
spontaneously

Grade III
prolapse but have to be
manually reduced

Fig. 2.34 Grading of haemorrhoids. Grade IV haemorrhoids are irreducible, and may be strangulated and thrombosed, presenting with severe perianal pain and a palpable perianal mass. (From Arulampalam THA, Biers SM, Quick CRG. *Essential Surgery: Problems, Diagnosis and Management*, 6th Edition. Elsevier; 2020.)

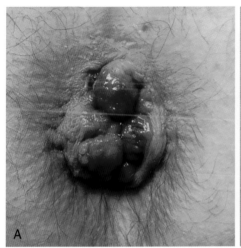
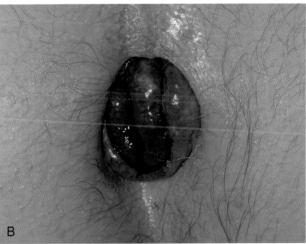

Fig. 2.35 External appearance of haemorrhoids. (A) Prolapsed grade III haemorrhoids. (B) Thrombosed haemorrhoids, with evidence of venous congestion and necrosis. (From A. Clark S. *Colorectal Surgery,* 6th Edition. Elsevier; 2019. B. Slater TA, Waduud MA, Ahmed N. *Pocketbook of Differential Diagnosis, 5th Edition.* Elsevier; 2022.)

- Sclerotherapy
- Cryotherapy

Surgical options are preferred for symptomatic grade III/IV haemorrhoids:

- Haemorrhoidectomy: haemorrhoid excision
- Haemorrhoidopexy: stapling for internal haemorrhoids

Anal fissure

An anal fissure is a superficial tear in the mucosa of the anal canal distal to the dentate line. Primary anal fissures arise at the posterior commissure and relate to anal trauma, commonly chronic constipation. Secondary fissures may occur laterally or anteriorly, relating to underlying disease, including anal surgery, IBD, infection or malignancy (Fig. 2.36).

Symptoms and signs

Symptoms include:

- Severe anorectal pain during defecation
- Bright red rectal bleeding
- Perianal pruritis

Management

Anal fissures are a clinical diagnosis. Treatment options include:

- Lifestyle modification: avoiding constipation, with dietary improvements and laxatives.
- Topical medications: antiinflammatory, analgesic, and topical vasodilator creams to reduce pain and anal sphincter spasm.

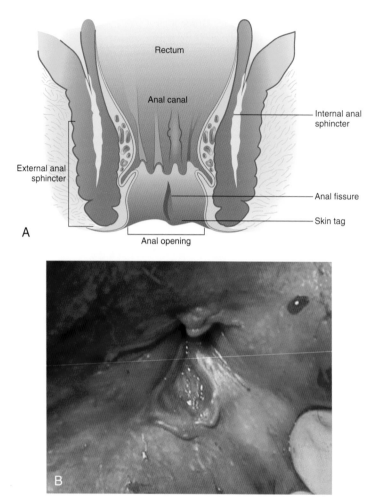

Fig. 2.36 Anal fissure. (A) Anal fissure in the posterior commissure with associated skin tag. (B) External appearance of an anal fissure. (From A. Tomkins Z. *Integrating Systems: Clinical Cases in Anatomy and Physiology.* Elsevier; 2021. Published January 1, 2022. B. From Koesterman JL. *Bucks 2020 Step-by-Step Medical Coding.* Elsevier; 2020.)

DIFFERENTIAL

Refractory or recurrent anal fissures with >8 weeks of unresolving symptoms is an indication for colonoscopy to exclude IBD or anal carcinoma.

If conservative measures fail, surgical management includes sphincterotomy or anal dilation. There is a risk of faecal incontinence, hence conservative measures are preferred first line.

Perianal abscesses and fistula

Perianal abscesses result from obstruction and bacterial infection of an anal crypt. They can also relate to IBD, intraabdominal infection, radiation proctitis or malignancy. Abscesses may progress to chronic fistula between the abscess and anal canal or perianal skin (Fig. 2.37).

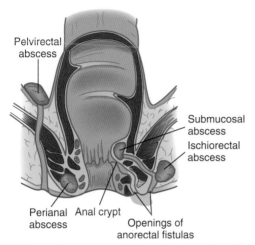

Fig. 2.37 Perianal abscess and fistula. Common sites of anorectal abscesses and fistula formation. (From Harding MM. *Lewis's Medical-Surgical Nursing: Assessment and Management of Clinical Problems,* 12th Edition. Elsevier; 2023.)

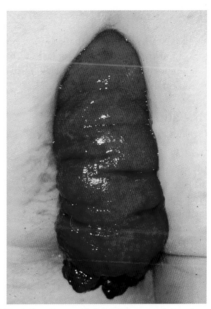

Fig. 2.38 Rectal prolapse. Full thickness rectal prolapse. (From Deakin PJ. *Essential Surgery: Problems, Diagnosis and Management,* 6th Edition. Elsevier; 2020.)

Symptoms and signs

Symptoms include:

- Anorectal pain and pruritis, worse on defecation
- Palpable subcutaneous mass
- Fever and rigors
- Purulent, mucoid, or bloody perianal discharge
- Chronic skin damage and faecal incontinence relating to fistulas
- Abscess and fistula can be very painful. DRE and investigations may only be possible with adequate analgesia or local anaesthesia.

Management

Abscesses and fistula are clinical diagnoses. CT or US imaging can be used to evaluate deep abscesses. Endoscopy may be required if there is suspicion of underlying IBD.
Management includes:

- Abscesses: Surgical incision and drainage
- Fistula: fistulotomy, with seton insertion or plugging, to promote drainage and fibrosis
- Supportive measures: including analgesia, laxatives and antibiotics

Rectal prolapse

A rectal prolapse is the partial or complete prolapse of the rectum through the anus. Partial prolapse of the rectal mucosa is common in children and typically resolves spontaneously. Full-thickness prolapse occurs in adults, typically relating to chronic constipation, excessive straining, and pelvic floor muscle weakness.

Symptoms and signs

Symptoms include:

- Painless rectal mass, appearing on straining
- Faecal incontinence and perianal pruritis
- Constipation
- Ulceration and rectal bleeding (Fig. 2.38)

Management

Rectal prolapse is a clinical diagnosis. Ulcerations should be biopsied to exclude malignancy. Management includes:

- Mucosal prolapse: manually reduction, with injection sclerotherapy if recurrent.
- Full-thickness prolapse: mesh rectopexy with sacral fixation. Sigmoidectomy can be performed simultaneously to relieve chronic constipation.
- Management of risk factors: avoiding constipation, by increasing dietary fibre, exercise and laxatives.

Anal carcinoma

Anal carcinoma is a rare malignancy that originates in the squamous mucosa of the lower anal canal. Risk factors include HPV infection, immunodeficiency (including HIV infection), anal intercourse, and smoking.

Symptoms and signs

Symptoms include:

- rectal bleeding
- palpable anal tumour
- anorectal pain
- rectal discharge and pruritus
- faecal incontinence

Investigations

Investigations include:

- DRE: large tumours may be externally visible or palpable within the anal canal.
- Anoscopy: to visualize tumours and take tissue samples or histology.
- CTTAP: for staging and identification of metastatic disease.

CLINICAL NOTES

Women with anal cancer should underlying evaluation for gynaecological malignancy (in particular cervical and vulval cancer), due to the association with HPV infection.

Management

Management involves radiochemotherapy, with surgical excision where possible for tumours of the anal margin. If complete excision is possible, the prognosis is improved, with a five-year survival rate of approximately 50%.

● Chapter Summary

- The classic causes of abdominal distension are the 6 F's: Fat, Fluid, Flatus, Faeces, Foetus and Fulminant mass.
- The most common cause of an acute lower GI bleed in older adults is diverticular bleeding.
- Refeeding syndrome is a life-threatening complication of chronic malnutrition, where rapid food introduction results in acute hypophosphatemia, hypokalaemia, and hypomagnesemia, with a risk of arrhythmias, seizures, and rhabdomyolysis.
- Small bowel obstruction is commonly related to adhesions or hernias. Large bowel obstruction typically relates to malignancy.
- Ulcerative colitis presents with profuse bloody diarrhoea, relating to continuous colonic mucosal inflammation and surface erosions. Crohn's disease presents with chronic diarrhoea and malabsorption, relating to transmural noncontinuous inflammation throughout the entire GIT.
- A volvulus is a closed-loop bowel obstruction relating to twisting of the bowel on the mesentery. Sigmoidoscopic decompression should be attempted, with bowel resection if refractory.
- Acute mesenteric ischaemia presents with severe abdominal pain, bloody diarrhoea, and atrial fibrillation.
- Unexplained anaemia in an older adult is a red flag for colorectal carcinoma.
- Peritonitis is diagnosed with a neutrophil count >250/mm^3 on peritoneal fluid analysis.
- Appendicitis presents with RIF pain, fever, and anorexia. Urgent laparoscopic appendectomy within 24 hours is indicated.

Chapter Summary—cont'd

UKMLA Conditions
Acid-base abnormality
Adverse drug effects
Anaemia
Anal fissure
Appendicitis
Arterial thrombosis
Cirrhosis
Coeliac disease
Colorectal tumours
Constipation
Dehydration
Diverticular disease
Family history of possible genetic disorder
Fever
Gastrointestinal perforation
Haemorrhoids
Human immunodeficiency virus
Human papilloma virus infection
Infectious colitis
Infectious diarrhoea
Inflammatory bowel disease
Intestinal ischaemia
Intestinal obstruction and ileus
Irritable bowel syndrome
Jaundice
Malabsorption
Malnutrition
Metastatic disease
Osteoporosis
Pallor
Perianal abscesses and fistulae
Peritonitis
Reactive arthritis
Sepsis
Shock
Viral gastroenteritis
Vitamin B_{12} and/or folate deficiency
Volvulus
Vomiting

UKMLA Presentations
Acute abdominal pain
Abdominal distension
Abdominal mass
Abnormal urinalysis
Bleeding from lower GI tract
Change in bowel habit
Change in stool colour
Chronic abdominal pain
Constipation
Decreased appetite
Disease prevention/screening
Dehydration
Diarrhoea
Electrolyte abnormalities
Faecal incontinence
Fatigue
Food intolerance
Fever
Human papilloma virus infection
Inflammatory bowel disease
Intestinal obstruction and ileus
Jaundice
Malnutrition
Massive haemorrhage
Melaena
Misplaced nasogastric tube
Nausea
Night sweats
Organomegaly
Pallor
Perianal symptoms
Rectal prolapse
Sepsis
Shock
Vomiting
Weight loss

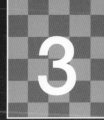

The anterior abdominal wall

3

CLINICAL ANATOMY

The abdominal wall is formed from skin, fascia, adipose tissue and muscle, beneath which layers of peritoneum enclose and protect the abdominal organs (Fig. 3.1).

Palpable surface landmarks on the abdominal wall guide the location of intra-abdominal structures. The line between the anterior superior iliac spine (ASIS) and the pubic tubercle delineates the inguinal ligament, formed from the aponeurosis of the external oblique muscle that forms the base of the inguinal canal.

The inguinal canal sits just superiorly to the medial part of the inguinal ligament. The deep inguinal ring forms the internal canal opening just superior to the mid-inguinal point. The superficial ring forms the external opening, at the medial end of the ligament, superior to the pubic tubercle (Fig. 3.2). The spermatic cord in men and round ligament of the uterus in women, alongside branches of the ilioinguinal and genitofemoral nerve, travel through the inguinal canal to the external genitalia (Fig. 3.3).

The femoral triangle is formed superiorly by the inguinal ligament, laterally by the sartorius muscle and medially by the adductor longus muscle. The femoral artery emerges at the mid-inguinal point medial to the femoral nerve, and the femoral vein lies medial to the artery. The femoral canal is a potential space just medial to the femoral vein, bordered anteriorly by the inguinal ligament. The canal contains lymphatics draining the deep inguinal nodes (Fig. 3.4).

HINTS AND TIPS

The order of vessels passing underneath the inguinal ligament laterally to medially can be remembered by the acronym **NAVY**

- **N**erve
- **A**rtery
- **V**ein
- **Y** fronts (groin creases)

ANTERIOR ABDOMINAL WALL PRESENTATIONS

History taking

Opening the consultation
Introduce yourself and confirm the patient details.

Presenting complaint (PC)
Ask an open question to identify the patient's presenting complaint.

History of presenting complaint (HPC)
Explore the presenting complaint using SOCRATES. Common symptoms of abdominal wall pathology include:

- Abdominal/groin swelling: a lump in the lower abdomen or groin that may come and go. May have gradually increased in size, or appeared suddenly.
- Groin pain: lower abdominal or groin pain or discomfort, exacerbated by standing, coughing or straining. May be associated with inner thigh pain or loss of sensation.
- Change in bowel habit (CIBH): obstructed hernias may present with constipation, and chronic constipation is a risk factor for hernia development.
- Nausea and vomiting: associated with incarcerated or strangulated hernias.
- Dysuria: difficulty or pain when passing urine can relate to compressive effects or suggest alternative differentials for groin swelling.

CLINICAL NOTES

Explore the history of a lump thoroughly:
- Site: where is the lump?
- Onset: when and how did you first notice it?
- Character: has the lump changed since you first noticed it?
- Radiation: are there any other lumps or swellings?
- Associated symptoms: pain, CIBH, dysuria, nausea and vomiting.
- Timing: does the lump ever come and go? Is it reducible?
- Exacerbating factors: does anything trigger the lump to appear or disappear?
- Severity: has the lump got worse over time? Does it trouble you?

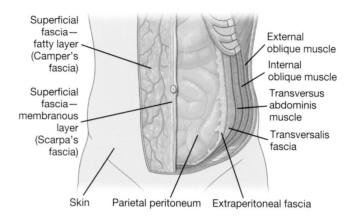

Fig. 3.1 The abdominal wall. (From Drake RL, Vogl AW, Mitchell AWM. *Gray's Basic Anatomy*. Churchill Livingstone, Elsevier Inc. 2013.)

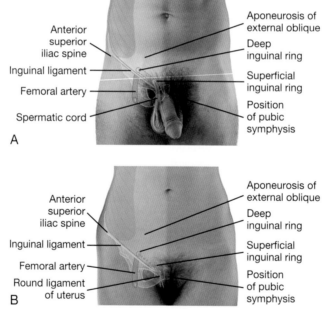

Fig. 3.2 Surface anatomy. (From Drake RL, Vogl AW, Mitchell AWM. *Gray's Basic Anatomy*. Churchill Livingstone, Elsevier Inc. 2013.)

HINTS AND TIPS	DIFFERENTIAL
There may be an identifiable trigger (i.e., heavy lifting) for appearance of the lump.	• Constitutional features including fever, lethargy, appetite and weight loss, and night sweats suggest malignant or immunological pathology. • Presentations include a solid groin lump or generalized lymphadenopathy.

Systemic screen

Screen for associated symptoms from other body systems.

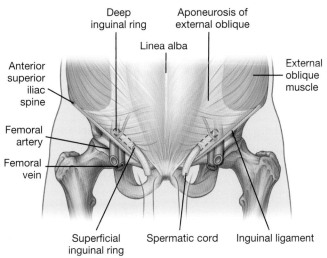

Deep inguinal ring
Aponeurosis of external oblique
Linea alba
Anterior superior iliac spine
External oblique muscle
Femoral artery
Femoral vein
Superficial inguinal ring
Spermatic cord
Inguinal ligament

Fig. 3.3 Inguinal canal. (From Drake RL, Vogl AW, Mitchell AWM. *Gray's Basic Anatomy*. Churchill Livingstone, Elsevier Inc. 2013.)

Past medical history

There may be relevant past medical history and surgical history that increase the risk of abdominal wall pathology, including abdominal surgery or trauma, stomas, previous hernias, or respiratory disease associated with chronic cough.

Drug history

Obtain a complete drug history, assessing compliance, side effects and allergy status.

HINTS AND TIPS

Drug related risk factors for hernias include:
- Ace inhibitors: chronic cough
- Opioids: constipation
- Immunosupressants: impaired wound healing

Family history

There may be a family history of hernias or associated conditions.

Social history

Screen for risk factors in the patient's history:

- Smoking: associated with chronic cough and impaired wound healing.
- Alcohol: excess use can exacerbate symptoms from hiatal hernias.
- Obesity: chronically raised intra-abdominal pressure increases the risk of hernias.

- Occupation: there may be an occupational history of heavy lifting.
- Hobbies and activities: weight-bearing exercise can precipitate hernia development.

Closing the consultation

Summarize the history, thank the patient and answer any questions.

DIFFERENTIAL DIAGNOSES

Groin swelling

Groin swelling can relate to urological pathology, infective disorders or pathology of the anterior abdominal wall (Fig. 3.5).

CLINICAL NOTES

- Fully examine the abdomen, hernial orifices and external genitalia before investigating further.
- The diagnosis may be reached on clinical features alone.

Investigation of a groin swelling

1. Bedside
   - Observations: fever suggests acute inflammation or infection.
   - Urinalysis: send for MC&S, to exclude urinary infection.
   - STI testing: groin swelling and regional lymphadenopathy can relate to STIs.

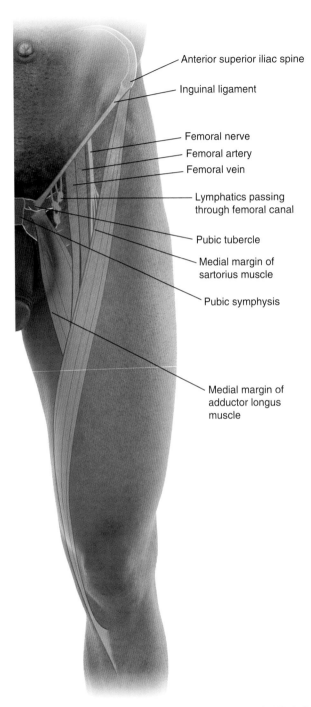

Anterior superior iliac spine

Inguinal ligament

Femoral nerve

Femoral artery

Femoral vein

Lymphatics passing through femoral canal

Pubic tubercle

Medial margin of sartorius muscle

Pubic symphysis

Medial margin of adductor longus muscle

Fig. 3.4 The femoral triangle. (From Drake RL, Vogl AW, Mitchell AWM. *Gray's Anatomy for Students,* 5th Edition. Elsevier; 2024.)

2. Bloods
   • FBC: ↑ white blood cell (WBC) suggests acute infection or inflammation.
   • HIV testing: HIV seroconversion can result in tender inguinal lymphadenopathy.
3. Imaging
   • Groin US: to differentiate a solid groin lump from a hernia containing bowel.
   • Doppler US: to demonstrate venous incompetence in suspected saphena varix.
   • CT abdomen/pelvis: to exclude suspected hernia if the US is negative.

HERNIA EXAM

Prepare for the examination and gain consent to proceed with a chaperone present.

HINTS AND TIPS

• Prepare for the examination using the **WIPER** structure:
  • **W** – **W**ash your hands
  • **I** – **I**ntroduce yourself
  • **P** – **P**atient details
  • **E** – **E**xplain the procedure and **E**xpose appropriately
  • **R** – **R**eposition patient
• A chaperone is essential for any intimate examination.

General inspection

Inspect the patient from the end of the bed:

• Abdominal scars: suggest previous abdominal surgery, risking incisional hernias.
• Pain: locate any obvious pain which may relate to underlying pathology.
• Abdominal distention: swelling is associated with hernias and bowel obstruction.
• Pallor: suggests anaemia, relating to chronic bleeding or malignancy.
• Equipment: objects around the bed including stoma bags and surgical drains may hint at underlying comorbidities.

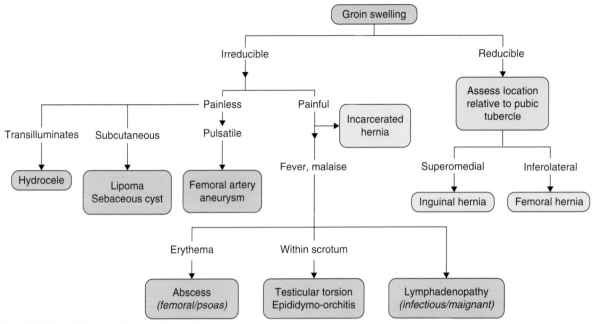

Fig. 3.5 Differential diagnosis of groin swelling.

Examination of the lump

Assess the lump thoroughly with the patient standing and sitting.

- Position: inguinal hernias are superomedial to the pubic tubercle, and femoral hernias inferolateral (Fig. 3.6).
- Reducibility: ask the patient to lay flat and assess for spontaneous reduction. If the lump remains present, attempt manual reduction. A reducible hernia may reappear on standing or removal of pressure.
- Cough impulse: to differentiate between direct and indirect hernias, manually reduce the hernia and ask the patient to cough. Reappearance suggests direct hernia.
- Scrotal examination: palpate the scrotum to assess the extension of a hernia. If you can get above the mass, it is likely scrotal in origin.

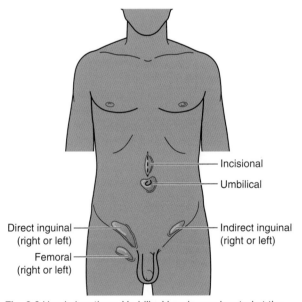

Fig. 3.6 Hernia locations. Umbilical hernias are located at the umbilicus, and incisional hernias associated with the lesion. (From Cooper K, Gosnell K. *Foundations of Nursing*, 9th Edition. Elsevier; 2023.)

- Transilluminate: a transilluminating mass suggests a scrotal hydrocele.
- Lymphadenopathy: palpate for tender, firm or rubbery groin lymph nodes.
- Auscultation: audible bowel sounds suggest hernia, and bruits a femoral aneurysm.

DIFFERENTIALS

- Inguinal hernias present with classical clinical features:
  - Inguinal lump
  - Reducible
  - Soft and painless
  - Positive cough impulse (direct)
  - Unable to get above the lump (indirect)
  - Bowel sounds on auscultation
- Lumps that are hard, multiple or transilluminate suggest alternative a scrotal.

RED FLAG

A tender, irreducible hernia may be incarcerated.

CLINICAL NOTES

- A parastomal hernia is an incisional hernia where abdominal contents prolapse into the superficial abdominal layers associated with the stoma incision.
- They are most common with colostomies.
- Symptoms include stoma enlargement, a positive cough impulse and a reducible parastomal mass.
- There is a risk of bowel obstruction and strangulation.

Completing the examination

Further tests include:

- Abdominal examination: to assess for stigmata of chronic disease, abdominal masses and ascites.
- Testicular examination: to identify features of associated pathology.
- External genitalia examination: examine the perineum and rectum, to identify urological or anorectal infective and malignant pathology.
- Imaging studies: US or CT imaging can be considered to identify pathology if there is high clinical suspicion but a negative examination.

ANTERIOR ABDOMINAL WALL DISORDERS

Hernias

A hernia is the protrusion of a viscus into an abnormal space. They occur at natural points of weakness, commonly the inguinal or femoral canal, or umbilicus. Risk factors include neuropathy, muscle weakness, low body mass index (BMI) and conditions that increase intra-abdominal pressure, such as heavy lifting, chronic cough, constipation, urinary outflow obstruction and ascites. Abdominal hernias manifest at areas of fascial weakness or through an existing potential space and contain bowel within a sack of parietal peritoneum. Reducible hernias can be manipulated back into their original position through the defect. Irreducible or incarcerated hernias remain stuck in their protruded position.

Inguinal hernias

An inguinal hernia is the protrusion of abdominal contents into the inguinal canal. Indirect inguinal hernias protrude via the deep inguinal ring. A direct inguinal hernia results from direct protrusion of the abdominal contents through an acquired weakness in the posterior wall of the inguinal canal (typically at Hesselbach's triangle) (Fig. 3.7).

CLINICAL NOTES

- You can differentiate between a direct and indirect hernia by reducing the hernia and placing a finger over the deep inguinal ring.
- If the hernia reappears, this suggests an abdominal wall defect resulting in *direct* herniation of the bowel into the inguinal canal.

Femoral hernias

A femoral hernia is the protrusion of abdominal contents into the femoral canal. They are much more common in women, and have a higher risk of complications compared to inguinal hernias, due to the narrowness of the femoral canal and associated ligamentous borders (Fig. 3.8).

HINTS AND TIPS

Femoral hernias are differentiated clinically inguinal hernias based on their position below and lateral to the pubic tubercle.

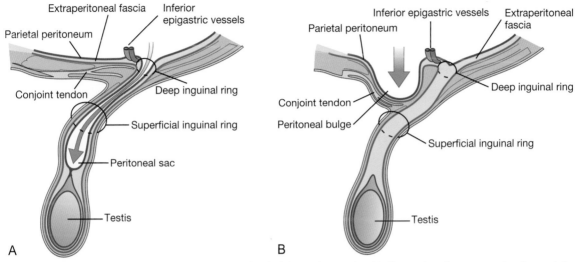

Fig. 3.7 (A) Indirect inguinal hernias pass through the deep inguinal ring and may extend to the scrotum, known as an inguinoscrotal hernia. (B) Direct inguinal hernias protrude directly through the abdominal wall into the inguinal canal. (From Drake RL, Vogl AW, Mitchell AWM. *Gray's Basic Anatomy*. Churchill Livingstone, Elsevier Inc. 2013.)

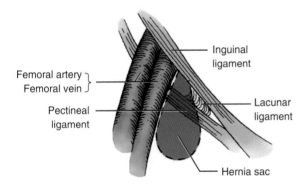

Fig. 3.8 Femoral hernias protrude into the femoral canal, medial to the femoral artery and vein. (From Gershenson DM, Lentz GM, Valea FA, Lobo RA. *Comprehensive Gynecology*, 8th Edition. Elsevier; 2022.)

Symptoms and signs

Both inguinal and femoral hernias present with an intermittent groin lump, or sudden appearance of a lump after heavy lifting. They may be otherwise asymptomatic or associated with mild groin discomfort or altered sensation, CIBH or urinary symptoms.

HINTS AND TIPS

- Femoral hernias can present suddenly as an irreducible groin lump with no previous presence of a lump.
- Many present initially with acute bowel obstruction.

Management

Hernias are a clinical diagnosis. In diagnostic uncertainty, groin US can be performed.

Management includes:

- Elective surgical repair: for symptomatic hernias. Usually required eventually due to gradual increasing hernia size and development of symptoms. Mesh repair is the gold standard, performed openly or laparoscopically (Fig. 3.9).
- Emergency surgical repair: for incarceration, obstruction or strangulation.

CLINICAL NOTES

All femoral hernias should be repaired, due to the risk of complications including incarceration, strangulation and bowel obstruction.

Complications

Severe pain or an irreducible lump suggests complications (Fig. 3.10):

- Incarceration: an irreducible hernia. Chronic incarceration occurs due to gradual adherence of the bowel to the herniated peritoneum, preventing spontaneous reduction. Acute incarceration risks bowel obstruction and strangulation.

- Obstruction: compression of the bowel lumen can result in obstruction, manifesting with colicky abdominal pain and distension, obstipation, nausea and vomiting.
- Strangulation: ischaemia of an incarcerated hernia, leading to infarction and necrosis, presenting with severe pain, systemic illness and sepsis.

Other hernias

There are several other types of hernia, with a range of aetiologies (Table 3.1).

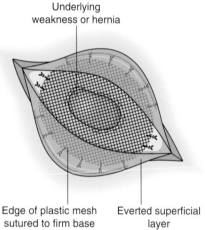

Underlying weakness or hernia

Edge of plastic mesh sutured to firm base   Everted superficial layer

Fig. 3.9 Mesh hernia repair. Mesh placement over the underlying abdominal wall weakness. (From Myint F. *Kirk's Basic Surgical Techniques*, 7th Edition. Elsevier; 2019.)

HINTS AND TIPS

- Obturator hernias predominantly affect elderly, multiparous women following weight loss.
- Paraumbilical and epigastric hernias affect those with a high BMI or chronically increased intra-abdominal pressure (i.e., ascites).
- Acquired diaphragmatic hernias typically follow abdominal trauma.

Incisional hernias may occur at any surgical incision; however, midline lesions are most common, as only one fascial layer prevents the abdominal contents from herniation (Fig. 3.12).

CLINICAL NOTES

Smoking, vascular, kidney or liver disease and immunosuppressant medications increase the risk of incisional or parastomal hernias due to impaired wound healing.

Stomas

A stoma is a surgically created artificial opening in the bowel or urinary tract for the passage of faeces (colostomy/ileostomy) or urine (urostomy) (Fig. 3.13). End colostomies/ileostomies are created following bowel resection for intra-abdominal pathology, to allow faeces excretion via the abdominal wall. Urostomies drain urine directly from the kidney, typically created

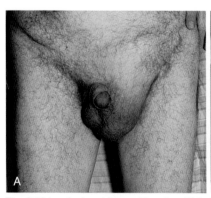
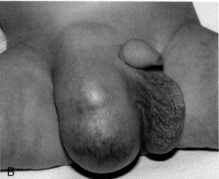
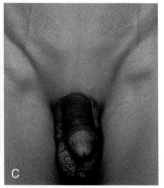

Fig. 3.10 Inguinal and femoral hernias. (A) Left indirect inguinal hernia extending into the scrotum. (B) Strangulated inguinal hernia in a child, with evidence of ischaemia and necrosis. (C) Right-sided groin swelling below the inguinal ligament, suggestive of femoral hernia. (From A. Swartz MH. *Textbook of Physical Diagnosis: History and Examination*, 8th Edition. Elsevier; 2021. B. Deakin PJ, Quick CRG, Biers S, Arulampalam T. *Essential Surgery: Problems, Diagnosis and Management*, 6th Edition. Elsevier; 2020. C. Zitelli BJ, McIntire SC, Nowalk AJ, Garrison J. *Zitelli and Davis' Atlas of Pediatric Physical Diagnosis*, 8th Edition. Elsevier; 2023.)

Table 3.1 Other types of hernias

Hernia	Aetiology	Clinical features	Management
Umbilical	Congenital persistence of the umbilical ring	'Outie' belly button palpable umbilical lump/distension Breakdown of overlying skin	Conservative Open mesh repair
Paraumbilical	Acquired defect in the umbilical linea alba		
Incisional	Bowel protrusion through previous surgical incision	Most commonly midline Palpable painful lump close to incision	Conservative Open mesh repair High recurrence rate
Parastomal	Incisional hernia at stoma site	Common with colostomy	Reverse/move stoma Mesh hernia repair
Hiatal	Intermittent stomach protrusion through oesophageal hiatus	Heartburn/reflux Para oesophageal – chest pain, early satiety	Conservative Acid reducing therapy
Diaphragmatic	Herniation through congenital/acquired diaphragm defect (Fig. 3.11)	Respiratory distress Absent ipsilateral breath sounds	Inotropic support Ventilation Urgent repair
Obturator	Widening of the pelvis with age/parity	No palpable lump Pain and altered sensation along the thigh	Urgent repair due to risk of complications
Epigastric	Epigastric defect in linea alba	May be asymptomatic Upper abdominal lump	Conservative/open mesh repair
Spigelian	Defect in the spigelian fascia	Pain/abdominal tightness Lateral abdominal lump	Urgent repair due to risk of complications

The linea alba is the fibrous band of tissue that runs down the anterior abdominal wall, from the xiphoid process to the pubic bone. The spigelian fascia lies between linea semilunaris and the rectus sheath.

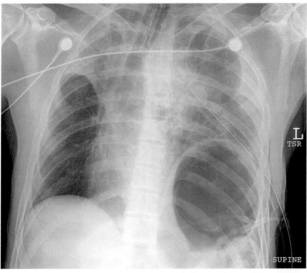

Fig. 3.11 Diaphragmatic hernia. X-ray demonstrating large diaphragmatic laceration and herniation of the stomach into the chest. (From Townsend CM, et. al. *Sabiston Textbook of Surgery: The Biological Basis of Modern Surgical Practice*, 21st Edition. Elsevier; 2022.)

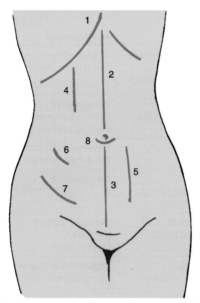

Fig. 3.12 Common surgical incisions. 1. Kocher incision. 2. Upper abdominal midline incision. 3. Lower abdominal midline incision. 4. Upper paramedian incision. 5. Lower paramedian incision. 6. McBurney incision. 7. Inguinal incision. 8. Infraumbilical. (From Odom-Forren J. *Drain's Perianesthesia Nursing: A Critical Care Approach*, 8th Edition. Elsevier; 2024.)

following cystectomy. A stoma bag is attached to the stoma to collect waste and emptied as required (Table 3.2).

HINTS AND TIPS

- Location only should not be relied up to identify a stoma, as this can vary.
- Stoma types hould be identified by the presence of a spout and contents of the collection bag.

CLINICAL NOTES

A Percutaneous Endoscopic Gastrostomy (PEG) involves endoscopic exteriorization of the gastric wall and provision of nutrition directly into the stomach, where the oral route is not possible.

A loop colostomy/ileostomy is a temporary stoma that is made to allow bowel and anastomoses to heal following surgery. They are typically reversed in 6 to 8 weeks. The proximal end forms a spout, to protect the skin, and the distal end is flat (Fig. 3.15).

Management
Patients should be educated about managing their stoma and followed up regularly by a specialized stoma nurse.

CLINICAL NOTES

- In colostomies, bowel lavage via the stoma and controlled faecal drainage is possible.
- This facilitates removal of the collection bag with a stoma cap put in place for 24-48 hours, enabling patients to live without the bag for this period.

Complications
Complications of stomas include:

- Skin irritation: the most common complication, resulting in dermatitis and ulceration. Bag change and skin care with emollients or barrier creams are required.
- High-output stoma: daily output >1.5 L, frequently occurring in ileostomies.

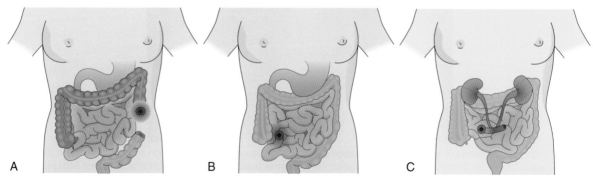

Fig. 3.13 (A) Colostomy. (B) Ileostomy. (C) Urostomy. (From A and B. Potter PA, Perry AG, Stockert PA, Hall AM. *Fundamentals of Nursing*, 11th Edition. Elsevier; 2023. C. Potter PA, Perry AG, Ostendorf WR, Laplante N. *Clinical Nursing Skills & Techniques*, 10th Edition. Elsevier; 2022.)

Table 3.2 Features of stomas

	Anatomy	Clinical features
Colostomy	Colon exteriorized	Flush to skin, contain semi-solid faeces Typically LIF
Ileostomy	Ileum exteriorized	Spouted, contain liquid bowel contents Typically RIF
Urostomy	Ileal conduit with end-to-end anastomosis Ureters anastomosed to conduit Conduit brought to skin	Spouted, contain urine Typically RIF

Urostomies and ileostomies are spouted, to prevent irritation of the abdominal skin by their contents (Fig. 3.14). LIF, Left iliac fossa; RIF, right iliac fossa.

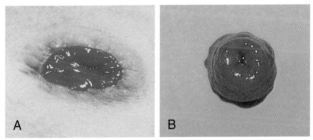

Fig. 3.14 Flat and spouted hernias. (A) Colostomy, flush to the skin. (B) Ileostomy or urostomy, spouted to prevent skin irritation. (From A. Shiland BJ. *Medical Assistant: Digestive System, Nutrition, Financial Management and First Aid*, 2nd Edition. St. Louis: Elsevier; 2015. B. Evans S. *Surgical pitfalls*, Philadelphia: Saunders; 2009.)

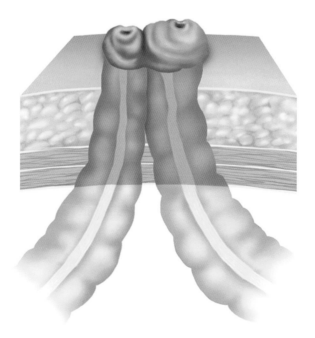

Fig. 3.15 Loop colostomy. (From Kuipers EJ. *Encyclopedia of Gastroenterology*, 2nd Edition. Elsevier; 2020.)

Management includes fluid resuscitation and anti-motility drugs. Most resolve spontaneously.

- Stoma necrosis: ischaemia of the exterior bowel segment, relating to operative vascular trauma or venous outflow obstruction. Presents with site discoloration and pain.
- Psychosocial: the psychosocial implications of a stoma can be significant, and patients need dedicated social and psychological support.
- Parastomal hernia: protrusion of the abdominal contents through the abdominal incision, presenting with stoma enlargement and a reducible mass. Risks incarceration and strangulation. Most common with colostomies.
- Stoma prolapse: the extension of the stoma when coughing, standing or straining. Can lead to ischaemia if chronically prolapsed.
- Stoma retraction: concave retraction of the stoma below the skin, resulting in poor bag attachment and associated skin irritation.
- Stoma haemorrhage: bleeding from the stoma resulting from bag change, or underlying gastrointestinal (GI) pathology.

Chapter Summary

- Risk factors for hernias include factors increasing intra-abdominal pressure, including heavy lifting, chronic cough or obesity.
- An incarcerated hernia is at risk of strangulation, presenting with severe pain and sepsis due to bowel necrosis.
- Hernias are a common cause of bowel obstruction, presenting with colicky abdominal pain, abdominal distention and obstipation.
- Indirect inguinal hernias protrude through the deep inguinal ring, and direct hernias directly through the abdominal wall.
- Femoral hernias are at high risk of strangulation. All require surgical repair.
- A colostomy is flat to the skin, and ileostomy/urostomy spouted.

UKMLA Conditions
Ascites
Constipation
Contact dermatitis
Gastro-oesophageal reflux disease
Hernias
Hiatus hernia
Lymphadenopathy
Lymphoma
Malnutrition
Obesity
Scrotal/testicular pain and/or lump/swelling
Urinary symptoms
Vomiting

UKMLA Presentations
Abdominal distension
Abdominal mass
Acute abdominal pain
Altered sensation, numbness and tingling
Ascites
Change in bowel habit
Chronic abdominal pain
Congenital abnormalities
Constipation
Fever
Gastro-oesophageal reflux disease
Hernias
Lump in groin
Lymphadenopathy
Lymphoma
Malnutrition
Nausea
Scrotal/testicular pain and/or lump/swelling
Urinary symptoms
Vomiting

Endocrine surgery | 4

CLINICAL ANATOMY

The endocrine glands are hormone-secreting glands that have vital roles in homeostasis and organ function.

The pituitary gland is a pea-sized gland located in the midline depression of the sphenoid bone (Fig. 4.1). It is connected to the hypothalamus by the infundibulum and lies adjacent to the optic chiasm.

The thyroid gland is a butterfly-shaped gland in the anterior neck that extends from C5-T1 and lies inferior and lateral to the cricoid cartilage (Fig. 4.2). It is composed of two lobes, joined by a central isthmus that crosses the anterior surface of the trachea (Fig. 4.3).

The parathyroid glands are four, small circular glands located on the posterior aspect of the thyroid gland, with two superior and two inferior parathyroid glands located at the superior and inferior poles of the thyroid (Fig. 4.4).

The adrenal glands sit above the kidneys and consist of an outer cortex and an inner medulla (Fig. 4.5). The right adrenal gland lies close to the right lobe of the liver and inferior vena cava, and the left adrenal gland lies posteriorly to the stomach, pancreas and spleen. They are surrounded by perinephric fat and enclosed within the renal fascia.

The neck can be divided into anterior and posterior triangles (Fig. 4.6). The anterior triangle is bounded by the anterior border of the sternocleidomastoid, the inferior border of the mandible, and the neck midline. It contains the thyroid and the parathyroid glands, as well as the larynx, trachea, oesophagus and vasculature including carotid arteries, jugular veins, Vagus and hypoglossal nerves, part of the sympathetic trunk, and lymphatics. The posterior triangle is bounded by the posterior border of the sternocleidomastoid, the anterior border of the trapezius, and the middle one-third of the clavicle, and contains the subclavian artery, external jugular vein, accessory nerve and fibres of the cervical plexus, and lymphatics.

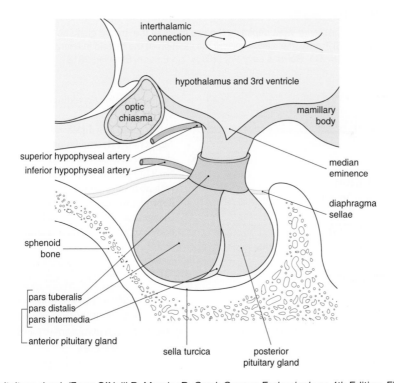

Fig. 4.1 The pituitary gland. (From O'Neill R, Murphy R. *Crash Course: Endocrinology,* 4th Edition. Elsevier; 2016.)

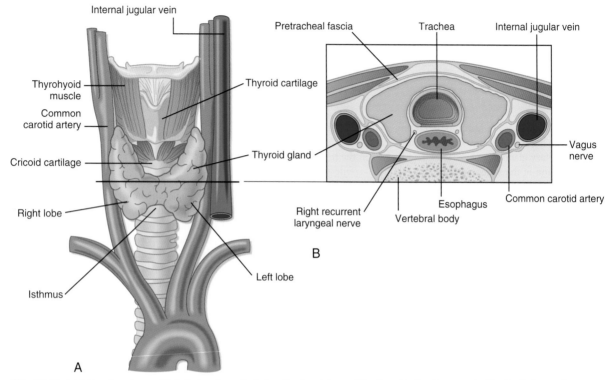

Fig. 4.2 Thyroid gland anatomy. (A) Anterior view, depicting the two lobes of the thyroid gland connected by the isthmus, just posterior to the cricoid cartilage. (B) Transverse view, showing the location of the thyroid in relation to the oesophagus and trachea. (From Koeppen BM, Stanton BA. *Berne & Levy Physiology,* 7th Edition. Elsevier; 2018.)

ENDOCRINE SURGERY PRESENTATIONS

History taking

Opening the consultation
Introduce yourself and confirm the patient's details.

Presenting complaint (PC)
Identify the chief complaint using an open question.

History of presenting complaint (HPC)
Explore the presenting complaint and obtain a timeline of symptoms. Common presentations in endocrine surgery are:

- Changes in appetite and weight: weight gain or loss, and changes in appetite.
- Change in bowel habit (CIBH): both diarrhoea and constipation are common.
- Fatigue/malaise: exceedingly common in endocrine dysfunction.
- Polyuria and polydipsia: excessive urination and thirst.
- Temperature dysregulation: heat or cold intolerance, and excessive or absent sweating.
- Neck lumps: may be painful, painless and if large, associated with hoarseness, shortness of breath and dysphagia.
- Reproductive dysfunction: menstrual irregularity, breast changes and discharge, erectile dysfunction, changes in body hair and loss of libido can all occur.

HINTS AND TIPS

- Nonspecific symptoms may include malaise, dizziness, nausea, generalized pain or weakness, or skin signs.
- Explore each symptom using SOCRATES to identify important features.

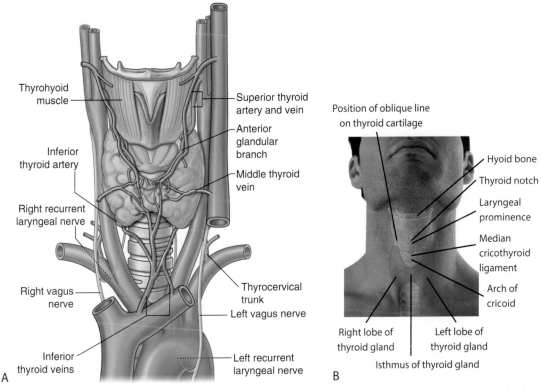

Fig. 4.3 (A) Vasculature of the thyroid gland. Note the close anatomical location of the recurrent laryngeal nerves and the Vagus nerve. The sympathetic trunk lies in close proximity, running just lateral to the vertebral bodies. (B) External view of the thyroid gland. (From A. Vogl AW, Mitchell AWM, Drake RL. *Gray's Anatomy for Students,* 5th Edition. Elsevier; 2024. B. Vogl AW, Mitchell AWM, Drake RL. *Gray's Basic Anatomy,* 3rd Edition. Elsevier; 2023.)

CLINICAL NOTES

Clarify each symptom fully, for example:
- Kilos of weight gained or lost over what period
- Quantity and type of fluid drank
- Number of episodes of urination

And so on. A diary can be used to track symptoms.

HINTS AND TIPS

Endocrine disease presents with a range of symptoms affecting many bodily systems. A brief systemic screen can provide invaluable diagnostic insights.

CLINICAL NOTES

In females, take a brief menstrual history including last menstrual period, recent cycle changes, and any history of pregnancy or fertility issues.

Systemic screen

A systemic screen early in the history can help formulate the differential diagnosis.

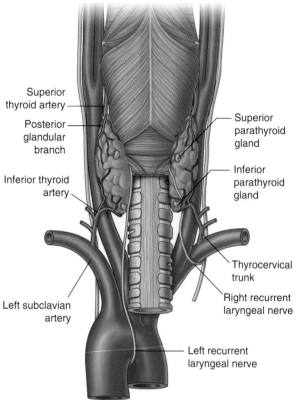

Fig. 4.4 The parathyroid glands. (From Vogl AW, Mitchell AWM, Drake RL. *Gray's Basic Anatomy,* 3rd Edition. Elsevier; 2023.)

Past medical history

Enquire about past medical history and current comorbidities, and ask specifically about past surgeries, investigations or imaging procedures.

> **DIFFERENTIALS**
>
> Comorbidities may hint at underlying endocrine disease.
> - New-onset diabetes? Consider Cushing syndrome.
> - Unexplained hypertension? Consider primary hyperaldosteronism or pheochromocytoma.
> - Recurrent fractures? Consider Cushing syndrome, hyperthyroidism or hyperparathyroidism.
> - A history of infertility or erectile dysfunction may relate to many endocrine disorders.

Drug history

A thorough drug history should be taken, including over-the-counter medications and allergies. Assess for medication compliance and any side effects.

Family history

Family history may point toward hereditary endocrine disease.

Social history

Explore the patient's social context:

- Baseline functional status: to assess independence and ability to cope at home.

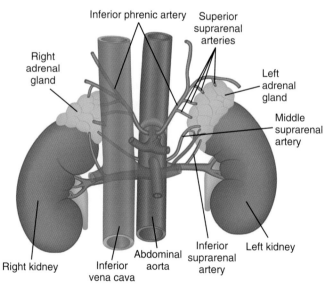

Fig. 4.5 The adrenal glands, located at the superior pole of the kidneys. (From Lough ME, Stacy KM, Urden LD. *Critical Care Nursing: Diagnosis and Management,* 9th Edition. Philadelphia, Elsevier; 2022.)

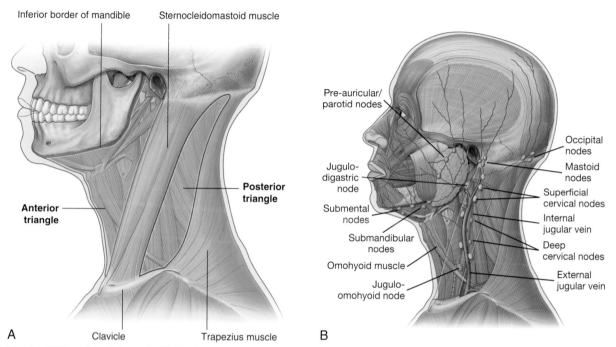

Fig. 4.6 (A) Triangles of the neck. (B) The lymphatic system in the neck. The superficial nodes drain into the deep nodes or directly into the supraclavicular trunk via the efferent lymphatic vessels. The deep nodes include the thyroid nodes. (From A. Mitchell AWM, Vogl AW, Drake RL. *Gray's Anatomy for Students,* 5th Edition. Elsevier; 2024. B. Drake RL, Vogl AW, Mitchell AWM. *Gray's Basic Anatomy*, 3rd Edition. Elsevier; 2023.)

- Alcohol, smoking and drug use: excess use may increase risk of several diseases.
- Exercise, diet and weight: may provide a simple explanation to weight changes!

Ideas, Concerns and Expectations

Eliciting ideas, concerns and expectations is helpful, as they may provide diagnostic clues, reveal other relevant symptoms, and highlight the goals of the consultation.

Closing the consultation

Summarize the key history, offer a chance to ask questions, and thank the patient for their time.

DIFFERENTIAL DIAGNOSIS

Appetite and weight change

Polyphagia describes excessive hunger, and anorexia describes loss of appetite. The differential diagnosis of appetite and weight change includes several endocrine diseases but is also a common symptom of other systemic diseases, as well as simple lifestyle

factors (Fig. 4.7). Appetite and weight change most commonly relate to lifestyle factors, so be sure to exclude this in the history.

CLINICAL NOTES

- Appetite is regulated by ghrelin and leptin.
- Ghrelin is released in response to fasting states and increases appetite and triggers growth hormone release.
- Leptin is released in response to fed states, and increases satiety and decreases appetite.

HINTS AND TIPS

- Water retention may also present with weight gain.
- Consider the possibility of free fluid in the abdomen, lungs or limbs.
- Screen for abdominal distension, peripheral oedema and dyspnoea.

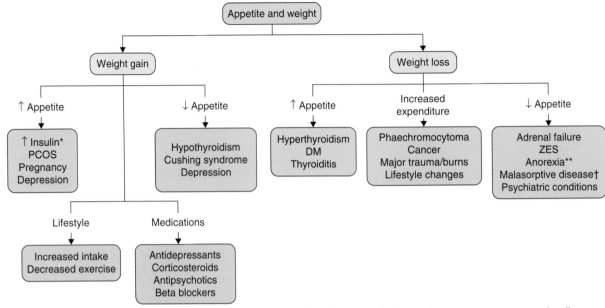

Fig. 4.7 Differentials for appetite and weight changes. *Hyperinsulinemia can result from an insulinoma or exogenous insulin therapy. †Malabsorptive disease includes IBD, coeliac, pancreatic insufficiency or cholestatic liver disease. **The aetiology of anorexia can be psychiatric (anorexia nervosa), related to medications, or chronic disease, including CKD, COPD, cancer or chronic infections. *DM*, Diabetes mellitus; *PCOS*, polycystic ovarian syndrome; *ZES*, Zollinger-Ellison syndrome.

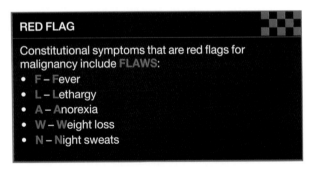

RED FLAG

Constitutional symptoms that are red flags for malignancy include FLAWS:
- F – Fever
- L – Lethargy
- A – Anorexia
- W – Weight loss
- N – Night sweats

Investigations for appetite and weight change

1. Bedside
   - Weight: as a baseline measurement and to track further weight changes.
   - Observations: fluctuations in heart rate and blood pressure may indicate adrenal or thyroid dysfunction.
   - ECG: considerable weight loss can cause skeletal muscle wasting and affect cardiac physiology. Thyroid and adrenal disorders can cause ECG changes.
   - CBG: hyperglycaemia may relate to diabetes or steroid use. Bedside ketones can be performed at the same time to screen for diabetic ketoacidosis (DKA).
   - Stool sample: if malabsorptive disease is suspected.

2. Bloods
   - FBC: anaemia can occur malabsorptive disease or malignancy.
   - U&Es: adrenal insufficiency or extreme weight loss, can cause deranged electrolytes. In malnutrition, electrolytes must be closely monitored, due to the risk of refeeding syndrome.
   - TFTs: to detect thyroid dysfunction.
   - Insulin: inappropriate hyperinsulinemia suggests insulinoma.
   - Cortisol: ↑ in Cushing's syndrome, ↓ in adrenal insufficiency.
   - FSH/LH: ↑ LH and ↑ LH:FSH ratio is typical of PCOS.

3. Imaging
   - CXR: unexplained weight loss in a smoker is a red flag for lung cancer.
   - Thyroid ultrasound (US): to detect thyroid nodules or goitres.
   - CTCAP: a full body CT can be done in unexplained symptoms to identify neuroendocrine tumours or a malignancy.

CLINICAL NOTES

Beware of the risk of incidentalomas with full body imaging. Only do full body imaging if there are red flag features of malignancy associated with weight loss.

Polyuria and polydipsia

The term polyuria refers to passing over 3 L of urine in 24 hours. Polydipsia is excessive thirst and is commonly associated with polyuria.

Investigations for polyuria and polydipsia

A systematic approach to polyuria and polydipsia can help identify the underlying aetiology (Fig. 4.8).

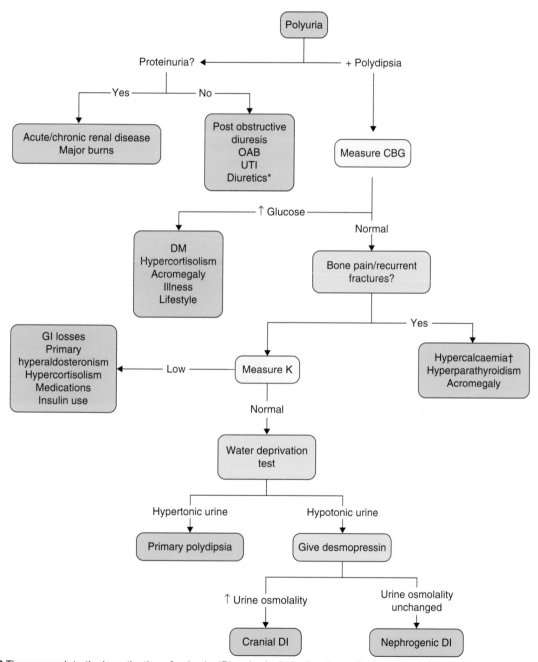

Fig. 4.8 The approach to the investigation of polyuria. *Diuretics include diuretic medications, alcohol and caffeine.
†Hypercalcaemia can be caused by steroid use, malignancy or iatrogenically through medications as well as secondary to excess PTH. *CBG*, Capillary blood glucose; *DI*, diabetes insipidus; *DM*, diabetes mellitus; *OAB*, overactive bladder.

Additional investigations include:

1. Bedside
   - Fluid chart: to accurately determine intake and output.
   - CBG: a vital first step. Random blood glucose >11 mmol with osmotic symptoms is diagnostic of diabetes.
   - Urinalysis: elevated leukocytes and nitrates indicate infection. Glucose and ketones may be elevated in diabetes. Proteinuria indicates renal disease.
   - Urine osmolality: very dilute urine may indicate excessive fluid intake and can be repeated after deprivation, to identify diabetes insipidus (DI).
   - Observations: hypotension can occur in significant fluid loss. Hypertension can result in nephropathy, which can present with polyuria and proteinuria.
2. Bloods
   - U&Es: ↑ Urea and creatinine indicate renal dysfunction, which may be acute or chronic. Diabetic nephropathy is important to screen for in patients with hyperglycaemia. ↓ K$^+$can cause polyuria and polydipsia.
   - Bone profile: ↑ Ca^{2+}may indicate underlying parathyroid or malignant disease.
   - PTH: if parathyroid pathology is suspected.
   - Serum osmolality: to detect dehydration.
   - Cortisol: ↑ cortisol levels can result in hyperglycaemia, polyuria and polydipsia.
   - Serum IGF-1: ↑ IGF-1 indicates acromegaly, which can cause hyperglycaemia and associated polyuria and polydipsia.

- Aldosterone/renin ratio (ARR): ↑ ARR *is* diagnostic of primary hyperaldosteronism.
3. Imaging
   - AXR: hypercalcemia can cause renal stones, constipation and bowel obstruction if severe, all of which can be seen on an abdominal film.
   - CTKUB: imaging of the renal and urological tract can diagnose renal pathology.
   - Adrenal CT: if adrenal adenoma is suspected as a cause of hyperaldosteronism.

Temperature dysregulation

Temperature dysregulation is relatively common and can relate to several endocrine diseases. Patient demographics and related symptoms can help identify the underlying diagnosis (Fig. 4.9).

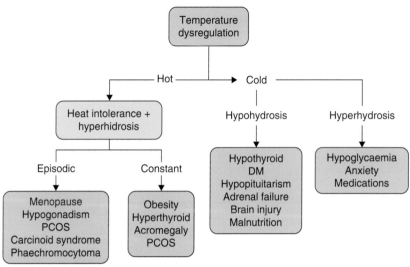

Fig. 4.9 Differentials for temperature dysregulation. *DM*, Diabetes mellitus; *PCOS*, polycystic ovarian syndrome.

DIFFERENTIALS

- In older women, hot flushes typically relate to menopause.
- Associated anxiety, diarrhoea, oligomenorrhea and palpitations suggest hyperthyroidism.
- In the cold, constipated, tired patient, suspect hypothyroidism. Other causes of temperature dysregulation are rare.

Investigations for temperature dysregulation

 CLINICAL NOTES

- Thermodysregulation can relate to body weight, dress, nutrition and mood.
- Avoid over investigating, unless symptoms are severe.

1. Bedside
   - Observations: baseline temperature should be assessed to determine whether there is objective derangement or subjective symptoms only.
   - CBG: hypoglycaemia is a common cause of transient sweating and coldness.
   - ECG: if thyroid dysfunction is suspected.

2. Bloods
   - TFTs: will quickly identify thyroid dysfunction.
   - Testosterone: ↓ in hypogonadism.
   - LH/FSH: ↑LH/FSH ratio may indicate underlying PCOS.
   - IGF-1: ↑ in acromegaly.
   - Cortisol: ↓ in adrenal insufficiency.
   - ACTH stimulation test: to diagnose the underlying cause of adrenal insufficiency.
   - Plasma 5-HIAA: ↑carcinoid syndrome, an exceedingly rare cause of hot flushes.
   - Plasma-free metanephrines: ↑ in pheochromocytoma, which is associated with.

3. Imaging
   - Thyroid US: further investigation of a goitre.
   - TVUSS: if PCOS is suspected.
   - Abdominal CT: to diagnosis pheochromocytoma or carcinoid syndrome.

Neck lumps

Neck lumps warrant thorough history and evaluation, due to the range of serious underlying causes. A good examination can often point toward the likely aetiology (Fig. 4.10).

Investigations for neck lumps

1. Bedside
   - ECG: thyroid dysfunction can cause ECG changes.
2. Bloods
   - FBC: anaemia is associated with malignancy. ↑ WBC suggests reactive lymphadenopathy.
   - TFTs: to identify thyroid dysfunction.

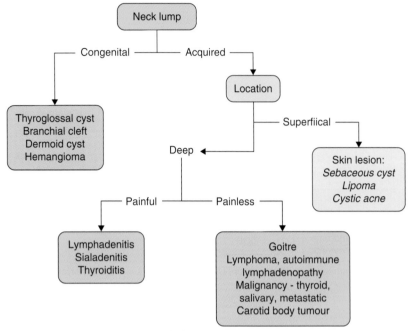

Fig. 4.10 Differential of a neck lump.

3. Imaging
   - Neck US: initial screening to determine the need for further imaging. Can be diagnostic in congenital lesions.
   - Thyroid US: to identify a goitre, or detect and characterize a thyroid mass.
   - CXR: if lung cancer is suspected as the cause of lymphadenopathy.
   - Biopsy: a biopsy is ultimately required if malignancy is suspected.

HINTS AND TIPS

- Transient, tender lymphadenopathy is very common with viral infections, particularly URTIs.
- Determine when the lump appeared, and its relation to recent illness.

RED FLAG

- Painless cervical lymphadenopathy is a red flag for malignancy.
- Lymphoma presents with a swollen, soft, rubbery lymph node.
- Several head and neck cancers drain into the cervical nodes, and can present with neck lumps.
- An urgent 2-week wait referral is indicated for suspected malignancy, without waiting for further diagnostic investigations.

Reproductive dysfunction

Reproductive dysfunction can be associated with many endocrine diseases. A good history is essential, to identify other related symptoms, and help narrow down the likely diagnosis (Fig. 4.11).

Investigations for reproductive dysfunction

Thorough investigation is required, as these symptoms can be very distressing for patients and have significant medical, psychological and social consequences.

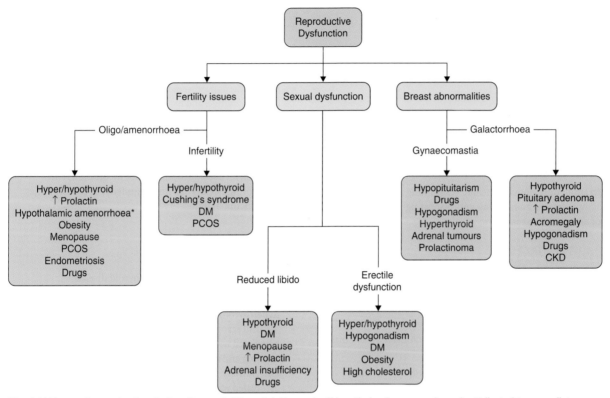

Fig. 4.11 Types of reproductive dysfunction and differential diagnosis. *Hypothalamic amenorrhoea is attributed to poor diet, malnutrition, chronic stress or excessive exercise, which may relate to psychological disorders. *CKD*, Chronic kidney disease; *DM*, diabetes mellitus; *PCOS*, polycystic ovarian syndrome.

1. Bedside
   - Weight: being both underweight and overweight can negatively affect fertility.
   - CBG: hyperglycaemia can suggest diabetes mellitus or Cushing's syndrome.
   - ECG: thyroid dysfunction can cause ECG changes.
   - Sperm count: low sperm count is the most common cause of male infertility.
2. Bloods
   - U&Es: to screen for acute and chronic renal impairment.
   - TFTs: thyroid dysfunction can cause a range of reproductive and sexual issues.
   - Oestrogen/testosterone: low levels can suggest hypogonadism, menopause or hypothalamic amenorrhoea.
   - FSH/LH: ↑ LH, and ↑ LH/FSH ratio, suggests PCOS.
   - Sex hormone binding globulin (SHBG): ↓ SHBG may indicate underlying PCOS.

   - Prolactin: hyperprolactinemia can cause reproductive dysfunction and breast abnormalities.
   - Cortisol: both ↑ and ↓ cortisol levels can affect fertility.
   - IGF-1: to diagnose acromegaly, which can cause reproductive issues as the result of ↑ growth hormone, and through the development of microprolactinomas.
   - Fasting lipids: hyperlipidaemia can cause erectile dysfunction, and is common in anorexia nervosa, PCOS and psychiatric medication use.
3. Imaging
   - Thyroid US: to detect goitre or nodules in suspected thyroid dysfunction.
   - TVUSS: to confirm a diagnosis of suspected PCOS or endometriosis.
   - Pituitary MRI: if prolactinoma, pituitary adenoma or hypopituitarism is suspected.

ENDOCRINE EXAMINATIONS

Examination should include examining the system where symptoms are manifesting and inspecting for peripheral signs of endocrine disease.

The thyroid exam

Introduction
Gather equipment and make appropriate introductions.

General inspection
A thorough inspection from the end of the bed can be invaluable in detecting thyroid pathology (Fig. 4.12):

- Weight: cachexia suggests thyrotoxicosis, and obesity suggests hypothyroidism.
- Clothing: the patient may be underdressed and hot and sweaty in hyperthyroidism, or overdressed and cold in hypothyroidism.
- Behaviour: hyperthyroid patients may be anxious, irritable and hyperactive, and hypothyroid patients may be low in mood and flat in affect.
- Vocal quality: a large goitre or malignant lesion can compress the larynx, causing vocal hoarseness. Speech may be slow and slurred in hypothyroidism.
- Equipment: bedside mobility aids, medications and monitoring devices can hint at underlying comorbidities and functional status.

Peripheral examination
Hands
Inspect the hands for stigmata of thyroid disease

- Palmar erythema: reddening of the palms, associated with hyperthyroidism.
- Thyroid acropachy: periosteal distal phalangeal overgrowth associated with Graves disease, presenting with digit swelling and nail clubbing.
- Onycholysis: detachment of the nail from the nail bed, associated with hyperthyroidism.
- Peripheral tremor: can be assessed for by placing a piece of paper over the outstretched palms. A sign of hyperthyroidism.

Radial pulse
Assess the rate and rhythm of the pulse. Hyperthyroid patients may be tachycardic, with an irregular pulse and hypothyroid patients may be bradycardic.

Face
Inspect the face for signs of thyroid disease

- Sweating: associated with hyperthyroidism.
- Dry, puffy skin: associated with hypothyroidism.
- Hair loss: loss of the outer third of the eyebrows is associated with hypothyroidism.

Eyes
Inspect the eyes from the front, side and from above to detect eye pathology

- Lid retraction: upper lid retraction is identified by the sclera being visible between the upper lids and iris border.
- Exophthalmos: the bulging of the eye out of the orbit.
- Eye inflammation: oedema and reddening of the eye can occur due to lid retraction and exophthalmos.

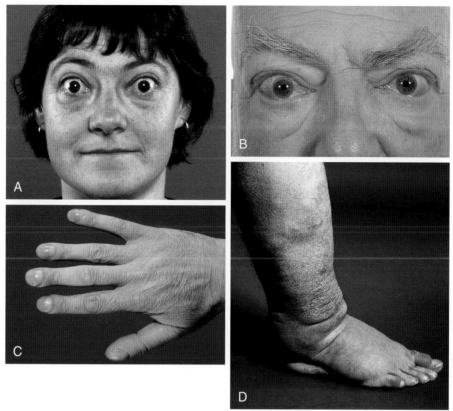

Fig. 4.12 Peripheral signs of hyperthyroidism. (A) Exophthalmos and lid retraction. (B) Eye inflammation, with chemosis and conjunctivitis. (C) Thyroid acropachy. (D) Pretibial myxoedema. (Modified from Strachan MWJ, Newell Price JDC. Endocrinology. In Ralston S, Penman I, Strachan MWJ, et al. (eds). *Davidson's Principles and Practice of Medicine*, 23rd Edition. Philadelphia: Elsevier; 2018.)

- Eye movements: ophthalmoplegia can be detected by the patient following an H-shaped movement of your finger with their eyes, with their head still, to assess for painful eye movement.
- Lid lag: a delay in the descent of the upper eyelid in relation to the eyeball when looking down.

CLINICAL NOTES

- Eye symptoms are associated with thyrotoxicosis, including Graves disease, secretory nodules and thyroiditis.
- There is a risk of long-term eye damage through exposure keratitis, infection, permanent double vision or change in the appearance of the eyes.

The thyroid gland
Inspection

Inspect the outer aspect of the thyroid gland. A normal thyroid is not visible.

- Scars: a midline neck scar may indicate previous thyroid surgery.
- Masses: a large goitre presents with symmetrical midline neck swelling. Nodules may be evident as asymmetrical, smaller lesions.

Assess a mass further by asking the patient to swallow water and protrude the tongue:

- Thyroid masses move upwards on swallowing, but not on tongue protrusion.
- Thyroglossal cysts move upwards on swallowing, and upwards on tongue protrusion.
- A lymph node will move minimally on swallowing or tongue protrusion.

- A thyroid malignancy may move asymmetrically on swallowing or not move at all if tethered to surrounding tissues, and will not move on tongue protrusion.

Palpation

Palpate the lobes and isthmus of the thyroid from behind and repeat swallowing water and tongue protrusion to assess the movement of the gland.

> **HINTS AND TIPS**
>
> - The isthmus of the thyroid gland overlies the cricoid cartilage, just superior to the first two rings of the trachea.
> - Each lobe of the thyroid lies a few centimeters out from the isthmus.

Note specific characteristics of the gland:

- Size: symmetrical or asymmetrical enlargement may suggest a goitre or a mass.
- Consistency: an irregular consistency may indicate a multinodular goitre.
- Masses: nodules or malignancy may be palpable as a distinct mass.

> **CLINICAL NOTES**
>
> - Note the position, size, shape, tethering or mobility of a mass during palpation.
> - Large masses may cause tracheal deviation.

Lymph nodes

Assess the regional lymph nodes systematically and thoroughly:

- Submental
- Submandibular
- Preauricular
- Postauricular
- Superficial and deep cervical
- Posterior cervical
- Supraclavicular

> **HINTS AND TIPS**
>
> Assess the size and texture of lymph nodes by rolling the fingers over the nodes in a circular motion in the regional lymph node areas.

Percussion

Percuss the sternum from the sternal notch downwards to assess for retrosternal dullness, which may indicate a large thyroid mass extending into the mediastinum.

Auscultation

Auscultate the lobes of the thyroid gland for bruits, which can occur secondary to increased vascularity of the thyroid gland. A palpable thrill may also be present.

> **HINTS AND TIPS**
>
> - A bruit is a continuous sound heard over a thyroid mass.
> - A systolic sound is more likely to represent a carotid bruit or radiation of a cardiac murmur.

Further tests

Further tests include:

- Reflexes: the biceps or knee jerk reflex can be used to assess for hyporeflexia, associated with hypothyroidism.
- Pretibial myxoedema: a waxy discolouration of the pretibial region associated with Graves disease.
- Proximal myopathy: ask the patient to stand from sitting with their arms crossed. The inability to do so suggests proximal myopathy, associated with Graves disease and multinodular goitre.

Completing the examination

Wash your hands, thank the patient and summarize your findings. Further tests include TFTs, ECG and thyroid US.

Examining a neck lump

Introduction
Prepare for the exam using the WIPER structure.

General inspection
Inspect the patient from the end of the bed for signs of underlying pathology.

- Vocal quality: large neck lumps can cause laryngeal compression and vocal hoarseness.
- Cachexia: underlying malignancy can cause muscle wasting.
- Shortness of breath: large neck masses may compress the upper respiratory tract.
- Behaviour: hyperthyroid patients may be anxious and hyperactive, and hypothyroid patients may be low in mood and flat in affect.
- Clothing: inappropriate dress for the weather indicates heat or cold intolerance, which may relate to thyroid pathology.
- Exophthalmos/lid lag: eye signs associated with Graves disease.

Examining the lump

Inspection
Inspect the lump from the front and side. The movement of the mass can be assessed by asking the patient to swallow and protrude their tongue.

Palpation
Palpate the neck lump systematically and note relevant features.

- Site: note the location of the lump in the midline, anterior or posterior triangle.
- Size: assess how large the lump is.
- Shape: assess whether there are irregular or regular borders.
- Consistency: soft lumps are more likely to represent benign lesions. Rubbery lumps are likely to be lymph nodes.
- Mobility: the lump may be mobile or tethered to surrounding tissues. Ask the patient to turn their head during palpation to assess whether the lump moves with muscle contraction.

- Fluctuance: a fluid-filled lump may bulge outward when compressed.
- Tenderness: a tender, warm mass suggests infective or inflammatory conditions.
- Skin changes: erythema around the mass indicates inflammation. A punctum may be seen in cystic lesions.

Lymph nodes
Lymphadenopathy is associated with several conditions that can present with a neck lump, and the lump itself may represent an enlarged lymph node. Thoroughly assess the regional lymph nodes in the neck, noting the site, size, shape and tenderness of any enlarged nodes.

CLINICAL NOTES

- Benign lymph nodes are painless, <1cm, smooth, mobile lumps.
- Reactive lymphadenopathy in infection presents with tender, smooth and mobile nodes.
- Haematological malignancies present with widespread lymphadenopathy and large, rubbery nodes.
- Metastatic cancer may cause regional lymphadenopathy with hard, firm and irregular nodes, tethered to underlying structures.

All relevant lymph node chains should be assessed:

- Submental
- Submandibular
- Preauricular
- Postauricular
- Superficial and deep cervical
- Posterior cervical
- Supraclavicular

Completing the examination
Wash your hands, thank the patient and summarize your findings.

Further tests include an examination of the oral cavity and thyroid exam if indicated, bloods including FBC and TFTs, and US scan of the mass

RED FLAG

- The red flags features of a neck lump on examination are:
  - A hard, fixed mass, that is tethered to the underlying tissue
  - A new neck lump in a patient over 35 years.
  - Persistent hoarseness or dysphagia
  - Shortness of breath, stridor
  - Trismus (lockjaw)
  - Unilateral ear pain
- Any of these features warrant an urgent 2-week wait referral to ENT for suspected head and neck malignancy.

PITUITARY DISORDERS

Pituitary hormone physiology

The pituitary gland is divided into an anterior and posterior gland, which function independently and regulate different hormones (Fig. 4.13).

The hypothalamic-pituitary axis

Hormone release from endocrine glands is regulated by the hypothalamic-pituitary-axes, a regulatory system which functions in response to negative feedback (Fig. 4.14). The hypothalamus centrally regulates hormone release. Secretion of releasing hormones from the hypothalamus triggers the release of tropic and nontropic hormones from the pituitary (Table 4.1). Tropic

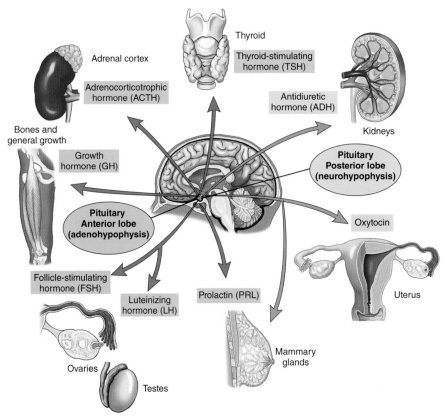

Fig. 4.13 The hormones released from the pituitary gland and the organs they act on. (From Brooks DL, Levinsky D, Brooks ML. *Exploring Medical Language: A Student-Directed Approach*, 11th Edition. Elsevier; 2022.)

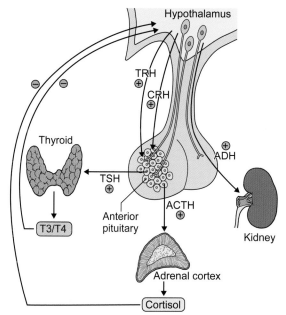

Fig. 4.14 Regulation of steroid and thyroid hormone by the hypothalamic-pituitary axes. ADH is released from the pituitary when hyperosmolarity is detected by the hypothalamic osmoreceptors. *CRH*, Corticotropin-releasing hormone; *T3/T4*, triiodothyronine/thyroxine; *TRH*, thyroid-releasing hormone.

hormones act on peripheral endocrine glands to trigger release of hormones into the systemic circulation. Nontropic hormones exert effects directly on target cells. Negative feedback occurs in response to increased levels of peripheral endocrine hormones or via the release of specific inhibitory hormones which inhibit hypothalamic hormone release.

Disruption at any stage can result in disease, and is classified according to location of pathology:

- Primary: disorder of the peripheral endocrine gland.
- Secondary: disorder of the pituitary gland.
- Tertiary: disorder of the hypothalamus.

Pituitary adenomas

Pituitary adenomas are neuroendocrine tumours that arise from the anterior pituitary gland. They are typically benign and classified based on size (microadenomas (<10 mm) or macroadenomas (>10 mm)), and by their ability to secrete hormones.

HINTS AND TIPS	

5% of pituitary adenomas relate to multiple endocrine neoplasia (MEN) conditions.

Table 4.1 Hormones produced by the pituitary gland

Anterior pituitary hormones				
Hormone	**Stimulation**	**Inhibition**	**Target**	**Effects**
Adrenocorticotropic hormone (ACTH)	CRH release from the hypothalamus in response to stress	Increased serum glucocorticoid	Adrenal glands	Stimulates steroid hormone release
Thyroid-stimulating hormone (TSH)	TRH release from the hypothalamus to regulate metabolic rate	Somatostatin release from hypothalamus	Thyroid gland	Stimulates T3/T4 release
Gonadotropins – follicle-stimulating hormone (FSH)/ luteinizing hormone (LH)	Pulsatile GnRH release from the hypothalamus to regulate reproductive function	GnRH release Inhibited by high prolactin	Ovaries Testes	FSH – germ cell maturation LH – female ovulation in females, male testosterone synthesis
Growth hormone (GH)	GHRH release from the hypothalamus to trigger bone, muscle and organ growth	Somatostatin release from hypothalamus	Nontropic hormone All tissues	Increased protein synthesis, insulin resistance, lipolysis. Decreased glucose uptake into cells
Prolactin	Enhancing factors: • TRH • Oxytocin • Oestrogen	Dopamine inhibits release	Nontropic hormone Lactotroph cells	Increased breast tissue growth and lactation Inhibits GnRH

continued

Table 4.1 Hormones produced by the pituitary gland–cont'd

Anterior pituitary hormones				
Hormone	Stimulation	Inhibition	Target	Effects
Posterior pituitary hormones				
Antidiuretic hormone (ADH)	Plasma hyperosmolality Hypovolaemia Hypotension ANG II	Atrial natriuretic peptide Cortisol	Renal collecting duct	Increased water reabsorption
Oxytocin	Nipple stimulation Vaginal or cervical stretch	Tocolytic agents Relaxin	Uterus Nipples	Promotes uterine contractions Facilitates milk ejection

Table 4.2 Features of secretory and nonsecretory pituitary adenomas

		Clinical features
Secretory	Prolactinoma (40%)	Hyperprolactinemia – galactorrhoea, amenorrhoea, reduced libido, infertility, gynaecomastia ↓ BMD in women due to oestrogen suppression.
	GH-secreting (10%–15%)	↑ Growth hormone – acromegaly/gigantism
	ACTH-secreting (5%)	Secondary hypercortisolism – Cushing's disease
	TSH-secreting (1%)	Secondary hyperthyroidism
	Gonadotroph adenoma (rare)	↑LH/FSH – fertility issues, menstrual irregularities, delayed or precocious puberty
Macroadenoma	Mass effect	Headache, visual field defects and diplopia
Features of hypopituitarism	GH deficiency	Short stature, weight gain, weakness and depression
	Prolactin deficiency	Lactation failure following childbirth
	FSH/LH deficiency	Primary amenorrhea, infertility, loss of libido and testicular atrophy
	TSH deficiency	Secondary hypothyroidism
	ACTH deficiency	Secondary adrenal insufficiency
	Central diabetes insipidus	Polyuria and polydipsia

Symptoms and signs

The clinical features depend on tumour size and associated hormone release:

- Secretory adenomas: symptoms relating to the hormone produced in excess.
- Nonsecretory microadenomas: typically asymptomatic.
- Macroadenomas: mass effects, including visual field defects and hypopituitarism due to local invasion and destruction of pituitary tissue (Table 4.2).

CLINICAL NOTES

- Most secretory adenomas produce one hormone, relating to their cell type of origin.
- Tumours which secrete multiple hormones should raise suspicion of pituitary carcinoma.

Investigations

Pituitary hormone assays should be performed in all patients:

- Serum prolactin
- TFTs
- 24-hour urinary cortisol
- IGF-1
- LH/FSH
- Testosterone/oestrogen

MRI Sella with IV contrast can be used to confirm a diagnosis following hormone assays (Figs. 4.15–4.16).

Visual field testing should be considered in all patients, even if asymptomatic.

Management

Conservative management is indicated for nonsecretory asymptomatic microadenomas.

Medical management includes:

- Prolactinomas: dopamine agonists (cabergoline/bromocriptine) inhibit prolactin secretion and cause adenoma shrinkage.
- ACTH/GH/TSH secreting adenomas: somatostatin analogues (octreotide) inhibit the peripheral effects of the hormones.

Transsphenoidal hypophysectomy is indicated first-line for symptomatic adenomas, involving surgical removal of pituitary tissue under endoscopic guidance through the sphenoidal sinus (Fig. 4.17). Removal may be partial (hemihypophysectomy) or complete (total hypophysectomy). Hypopituitarism may develop postoperatively, and lifelong hormone replacement therapy will be required.

Complications

The complications of pituitary adenomas relate to compressive effects of the tumour and alterations in hormone regulation.

- Pituitary apoplexy: bleeding of adenomas into the gland which results in gland infarction presenting with a severe headache, visual symptoms and acute adrenal insufficiency, which can be life-threatening. Patients will have subsequent hypopituitarism requiring life-long hormone replacement therapy.
- Acute hormonal imbalance: acute hyper or hypopituitarism or can result in severe hormonal alterations and acute illness, including secondary adrenal insufficiency, myxoedema coma and thyroid storm.

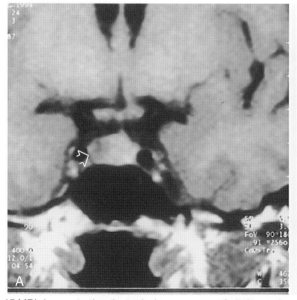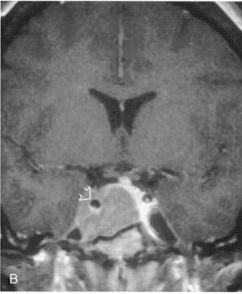

Fig. 4.15 MRI demonstrating the typical appearance of pituitary microadenoma. (A, B) There is a hypodense lesion on the right side of the gland. The infundibulum has deviated away from the lesion. (From Melmed S, Stewart PM, Kronenberg HM, Polonsky KS, Larsen PR. *Williams Textbook of Endocrinology,* 11th Edition. Elsevier; 2008.)

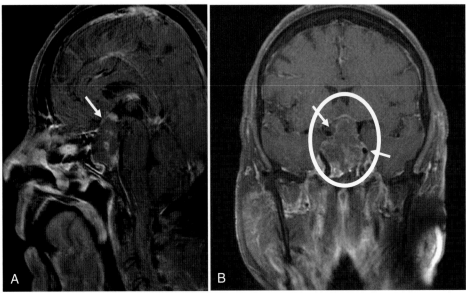

Fig. 4.16 MRI demonstrating large macroadenoma of the pituitary gland. (A) Sagittal view and (B) coronal view of large right-sided macroadenoma, with extension of the tumour above and below the Sella. (From Goldman L, Schafer AI, Weiss RE. *Goldman-Cecil. Tratado de medicina interna,* 26.ª Edición. Elsevier, Spain; 2021.)

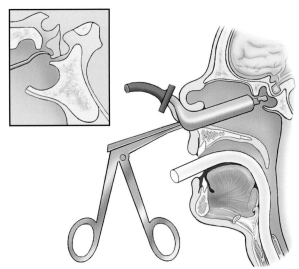

Fig. 4.17 Transsphenoidal surgery. Endoscopic entry via the sphenoidal sinus allows removal of neoplastic tissue from the pituitary gland. (From Harding, M., et al. *Lewis's medical-surgical nursing: Assessment and management of clinical problems*, 11th Edition. Mosby, Elsevier; 2020.)

- Visual field defects: large macroadenomas may compress the optic chiasm, resulting in bitemporal hemianopia, with bilateral temporal vision loss (Fig. 4.18).
- Acromegaly: relating to GH-secreting tumours.
- Diabetes insipidus: due to macroadenoma-related hypopituitarism or following surgery.
- SIADH: common following transsphenoidal hypophysectomy.

CLINICAL NOTES

- Acromegaly results from excess growth hormone release from a macroadenoma.
- Pathological growth of soft tissues and bone produces large extremities and facial features.
- Visual field defects relate to adenoma compression of the optic chiasm.
- Diabetes is common due to increased IGF-1 levels.
- Transphenoidal adenoma removal or medical therapy with somatostatin analgesics are the mainstays of treatment.

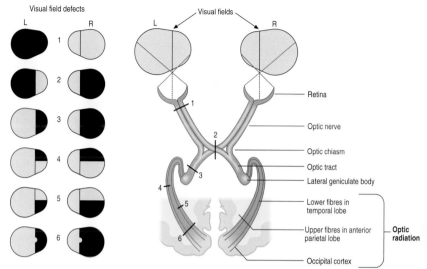

Fig. 4.18 Visual fields and related defects associated with the location of pathology. Bitemporal hemianopia most commonly occurs with a pituitary lesion. (From Innes JA, Tint NL, Dover A, Borooah S, Fairhurst K. *Macleod's Clinical Examination*, 15th Edition. Elsevier; 2024.)

DIFFERENTIALS

- SIADH can develop following transsphenoidal hypophysectomy.
- Excess ADH secretion results in dilutional hyponatremia.
- Symptoms include nausea, muscle cramps, lethargy and confusion, and seizures.
- A fluid status assessment should be performed to detect other causes of hyponatremia.
- Correction of sodium should be done slowly (max 10 mmol/24 hours), via fluid restriction (or desmopressin in severe cases), due to the risk of neurological complications including cerebral pontine myelinolysis with rapid correction.

Diabetes insipidus

Antidiuretic hormone

Antidiuretic hormone (ADH) is secreted by the posterior pituitary in response to hypovolemia, hypotension and plasma hyperosmolality (Fig. 4.19). It acts on the renal collecting duct to increase water reabsorption, decreasing osmolality and increasing blood pressure.

Diabetes insipidus

Diabetes insipidus (DI) is a condition where the kidneys are unable to concentrate urine. DI is classified as either central or nephrogenic. Central DI results from intracerebral pathology affecting the hypothalamus or pituitary gland, leading to reduced ADH secretion. Nephrogenic DI results from renal pathology, where ADH receptors are unable to respond to ADH. Primary polydipsia is a differential for DI, where patients have normal ADH physiology, however, are drinking excessive water leading to polyuria (Table 4.3).

THYROID DISORDERS

Thyroid hormone physiology

The thyroid gland is composed of follicular and parafollicular cells. Follicular cells produce thyroid hormones T_3 (triiodothyronine) and T_4 (tetraiodothyronine) that regulate cellular metabolism and growth. Parafollicular cells secrete calcitonin, which acts as a PTH antagonist, released in response to elevated serum Ca^{2+} levels.

The synthesis of thyroid hormone is regulated by the hypothalamic-pituitary-thyroid axis. Increased metabolic demand triggers the release of TRH from the hypothalamus, stimulating TSH secretion from the pituitary gland. TSH

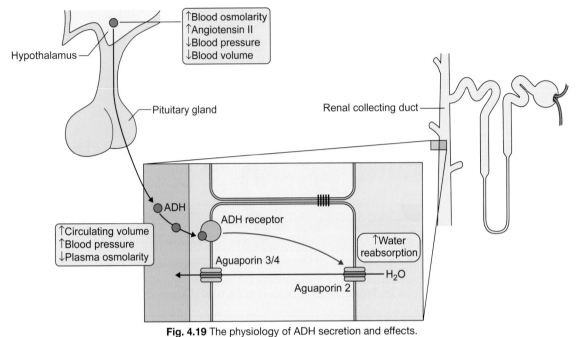

Fig. 4.19 The physiology of ADH secretion and effects.

Table 4.3 Comparison of diabetes insipidus and primary polydipsia

		Central DI	Nephrogenic DI	Primary polydipsia
Aetiology		Brain tumours Neurosurgery (post hypophysectomy) Pituitary apoplexy Intracerebral injury or bleed Brain malformations Infection (i.e., meningitis, encephalitis)	Hereditary Acquired – medications (lithium), ↓K, ↑Ca, renal disease, pregnancy, hyperaldosteronism	Psychiatric illness (schizophrenia, OCD, stress, anxiety) resulting in excessive water intake
Symptoms and signs		Polyuria, with excessive secretion of dilute urine Dehydration, and associated lethargy, hypotension, and altered mental state Polydipsia (excessive thirst) Nocturia Sleep deprivation and daytime somnolence Postural hypotension Hypernatraemia – muscle weakness, confusion, lethargy, irritability, seizures and coma if severe		Polyuria Polydipsia Hyponatremia – headache, muscular weakness, confusion, vomiting, irritability
Ix:	Na	↑	↑	↓
	ADH	↓	↑	↓
	Plasma osmolality	↑	↑	↓
	Urine osmolality	↓	↓	↓↓

Table 4.3 Comparison of diabetes insipidus and primary polydipsia–cont'd

	Central DI	Nephrogenic DI	Primary polydipsia
Water deprivation test	Plasma osmolality remains high Urine osmolality remains low		Plasma osmolality remains within normal limits Urine osmolality rises to normal range
Desmopressin administration	Plasma osmolality normalizes, urine osmolarity increases (renal ADH receptors able to respond to ADH)	Plasma osmolality remains high, urine osmolality remains low (renal ADH receptors unable to respond to ADH)	Not required
Treatment	Desmopressin (synthetic ADH)	Discontinue causative medication Thiazide diuretics (increase Na/H_2O reabsorption in PCT)	Management of acute hyponatremia Behavioural therapy Treatment of psychiatric disorders Water restriction

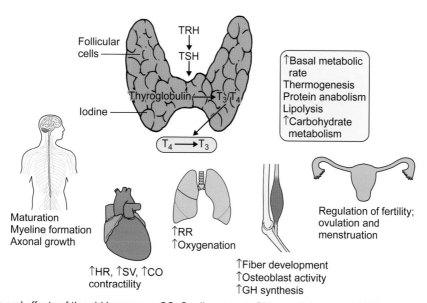

Fig. 4.20 Synthesis and effects of thyroid hormones. *CO*, Cardiac output; *GH*, growth hormone; *HR*, heart rate; *RR*, respiratory rate, *SV*, stroke volume.

triggers iodine uptake by follicular cells, allowing conversion of thyroglobulin (a thyroid hormone precursor) into T_3 and T_4, which are then secreted into the serum. T_3 is biologically active, but has a shorter half-life, and is secreted in small amounts. Biologically inactive T_4 is secreted in large amounts and metabolized to active T_3 in the peripheries (Fig. 4.20).

Goitres and thyroid nodules

A goitre is the abnormal enlargement of the thyroid gland. It can relate to both hypothyroidism and hyperthyroidism. In the developing world, it commonly relates to iodine deficiency. In the developed world, goitres relating to autoimmune thyroid disease are more common. Benign or malignant thyroid nodules are also described as goitres.

Signs and symptoms

Goitres can present as asymmetrical or symmetrical neck swellings (Figs. 4.21–4.22). Obstructive symptoms may occur secondary to a large goitre, including dyspnoea, stridor, wheeze or dysphagia.

Goitres can relate to both hyperthyroid and hypothyroid disease, with associated symptoms (Table 4.4):

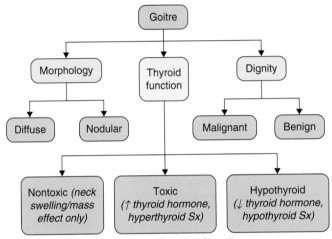

Fig. 4.21 Classification of a goitre.

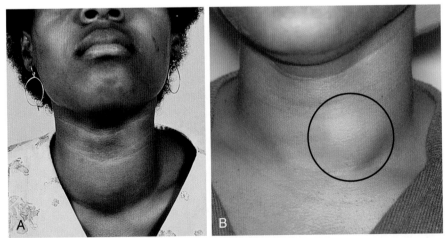

Fig. 4.22 External appearance of a goitre. (A) Patient with a symmetrical goitre. (B) Patient with an asymmetrical goitre relating to iodine deficiency. (From A. Fehrenbach MJ, Popowics T. *Illustrated Dental Embryology, Histology, and Anatomy*, 5th Edition. St. Louis: Elsevier; 2020. B. Lemmi FO, Lemmi CAE. *Physical assessment findings [CD-ROM]*, Philadelphia, Saunders; 2009.)

Table 4.4 Comparison of hyperthyroidism and hypothyroidism

		Hyperthyroidism	Hypothyroidism
Aetiology		Graves' disease TMG 'Hot' thyroid nodule TSH-secreting pituitary adenoma Thyroiditis (subacute, postpartum, drug-induced)	Hashimoto's thyroiditis Thyroiditis (subacute, postpartum) Pituitary adenoma -> TSH deficiency Iatrogenic (post thyroidectomy, radioiodine therapy, drugs) Iodine deficiency
Symptoms		Weight loss Appetite increase Fatigue, weakness, Heat intolerance Hyperhidrosis Diarrhoea Oligo/amenorrhoea, infertility Anxiety, agitation, insomnia Tremor, palpitations	Weight gain Appetite decrease Fatigue Cold intolerance Hypohidrosis Constipation Menorrhagia, infertility Depression, dementia
Signs		Goitre Eye signs – lid lag, retraction Onycholysis Tachycardia, irregular pulse Hypertension, chest pain Pretibial myxoedema	Goitre Hair loss, brittle nails, dry, doughy skin Bradycardia Hypertension Pretibial/periorbital oedema
TFTs	TSH	↓	↑
	T_3/T_4	↑	↓
Management		Antithyroid drugs – carbimazole/propylthiouracil RAIA Surgery Symptomatic – beta-blockers	Lifelong levothyroxine (synthetic T_4)
Complications		Thyrotoxic crisis Atrial fibrillation Heart failure Graves ophthalmopathy	Myxoedema coma Primary thyroid lymphoma Carpal tunnel syndrome Hyperlipidaemia

RAIA, *Radioactive iodine ablation;* TMG, *toxic multinodular goitre.*

HINTS AND TIPS

A handy mnemonic for the symptoms of hypothyroidism is **CHAMPS**:

- **C** – **C**onstipation
- **H** – **H**eat (cold intolerance, reduced sweating), hair loss
- **A** – **A**ppetite loss, weight gain
- **M** – **M**enorrhagia, muscle aches
- **P** – **P**ersonality – impaired memory and depression
- **S** – **S**kin changes

Investigations

The investigation of a goitre includes testing TFTs, thyroid antibodies and imaging:

- T_3/T_4: to objectively diagnose hypo or hyperthyroidism.
- TSH: suppressed in hyperthyroidism and elevated in hypothyroidism.
- Thyroid antibodies: thyroglobulin and thyroid peroxidase are associated with in Hashimoto thyroiditis, and SH receptor antibodies are associated with Graves disease.
- Thyroid imaging: US, CT or MRI to determine goitre size, and identify nodules suspicious for malignancy (Figs. 4.23–4.24).

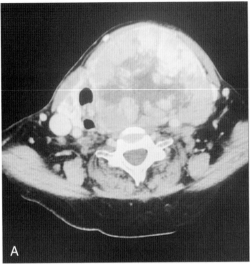
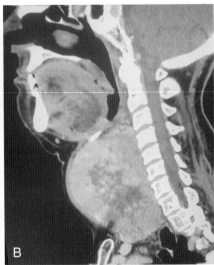

Fig. 4.23 Large goitre arising from the left thyroid lobe. (A) Axial view. (B) Sagittal view. There is significant anatomical distortion with tracheal deviation toward the right-hand side. (From Brennan PA, Standring SM, Wiseman SM. *Gray's Surgical Anatomy*. Elsevier; 2020.)

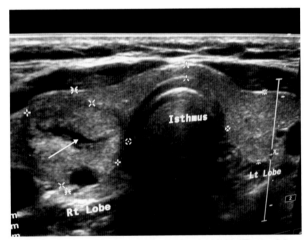

Fig. 4.24 Thyroid US with nodules in the right lobe. The nodule is predominantly solid, with a central cystic area. (From Sharma SK, Strachan MWJ, Sherif I, Hunter JAA. *Davidson's 100 Clinical Cases,* 2nd Edition. Churchill Livingstone, Elsevier; 2012.)

• Thyroid scintigraphy: if a nodule is detected, radioiodine uptake scans can determine whether a lesion is 'hot' (produces thyroid hormone) or cold (inactive).

If there are concerning US features or a nodule is cold on scintigraphy, fine-needle aspiration and cell cytology should be performed to evaluate for malignancy (Table 4.5).

Table 4.5 Benign and malignant thyroid nodules

Benign nodules (95%)	Malignant nodules (5%)
Thyroid adenoma • Follicular • Toxic* • Papillary • Thyroid cystMultinodular goitre* Hashimoto thyroiditis	Thyroid carcinoma • Papillary • Follicular • Medullary • AnaplasticThyroid lymphoma Metastatic disease

Represents the most common hot nodules.

CLINICAL NOTES

• TSH is sensitive to changes in levels of thyroid hormones, and therefore very reliable to assess thyroid derangement.
• TSH may be suppressed or elevated despite normal T_3/T_4 levels in subclinical thyroid derangement.

RED FLAG

A cold nodule has a 5% to 15% association with malignancy, and hence is a red flag for thyroid cancer. Malignancy is rare in hot nodules.

Management

Management options include:

- Conservative: for asymptomatic, nontoxic goitres or thyroid cysts.
- Medical: hot nodules should be treated with beta-blockers for symptomatic control and antithyroid medications.
- Surgical: large goitres with obstructive symptoms, toxic adenomas and multinodular goitres require surgical resection (hemithyroidectomy or thyroidectomy) or radioactive iodine ablation (RAIA).

CLINICAL NOTES

- Surgery is always indicated for a follicular or papillary thyroid adenoma, as fine-needle aspiration cannot definitively exclude malignancy.
- Hemithyroidectomy and histopathology should be performed.
- If malignancy is present, total thyroidectomy should follow.

Thyroid carcinoma

Thyroid carcinoma is a malignancy arising from the thyroid gland (Table 4.6). It is most common in women between 30 and 50 years. Risk factors include exposure to ionizing radiation and a family history of thyroid malignancy.

Symptoms and signs

Thyroid carcinoma may be asymptomatic and picked up incidentally. Other features include:

- A hard, painless, fixed, nodule, with tethering to adjacent tissues
- Hoarse voice
- Dyspnoea
- Dysphagia
- Cervical lymphadenopathy

CLINICAL NOTES

Diarrhoea and facial flushing may occur in advanced medullary carcinoma, due to excess calcitonin secretion.

HINTS AND TIPS

The differential of a mediastinal mass includes the 4 **Ts**:

- **T** – **T**hyroid carcinoma
- **T** – **T**hymoma
- **T** – **T**eratoma
- **T** – **T**errible lymphoma

Mediastinal masses risk superior vena cava (SVC) obstruction, which presents with distended chest wall veins, facial flushing and Pemberton's sign (facial congestion, cyanosis and respiratory distress after raising the arms above the head for 1 minute).

Urgent stenting of the SVC and debulking of the mass is required.

Investigations

All thyroid nodules should be investigated with TSH and US. Lesions suspicious of malignancy should be sampled with

Table 4.6	Classification of thyroid cancer		
	Epidemiology	**Characteristics**	**Prognosis**
Papillary	Most common (80%) 30–50 years	Well differentiated May be multifocal	Very good
Follicular	10% 40–60 years	Well differentiated Rarely multifocal	Good
Medullary	<10% 50–60 years Associated with MEN2	Poorly differentiated Arises from parafollicular cells Produces calcitonin	Moderate
Anaplastic	1%–2% >60 years	Poorly differentiated Rapid local growth and metastasis Compressive symptoms	Very poor

fine-needle aspiration cytology. Thyroid carcinoma will present as a cold nodule on thyroid scintigraphy (Fig. 4.25). Further imaging can be performed for staging and to evaluate for metastasis.

Management

Management includes:

- Follicular/papillary carcinoma: total thyroidectomy (+/– radical lymph node dissection) and radioactive iodine ablation (RAIA). High-dose thyroid hormone replacement therapy is given postoperatively to suppress TSH and reduce the risk of cancer recurrence.
- Medullary/anaplastic carcinoma: total thyroidectomy (+/– lymph node dissection) and radiochemotherapy, with thyroid hormone replacement therapy following surgery.

For unresectable or metastatic disease, the management is palliative.

CLINICAL NOTES

- Anaplastic carcinomas rapidly grow and invade local structures.
- They metastases via haematogenous and lymphatic spread to the lungs, bone and brain.
- The prognosis is terrible, with 5-year survival approximately 5%.
- Management is typically palliative.

Postoperative complications

Thyroid surgery is associated with a range of complications.

- Immediate haematoma: occurring hours after surgery, resulting in laryngeal oedema, stridor and dyspnoea. A surgical emergency, requiring urgent return to theatre to open the wound and control any haemorrhage.
- Recurrent laryngeal nerve injury: development of a hoarse voice and cough, with a risk of aspiration pneumonia. If the injury is bilateral, there will be immediate dyspnoea and stridor postoperatively, and emergency airway manoeuvres must be performed.
- Superior laryngeal nerve palsy: presents with vocal fatigability and loss of vocal pitch, which typically normalises spontaneously.
- Hypoparathyroidism: damage to the parathyroid glands may result in temporary or permanent hypoparathyroidism, presenting with signs of hypocalcaemia, including perioral numbness, tetany and seizures. It is essential to monitor calcium postoperatively and supplement where needed.
- Thyrotoxic crisis: if euthyroid status was not achieved preoperatively in hyperthyroid patients. A life-threatening status of hypermetabolism, that presents with pyrexia, agitation confusion and tachycardia, and can lead to acute heart failure and tachyarrhythmias.
- Myxoedema coma: postoperatively, hypothyroidism can develop, and without adequate thyroid hormone replacement, can decompensate into myxoedema coma, which presents with hypothermia, hypotension and ↓ GCS. It is a life-threatening medical emergency (Fig. 4.26).

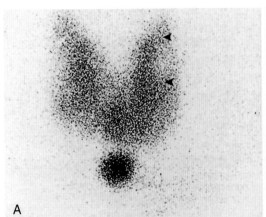
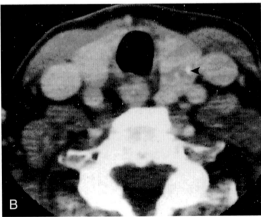

Fig. 4.25 Thyroid scintigraphy. (A) Cold nodule in the left thyroid lobe, with reduced radioiodine uptake. (B) A large lesion in the left lobe of the thyroid, extending medially into the mediastinum. (From Skarin AT. *Atlas of diagnostic oncology*, 3rd Edition. St Louis, Mosby; 2003.)

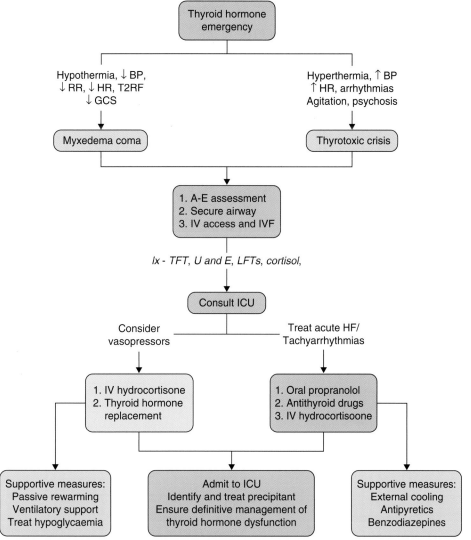

Fig. 4.26 Acute management of thyroid emergencies. *GCS*, Glasgow Coma Scale; *HF*, heart failure; *T2RF*, Type 2 respiratory failure.

PARATHYROID DISORDERS

Parathyroid hormone physiology

The parathyroid glands secrete parathyroid hormone (PTH) in response to reduced serum calcium levels and acts at the kidney, bones and GIT to increase serum calcium, reduce serum phosphate and activate vitamin D, which further increases gut calcium reabsorption (Fig. 4.27).

Hyperparathyroidism

Hyperparathyroidism is abnormally high PTH levels of PTH, due to overactive parathyroid glands. It is classified based on the underlying cause (Table 4.7).

Investigations

Investigations include:

- Calcium, phosphate and PTH levels: to diagnose and classify hyperparathyroidism.

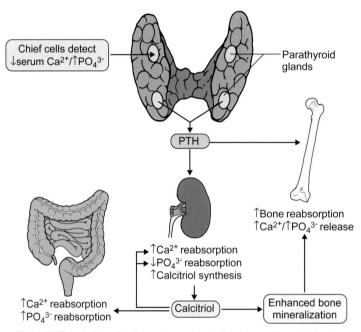

Fig. 4.27 Regulation of calcium homeostasis by the parathyroid glands.

Table 4.7 Overview of hyperparathyroidism

		Primary	Secondary	Tertiary
Aetiology		Parathyroid adenoma Parathyroid carcinoma	CKD Vitamin D deficiency Malabsorption	CKD Untreated secondary hyperparathyroidism
Pathophysiology		Abnormally active parathyroid glands	Reactive hyperplasia of parathyroid glands in response to chronic ↓ Ca^{2+}	Longstanding secondary hyperparathyroidism -> autonomous refractory ↑ PTH secretion
Ix	PTH	↑	↑	↑↑
	Ca^{2+}	↑	↓	↑
	PO_4^{3-}	↓	↑ in CKD ↓ in other causes	↑
Symptoms		Majority asymptomatic Symptoms of ↑ Ca^{2+} – bone pain, renal stones, constipation, nausea, polyuria, polydipsia, depression	Bone pain Symptoms relating to underlying cause (i.e., renal disease)	
Complications		↓ BMD, ↑ fracture risk Hypercalcaemic crisis	↓ BMD, ↑ fracture risk	↓ BMD, ↑ fracture risk Hypercalcaemic crisis

BMD, *Bone mineral density;* CKD, *chronic kidney disease.*

- X-rays: may show subperiosteal erosions, cortical thinning (acroosteolysis), erosions, decalcification and chondrocalcinosis (Fig. 4.28).

Management

Symptomatic patients with primary hyperparathyroidism should have surgery:

- Parathyroidectomy: for solitary adenoma confined to one gland.

- Total parathyroidectomy: for parathyroid gland hyperplasia.
- Tumour resection: for parathyroid carcinoma, including removal of the ipsilateral lobe of the thyroid gland and radical lymph node dissection.

Adjunctive medical therapy can be used postoperatively:

- Calcimimetics: modulate parathyroid gland calcium receptors and inhibit PTH release.
- Bisphosphonates: to treat osteoporosis.

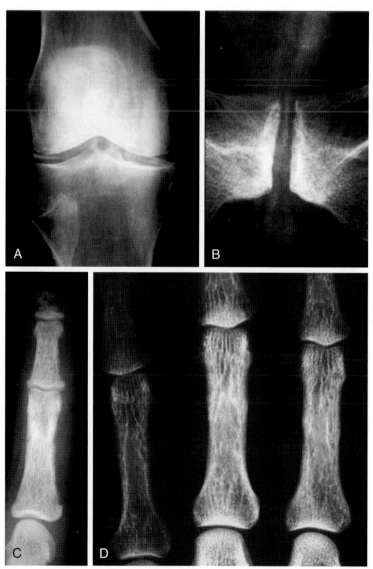

Fig. 4.28 Bone changes in hyperparathyroidism. (A) and (B) Chondrocalcinosis in the knee and pubic symphysis. (C) Subperiosteal erosions and acroosteolysis. (D) Cortical thinning in the proximal phalanges. (From Adam A, et al. *Grainger & Allison's diagnostic radiology*, 5th Edition. London, Churchill Livingstone; 2007. In Grant LA: *Grainger & Allison's diagnostic radiology essentials*, 2nd Edition. London, Elsevier; 2019.)

Management of secondary and tertiary hyperparathyroidism should focus on treating the underlying condition and management of hyperphosphatemia, with dietary phosphate restriction and phosphate binders to prevent GIT phosphate absorption.

Complications

Complications include:

- Hypercalcaemia (Fig. 4.29)
- Impaired renal function
- Osteoporosis and increased fracture risk

HINTS AND TIPS

- A hypercalcaemic crisis is a life-threatening condition presenting with dehydration, oliguria, ↓GCS and psychosis.
- It is a medical emergency and requires urgent treatment with aggressive fluid resuscitation and calcium-lowering medications.

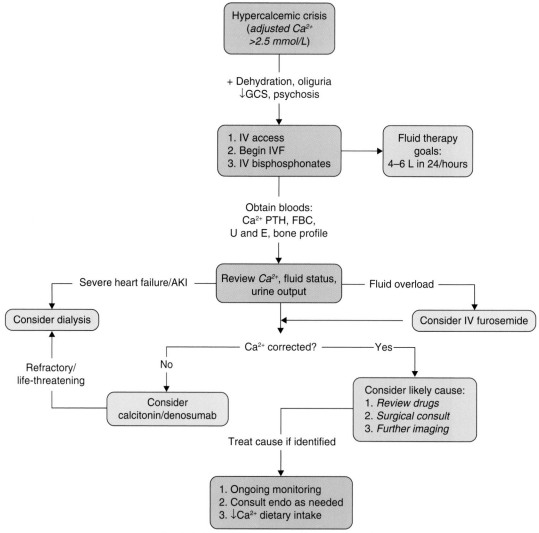

Fig. 4.29 Acute management of hypercalcaemia.

ADRENAL DISORDERS

Adrenal hormone physiology

The adrenal glands sit above the kidneys and consist of an outer cortex and an inner medulla. The adrenal medulla contains chromaffin cells which secrete catecholamines including noradrenaline, adrenaline and dopamine, as a sympathetic response to stress, increasing pulse, BP and sympathetic activity.

The adrenal cortex is split into three layers, which synthesize different steroid hormones from their common precursor, cholesterol (Fig. 4.30).

- Zona glomerulosa: responsible for mineralocorticoid secretion, regulated by the renin-angiotensin-aldosterone system (RAAS).
- Zona fasciculata: responsible for glucocorticoid secretion, regulated by the hypothalamic-pituitary-adrenal axis.
- Zona reticularis: responsible for androgen (sex hormone precursors) secretion, regulated by the hypothalamic-pituitary-adrenal axis.

Diseases of the adrenal gland can relate to insufficient or excess hormone secretion and can have devastating effects, due to the essential interaction of adrenal hormones with nearly every bodily system.

Cushing's syndrome

Cushing's syndrome describes the syndrome of hypercortisolism or excess circulating levels of glucocorticoids. It can relate to exogenous iatrogenic prescription of steroid hormones, or endogenous hypercortisolism (Table 4.8).

> **HINTS AND TIPS**
>
> Cushing's syndrome relating to an ACTH secreting pituitary adenoma is described as Cushing's disease.

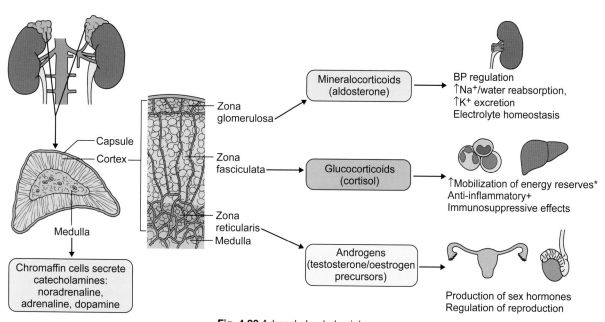

Fig. 4.30 Adrenal gland physiology.

Table 4.8 Classification of Cushing's syndrome

	Pathophysiology	Aetiology
Exogenous	Long-term, high-dose steroid prescriptions, ACTH suppression, bilateral adrenal atrophy	Iatrogenic
Primary	Autonomous overproduction of glucocorticoids from the adrenal gland	Adrenal adenomas, carcinomas or hyperplasia
Secondary	Excess pituitary ACTH secretion -> adrenal gland hyperplasia, ↑ glucocorticoid secretion	Pituitary adenoma (Cushing's disease)
Ectopic	Paraneoplastic secretion of ACTH -> adrenal gland hyperplasia, ↑ glucocorticoid secretion	SCLC RCC Carcinoid tumours Pheochromocytoma Medullary thyroid carcinoma

RCC, *Renal cell carcinoma;* SCLC, *small cell lung cancer.*

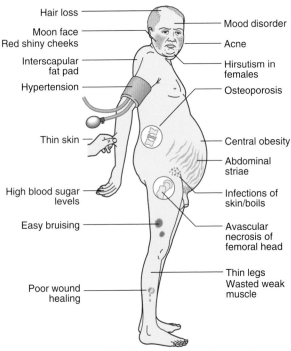

Fig. 4.31 Symptoms of Cushing's syndrome. Acne, baldness and hirsutism relate to the excess production of adrenal androgens stimulated by adrenal overactivity. (From Court DS, Hinson J, Naish J, Raven P. *Medical Sciences,* 3rd Edition. Elsevier; 2019.)

Symptoms and signs

Clinical features relate to excess circulating cortisol (Figs. 4.31–4.32).

HINTS AND TIPS

- Key features of Cushing's syndrome are remembered using the acronym **CUSHINGOID**:
  - **C** – **C**ataracts
  - **U** – **U**lcers, urinary symptoms
  - **S** – **S**triae, skin thinning
  - **H** – **H**ypertension, hirsutism, hair loss, hump (buffalo)
  - **I** – **I**nfections
  - **N** – **N**ecrosis (femoral head), neuropsychiatric changes
  - **G** – **G**lucose elevation (diabetes)
  - **O** – **O**steoporosis, obesity
  - **I** – **I**mmunosuppression
  - **D** – **D**epression, dyslipidaemia
- There are many other symptoms, and it can also be useful to picture the patient with Cushing's syndrome to remember some of the characteristic features.

RED FLAG

- Symptoms of Cushing's syndrome associated with headache, visual changes (bitemporal hemianopia) and cutaneous hyperpigmentation suggest a large pituitary adenoma exerting mass effect.
- Urgent assessment and treatment is required due to the risk of visual loss.

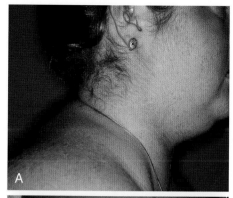

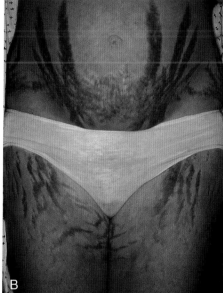

Fig. 4.32 Clinical features of Cushing syndrome. (A) Buffalo hump. (B) Central obesity and abdominal striae. (From Ko CJ, Schaffer JV, Duncan KO, Bolognia JL. *Dermatology Essentials,* 2nd Edition. Elsevier; 2022.)

Investigations

Diagnosis is made and the aetiology identified using the dexamethasone suppression test (Fig. 4.33). Imaging can be performed to identify malignant aetiologies (Fig. 4.34).

Management

The first-line management of endogenous Cushing's syndrome is surgical resection of the contributing tumour:

- Adrenal tumours: unilateral or bilateral adrenalectomy.
- Cushing's disease: transsphenoidal hypophysectomy.
- Ectopic ACTH: appropriate tumour resection.

CLINICAL NOTES

Anticoagulation may be required perioperatively, as Cushing's syndrome is an extremely hypercoagulable state with a high risk of venous thromboembolism (VTE).

Postoperative management includes:

- Management of comorbidities: diabetes, hypertension, hyperlipidaemia, osteoporosis and mood disorders should be screened for and treated where appropriate.
- Glucocorticoid replacement therapy: for postoperative adrenal insufficiency.
- Monitoring for recurrence: adrenal carcinoma has a high risk of recurrence.

HINTS AND TIPS

- Lifelong glucocorticoid replacement is required in bilateral adrenalectomy.
- In unilateral adrenalectomy or resection of an ectopic ACTH secreting tumour, glucocorticoid therapy should be reviewed annually, and stopped where possible.

Adrenal insufficiency

Adrenal insufficiency is the insufficient production of adrenal hormones, including glucocorticoids, mineralocorticoids and androgens (Table 4.9).

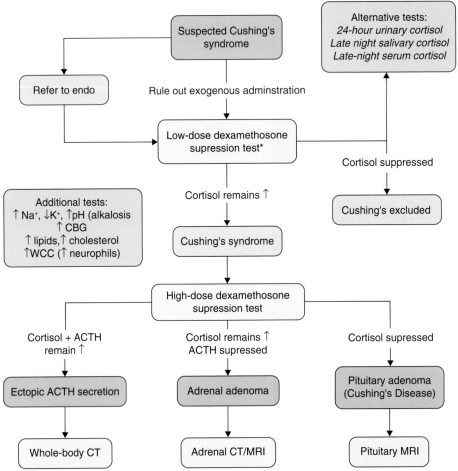

Fig. 4.33 Investigations for suspected Cushing's disease. *The dexamethasone suppression test is typically the preferred first line, as it is convenient to carry out, and indicates the underlying cause of symptoms. *CBG*, Capillary blood glucose; *RCC*, renal cell carcinoma; *SCLC*, small cell lung cancer.

 CLINICAL NOTES

Acute adrenal insufficiency relating to sudden cessation of glucocorticoids is significantly more common than primary adrenal disease

 HINTS AND TIPS

Waterhouse-Friderichsen syndrome describes adrenal haemorrhage and subsequent acute adrenal insufficiency in meningococcal sepsis

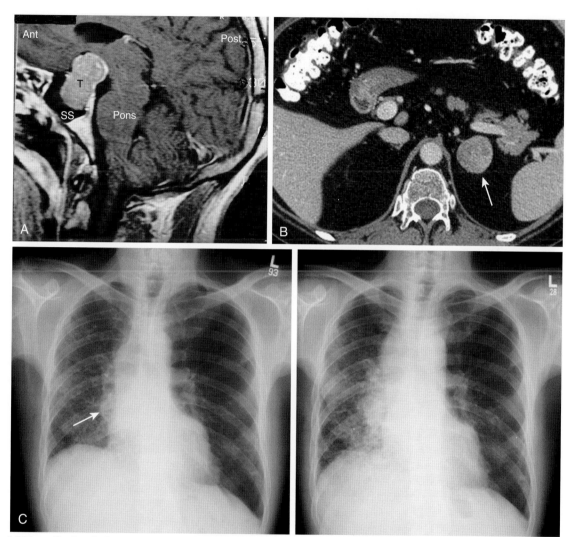

Fig. 4.34 Investigation findings in Cushing syndrome. (A) Pituitary adenoma (Cushing disease). (B) Adrenal adenoma. (C) Lung mass in left hilar region suspicious of small cell lung cancer. (From A. Mettler Jr FA. *Essentials of Radiology*, 3rd Edition. Philadelphia: Saunders; 2014. B. Korobkin M, Francis IR. *Adrenal imaging, Seminars in Ultrasound, CT and MRI*, Volume 16, Issue 4, August 1995, Pages 317-330. https://doi.org/10.1016/0887-2171(95)90036-5. C. Stapleton RD, Kotloff RM, Broaddus VC, et al. *Murray & Nadel's Textbook of Respiratory Medicine*, 7th Edition. Elsevier; 2022.)

Table 4.9 Classification of adrenal insufficiency

	Pathophysiology	Aetiology
Primary (Addison disease)	Acute or chronic destruction of the adrenal glands -> ↓hormone production and release	Autoimmune (80%–90%) Infectious – TB, CMV Adrenal haemorrhage – sepsis, DIC, VTE, trauma Infiltration – adrenal tumour, amyloidosis, haemochromatosis Adrenalectomy Pituitary apoplexy
Secondary	Decreased ACTH production	Chronic glucocorticoid therapy with sudden discontinuation Hypopituitarism
Tertiary	Decreased CRH production	Chronic glucocorticoid therapy with sudden discontinuation Hypothalamic dysfunction – trauma, mass, haemorrhage, anorexia

CMV, *Cytomegalovirus*; DIC, *disseminated intravascular coagulation*; TV, *tuberculosis*; VTE, *venous thromboembolism*.

Symptoms and signs

Clinical features relate to the underlying hormonal derangements (Fig. 4.35).

CLINICAL NOTES

- The anion gap is calculated from the difference between serum cations and anions:
- $(Na^+ + K^+) - (Cl^- + HCO_3^-)$
- Normal anion gap metabolic acidosis relates to an imbalance in serum cations and anions.
- Adrenal insufficiency causes a type 4 renal tubular acidosis relating to ↓ aldosterone, resulting in reduced K^+ and H^+ secretion and reduced HCO_3^- reabsorption in the collecting duct of the kidney, and acidosis.
- Loss of HCO_3^- is buffered by increased reabsorption of Cl^-, and hence the anion gap remains normal.
- Elevated anion gap metabolic acidosis is caused by the addition of unmeasured ions, such as lactate, ketones and urea.

HINTS AND TIPS

Subclinical adrenal insufficiency may only manifest when cortisol requirement is increased in stress, surgery or illness.

Investigations

Cortisol and ACTH should be measured to determine the aetiology (Fig. 4.36).

RED FLAG

- Acute adrenal insufficiency is immediately life threatening
- It is a clinical diagnosis, and investigations should not delay glucocorticoids administration.

Management

Acute adrenal insufficiency is a life-threatening medical emergency and should be managed with urgent assessment and treatment (Fig. 4.37).

HINTS AND TIPS

- Management of adrenal crisis can be remembered by the 5 S's:
  - S – Steroids (100 mg hydrocortisone IV)
  - S – Salt (0.9% saline
  - S – Sugar (50% dextrose)
  - S – Supportive – monitoring, fluid replacement, 200 mg hydrocortisone/24 hours
  - S – Search – for the underlying cause

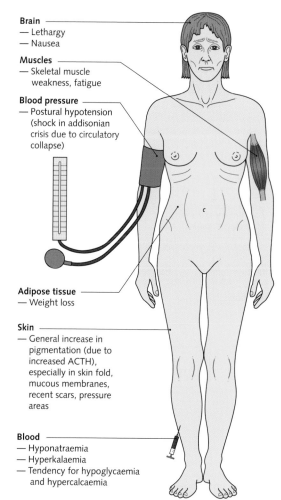

Brain
— Lethargy
— Nausea

Muscles
— Skeletal muscle weakness, fatigue

Blood pressure
— Postural hypotension (shock in addisonian crisis due to circulatory collapse)

Adipose tissue
— Weight loss

Skin
— General increase in pigmentation (due to increased ACTH), especially in skin fold, mucous membranes, recent scars, pressure areas

Blood
— Hyponatraemia
— Hyperkalaemia
— Tendency for hypoglycaemia and hypercalcaemia

Fig. 4.35 Clinical features of adrenal insufficiency. *Features of hypoaldosteronism and ↑ACTH are only present in primary adrenal insufficiency. *DHEA-S*, Androgen produced by the adrenal gland that is converted into active metabolites (DHEA/testosterone) in peripheral tissues; *MSH*, melanocyte-stimulating hormone; *NAG*, normal anion gap. (From Eiben I, et al. *Crash Course General Medicine*, 5th Edition. Elsevier; 2019.)

RED FLAG

- Severe hyperkalaemia is a medical emergency due to the risk of arrhythmias.
- Emergency management should be initiated at K⁺ >6.5 mmol/L, or in ECG changes:
  - Protecting the heart: IV calcium gluconate (to stabilize the myocardium).
  - Move K⁺ into cells: IV Insulin and dextrose +/– nebulized salbutamol.
  - Remove K⁺ from the body: treat AKI +/– sodium zirconium.
- Patients with K⁺ levels 5.5–5.9 can be managed by investigating and treating the underlying cause.

Once stable and the underlying cause diagnosed, medical replacement therapy can be given:

- Primary adrenal insufficiency: glucocorticoid and mineralocorticoid replacement, and androgen replacement if required.
- Secondary/tertiary adrenal insufficiency: glucocorticoid replacement and androgen replacement if required.

CLINICAL NOTES

- It is essential the patients are counselled on the Don't **STOP** criteria when starting steroids:
- Don't – stop steroids abruptly, due to the risk of adrenal crisis
- S – **S**ick day rules
- T – **T**reatment card
- O – **O**steoporosis prophylaxis (bisphosphonates and calcium/vitamin D supplementation)
- P – **P**PIs for gastro protection
- The sick day rules avoid development of adrenal crisis:
  - Double routine dose in intercurrent illness or for a minor surgical procedure
  - IV glucocorticoids in severe illness, trauma, fasting or over the perioperative period

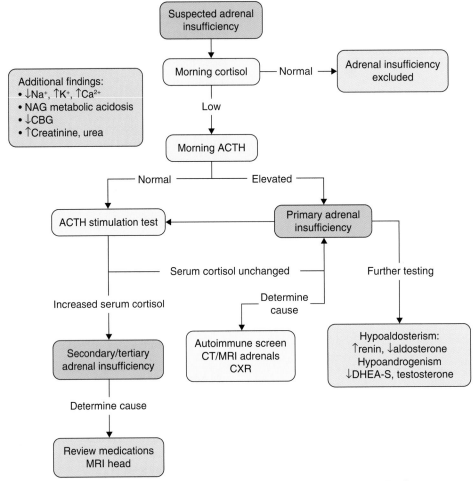

Fig. 4.36 Investigation of suspected adrenal insufficiency. *CBG*, Capillary blood glucose; *DHEA-S,* testosterone precursor.

Additional measures related to the underlying cause:

- Adrenal malignancy: tumour resection.
- Adrenal haemorrhage – surgical resection and angioembolization.
- Hypopituitarism – pituitary hormone substitution.
- Drug-induced – review medications.

Primary hyperaldosteronism

Primary hyperaldosteronism is an excess of aldosterone secretion from the adrenal glands. It is typically caused by bilateral adrenal gland hyperplasia or a unilateral adrenal adenoma. Rarer causes include adrenal carcinoma or paraneoplastic aldosterone secretion.

Symptoms and signs

The symptoms and signs relate to the systemic effects of excess aldosterone (Fig. 4.38).

Investigations

Investigations include:

- Screening tests: ↑ Aldosterone:renin ratio (↑ aldosterone and ↓ renin).
- Confirmatory tests: oral sodium loading test, which involves 3 days of high sodium intake, and 24-urine aldosterone collection on the final day. ↑ Aldosterone confirms a diagnosis of primary hyperaldosteronism.
- Diagnostic imaging: adrenal CT will diagnose the lesion (Fig. 4.39).

DIFFERENTIALS

Screen for primary hyperaldosteronism in drug-resistant hypertension (combination therapy with three different antihypertensives) or hypertension <40 years of age.

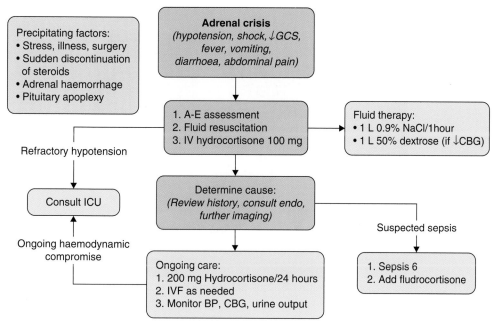

Fig. 4.37 Acute management of adrenal crisis. *CBG,* Capillary blood glucose.

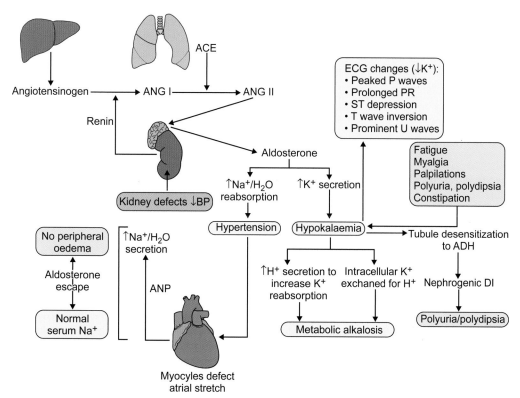

Fig. 4.38 Overview of the renin-angiotensin-aldosterone-system and systemic effects of hyperaldosteronism. Aldosterone escape is a compensatory mechanism that explains an absence of oedema and hypernatraemia in patients with primary hyperaldosteronism.

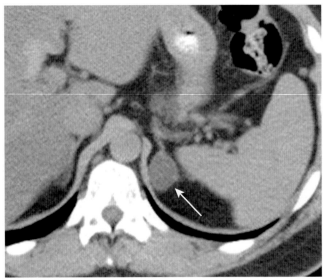

Fig. 4.39 Adrenal CT. Left adrenal adenoma. (From Lin DS, Caoili EM, Wong KK, et al. *DeGroot's Endocrinology: Basic Science and Clinical Practice,* 8th Edition. Elsevier; 2023.)

Management

Management includes antihypertensive medications and treating the underlying cause:

- Unilateral adenoma/carcinoma: laparoscopic adrenalectomy.
- Bilateral hyperplasia: aldosterone receptor antagonists (spironolactone/eplerenone).

Complications

Complications are related to systemic effects of chronic hypertension:

- Cardiovascular disease (stroke/myocardial infarction)
- Heart failure
- Atrial fibrillation
- Impaired renal function
- Hypertensive retinopathy
- Vascular dementia

Pheochromocytoma

A pheochromocytoma is a catecholamine-secreting tumour that develops from the chromaffin cells in the adrenal medulla. A small percentage develop in the sympathetic ganglia, and they may be multiple. The majority are benign.

CLINICAL NOTES

- 25% of pheochromocytomas are hereditary, associated with the MEN (Multiple Endocrine Neoplasia) conditions, neurofibromatosis type 1 and Von-Hippel-Lindau disease.
- If this is suspected, genetic testing should be performed.

Symptoms and signs

A pheochromocytoma may be asymptomatic. Other symptoms relate to paroxysmal catecholamine secretion:

- Malignant hypertension: episodic blood pressure crises with extreme hypertension, headaches, sweating, palpitations and pallor.
- Persistent hypertension: chronic, unexplained, drug-resistant hypertension.
- Abdominal pain and nausea: mass effect of the tumour.
- Anxiety: related to sympathetic nervous system overactivity.
- Weight loss: increased basal metabolism results in weight loss despite normal or increased dietary intake.
- Hyperglycaemia: catecholamines trigger increased insulin resistance and increased serum glucose.

Pheochromocytomas may also secrete EPO, resulting in polycythaemia and hypercoagulability.

- The symptoms of pheochromocytoma can be remembered by the 5 **P's**:
  - **P** – Increased blood **P**ressure
  - **P** – **P**ain (headache)
  - **P** – **P**alpitations
  - **P** – **P**allor
  - **P** – **P**erspiration

CLINICAL NOTES

Triggers for malignant hypertension include foods high in tyramine (the tyramine cheese reaction!), surgery, tumour palpation, and drugs, including beta-blockers and monoamine-oxidase inhibitors.

DIFFERENTIALS

Pheochromocytoma and primary hyperaldosteronism are key causes of secondary hypertension and hypertensive crises.

Investigations

Investigations include:

- Plasma-free metanephrines: catecholamines metabolites that will be significantly elevated.
- 24-hour urinary metanephrines/catecholamines: to confirm the diagnosis.
- Abdominal CT/MRI: to locate the tumour (Fig. 4.40).

Management

Management includes:

- Blood pressure control: with combined alpha and beta-blockade.

- Surgical resection: with additional antihypertensives if hypertension persists.
- Inoperable disease: alpha-blockade if benign, or radiotherapy/chemotherapy with tumour embolization if malignant.

CLINICAL NOTES

- It is essential to give alpha-blockers before beta-blockers.
- Unopposed alpha-adrenoceptor stimulation may lead to systemic vasoconstriction and a profound hypertensive crisis.

HINTS AND TIPS

- There is a 15% chance of recurrence of a benign pheochromocytoma within 5 to 15 years.
- Consider recurrence in those with previous pheochromocytoma and new hypertension.

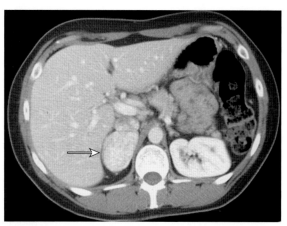

Fig. 4.40 Abdominal CT demonstrating large right-sided pheochromocytoma. Large right-sided pheochromocytoma. (From Goldman L, Schafer AI, Young Jr WF. *Goldman-Cecil Medicine, 2-Volume Set,* 26th Edition. Elsevier; 2020.)

Complications

Hypertensive crises require urgent assessment and treatment to prevent end-organ damage (Table 4.10, Fig. 4.41).

Lymphadenopathy

The lymphatic system is made up of primary and secondary lymphatic organs, lymphatic vessels and lymph. The lymphatic system functions to remove excess interstitial fluid and waste products from the bloodstream, so they can be excreted (Fig. 4.42).

Lymphadenopathy is enlargement of one or multiple lymph nodes. It commonly occurs in the cervical region, presenting as a neck lump (Fig. 4.43).

- Benign lymphadenopathy (lymphadenitis): proliferation of immune cells in the gland, secondary to localized or systemic inflammation. Common in infectious conditions or autoimmune disease. Typically soft, mobile and tender.

Table 4.10 Manifestations of end-organ dysfunction hypertensive crisis

System	End-organ dysfunction	Clinical features
Cardiac	Acute heart failure	Dyspnoea, pulmonary oedema
	Myocardial infarction	Chest pain, diaphoresis
	Aortic dissection	Chest pain, asymmetrical pulses
Neurological	Hypertensive encephalopathy	Headache, vomiting, confusion, seizures, papilloedema
	Stroke	Focal neurology, ↓GCS
Renal	Acute nephrosclerosis	AKI, oliguria, haematuria
Ophthalmic	Acute hypertensive retinopathy	Reduced visual acuity, flame haemorrhages, papilloedema
Haematological	Microangiopathic haemolytic anaemia	Fatigue, pallor, bleeding, jaundice

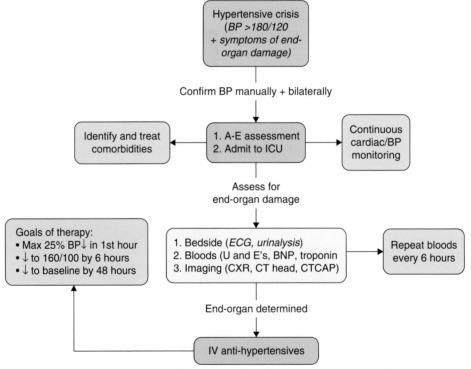

Fig. 4.41 Acute management of hypertensive crisis. The choice of IV antihypertensive is based on the organ system affected. *BNP*, Brain natriuretic peptide; *CTCAP*, CT chest, abdo, pelvis.

- Malignant lymphadenopathy: proliferation of malignant cells in a lymph node, presenting with painless, progressively enlarging, firm, fixed, nodes. Typically relates to haematological malignancy or systemic metastasis.

Investigation

Benign nodes require no investigations. Malignant nodes should be investigated further:

- Bloods: FBC, U&E, LFTs.
- Peripheral blood smear, reticulocytes and LDH: to identify haematological malignancy.

- Lymph node US: malignant nodes are irregular lesions with increased vascularity.
- CT/MRI: for detailed assessment of nodes (Fig. 4.44).
- Biopsy and histology: for definitive diagnosis of underlying pathology.

HINTS AND TIPS

Have a low threshold for HIV testing in patients with persistent, generalized, tender lymphadenopathy.

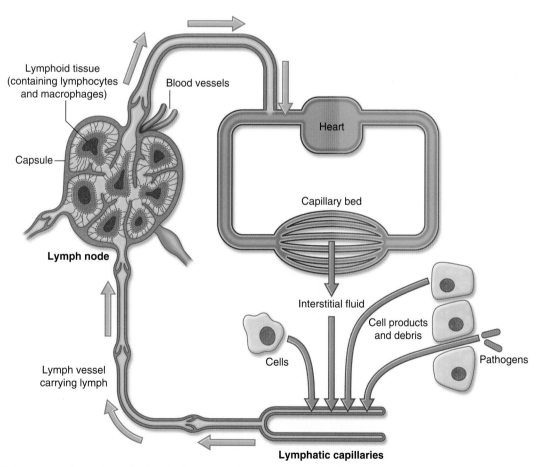

Fig. 4.42 Structure and function of the lymphatic system. (From Drake RL, et al. *Gray's Anatomy for Students,* 5th Edition. Elsevier Inc. 2024.)

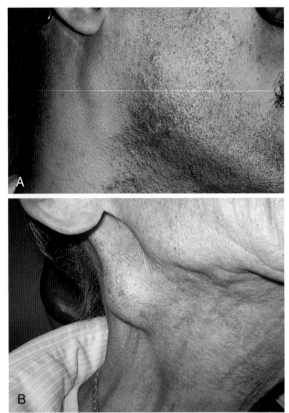

Fig. 4.43 Cervical lymphadenopathy (A) Posterior cervical chain. (B) Deep cervical/anterior cervical chain. Massive lymphadenopathy, as seen in (B), is commonly associated with malignancy. (From A. Damm DD, Allen CM, Chi AC, Neville BW. *Oral and Maxillofacial Pathology,* 5th Edition. Elsevier; 2024. B. Talley N, O'Connor S. *Talley and O'Connor's Clinical OSCEs.* Elsevier; 2022.)

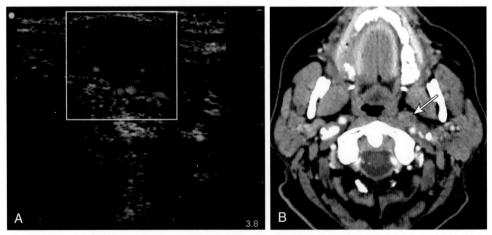

Fig. 4.44 Imaging features of malignant lymphadenopathy. (A) Colour flow Doppler of a malignant supraclavicular lymph node. Note the irregular, blurred border and increased peripheral vascularity. (B) Malignant lymph node on CT scan. Note the large size, necrotic centre and round shape. (From A. Soni AN, Franco-Sadud R, Soni NJ, Kory P, Arntfield R. *Point-of-Care Ultrasound,* 2nd Edition. Elsevier; 2020. B. Tamimi D. *Specialty Imaging: Temporomandibular Joint and Sleep-Disordered Breathing,* 2nd Edition. Elsevier; 2023.)

Benign neck lumps

Neck lumps have a range of benign aetiologies (Table 4.11, Fig. 4.45).

Management is typically conservative in asymptomatic lesions. Surgical resection can be considered for cosmetic reasons, symptomatic lumps or those associated with infection. For lesions with malignant potential, prophylactic resection may be indicated.

NEUROENDOCRINE TUMOURS

A neuroendocrine tumour is a tumour derived from neuroendocrine cells. They may be malignant or benign. Tumours most commonly arise from the GIT, including the stomach, pancreas and bowel.

HINTS AND TIPS

- Neuroendocrine tumours may arise sporadically or in association with an underlying genetic condition, including multiple endocrine neoplasia (MEN), Neurofibromatosis type 1 and Von-Hippel-Lindau syndrome.
- The conditions associated with each MEN syndrome include
  - MEN1 – 3 P's – parathyroid adenoma, pancreatic tumour, pituitary adenoma
  - MEN2a – 1 M, 2 P's – medullary thyroid carcinoma, parathyroid adenoma, pheochromocytoma
  - MEN2b – 2 M's, 1 P – Medullary thyroid carcinoma, Multiple neuromas, pheochromocytoma

Table 4.11 Aetiology and clinical features of common neck lumps

	Lump	Aetiology	Clinical features
Congenital	Thyroglossal cyst	Remnant of embryological thyroglossal duct	Painless, firm, midline mass near hyoid bone Elevates with swallowing and tongue protrusion
	Branchial cleft	Remnant of embryological branchial cleft	Painless, firm mass, lateral to midline No movement on swallowing
	Haemangioma	Benign vascular tumour	Red papule/macule May involute slowly
	Dermoid cyst	Germ cell tumour (teratoma) containing somatic tissue	Mostly asymptomatic May exert pressure effects
Acquired	Sebaceous cyst	Formed by blockage of a sebaceous gland, contains sebum	Slow growing, mobile, firm, painless Infection – painful, red, exudative mass
	Lipoma	A benign tumour of mature adipocytes	Slow growing, soft, painless, mobile, rubbery nodule May be multiple
	Sialadenitis	Acute inflammation of the salivary gland	Unilateral painful swelling and erythema, purulent discharge

Neuroendocrine tumour release hormones relating to their cellular origin, which result in their clinical features. Positive screening tests warrant CT/MRI imaging to detect the primary tumour, evaluate for metastasis, and guide ongoing management. Rarely, tumours can be nonfunctioning, and produce symptoms relating to compression of surrounding structures (Table 4.12).

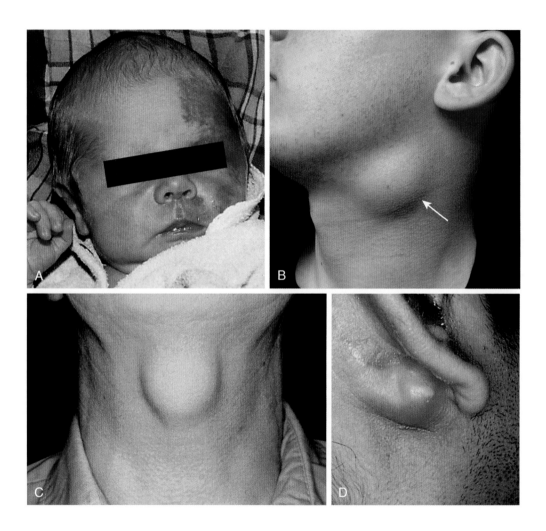

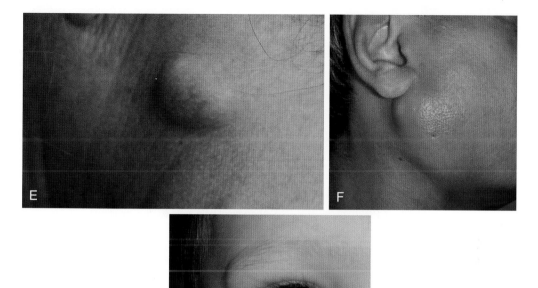

Fig. 4.45 Typical appearance of common neck lumps. (A) Haemangioma. (B) Branchial cleft. (C) Thyroglossal cyst. (D) Sebaceous cyst. (E) Neck lipoma. (F) Salivary calculi. (G) Dermoid cyst. (From A. Cameron P, et al. *Textbook of Paediatric Emergency Medicine*, 3rd Edition. Elsevier; 2019. B. Gurgel RK, Harnsberger HR. *Imaging in Otolaryngology*. Elsevier; 2018. C. Innes JA, Hathorn I, Dover A, Fairhurst K. *Macleod's Clinical Examination,* 15th Edition. Elsevier; 2024. D. Solomon BS, Ball JW, Dains JE, Flynn JA, Stewart RW. *Seidel's Guide To Physical Examination: An Interprofessional Approach,* 9th Edition. Elsevier; 2019. E. Courtesy, Ian Odell, MD. F. Zanation A, Patel S, Yarbrough WG, et al. *Sabiston Textbook of Surgery: The Biological Basis of Modern Surgical Practice,* 21st Edition. Elsevier; 2022. G. Palay DA, Krachmer JH. *Cornea Atlas: Expert Consult – Online and Print,* 3rd Edition. Elsevier; 2014.)

HINTS AND TIPS

- Carcinoid tumours are typically asymptomatic, as serotonin is metabolized by the liver before it can exert systemic effects.
- Tumours that have metastasized to liver produce symptoms, which can be remembered by the mnemonic **FIVE-HT**:
  - **F** – **F**lushing
  - **I** – **I**ntestinal complaints (diarrhoea)
  - **V** – **V**alvular lesions
  - **E** – wh**EE**zing
  - **H** – **H**epatic involvement
  - **T** – **T**ryptophan deficiency
- Tryptophan deficiency can result in pellagra, a disease of niacin deficiency, that presents with the 4 D's – **D**ermatitis, **D**iarrhoea, **D**ementia and **D**eath.

CLINICAL NOTES

- Serum chromogranin A (CgA) is a useful broad-spectrum marker for neuroendocrine tumours.
- It is almost always raised in gastrointestinal and pancreatic neuroendocrine tumours, as well as SCLC.

CLINICAL NOTES

- Octreotide is a somatostatin analogue that inhibits the secretion of many hormones
- It is often used in management of neuroendocrine tumours, as an adjunctive treatment or as an alternative to surgery.

Table 4.12 Overview of neuroendocrine tumours

	Tumour	Investigation findings	Clinical features	Treatment
PNETs	Insulinoma (β cells)	↑ **Insulin** ↑ Proinsulin ↑ C-peptide ↓CBG	Whipple's triad – ↓CBG, hypoglycaemia symptoms, relief upon administering glucose Weight gain	Tumour resection Octreotide
	Glucagonoma (α-cells)	↑**Glucagon** ↑CBG ↓ Hb	Diarrhoea Weight loss Hyperglycaemia, diabetes mellitus Necrolytic migratory erythema	Tumour resection Glycaemic control Octreotide
	VIPoma (Innervating nerve fibres)	↑**VIP** ↓K$^+$ ↑Ca^{2+} ↑CBG ↓Hb	Watery diarrhoea ++ Hypokalaemia Weight loss Abdominal pain, nausea and vomiting Hyperglycaemia Anaemia	Tumour resection Octreotide
	Somatostatinoma (δ-cells)	↑**Somatostatin** ↓Insulin, glucagon, gastrin, CCK ↑CBG ↓Hb	Triad – diabetes, cholelithiasis, steatorrhea Abdominal pain Weight loss Anaemia	Surgical resection Octreotide Chemotherapy
Gastrinoma (Zollinger-Ellison syndrome)		↑ **Gastrin** ↓ Gastric pH	Drug-resistant PUD Diarrhoea Often malignant	Surgical resection PPIs Octreotide
Carcinoid tumour		↑**Serotonin** ↑Urinary 5-HIAA	May be asymptomatic. Cutaneous flushing, diarrhoea, abdo pain Palpitations Dyspnoea and wheeze Right heart failure	Surgical resection Octreotide Radiotherapy

CBG, *Capillary blood glucose;* PNETs, *pancreatic neuroendocrine tumours;* PUD, *peptic ulcer disease;* VIP, *vasoactive intestinal polypeptide. Other key examples of neuroendocrine tumours include small cell lung cancer, medullary thyroid cancer, parathyroid tumours and pheochromocytomas.*

● Chapter Summary

- Unexplained weight loss should always raise suspicion of underlying malignancy.
- Polyuria and polydipsia most commonly relate to uncontrolled diabetes mellitus.
- Unexplained hoarseness in a smoker is a red flag for head and neck malignancy.
- A new bitemporal hemianopia is likely to represent a pituitary adenoma.
- Hyponatraemia should be normalised slowly to prevent development of cerebral pontine myelinolysis.
- Immediate haematoma post-thyroid surgery is immediately life threatening and warrants urgent return to theatre.
- Hypercalcemia presents with 'bones, stones, groans, thrones and moans'. Urgent aggressive fluid resuscitation is required.
- Differentiating between Cushing's syndrome and Cushing's disease can be done with the dexamethasone suppression test, with suppression of cortisol indicating Cushing's disease.
- Steroids must never be stopped suddenly, due to the risk of acute life-threatening adrenal insufficiency.
- Hyperkalaemia with ECG changes is an emergency, and should be treated with IV calcium gluconate and insulin and dextrose.

UKMLA Conditions

Addison disease
Cushing syndrome
Diabetes insipidus
Essential, or secondary hypertension
Hypercalcaemia of malignancy
Hyperlipidaemia
Hyperparathyroidism
Hyperthermia and hypothermia
Hypoglycaemia
Hypoparathyroidism
Hypothyroidism
Obesity
Osteoporosis
Pituitary tumours
Thyroid eye disease
Thyroid nodules
Thyrotoxicosis

UKMLA Presentations

Amenorrhoea
Bone pain
Confusion
Electrolyte abnormalities
Erectile dysfunction
Fatigue
Gynaecomastia
Hoarseness and voice change
Hypertension
Menstrual problems
Nausea
Neck lump
Nipple discharge
Palpitations
Polydipsia (thirst)
Pubertal development
Subfertility
Urinary symptoms
Weight gain
Weight loss

Breast surgery 5

CLINICAL ANATOMY

The breasts are located on the anterior chest wall, from the lateral sternal border to the mid-axillary line. The central nipple is surrounded by pigmented areolar skin, which contains sebaceous oil-secreting glands which lubricate and protect the nipple during breastfeeding. The axillary tail is a projection of mammary tissue extending into the axilla (Fig. 5.1).

The breasts contain mammary glands, adipose and connective tissue. The mammary glands contain ducts and secretory lobules which form secretory lactiferous ducts. The breast is supplied and drained from branches of the axillary, internal thoracic and intercostal arteries, and veins, and innervated via cutaneous branches of the intercostal nerves. The lymphatic drainage of the breast is predominantly to the axillary nodes, with the remainder draining to the parasternal and posterior intercostal nodes (Fig. 5.2).

At puberty increased circulating oestrogen and progesterone cause duct and lobule development, and fat and connective tissue growth. During pregnancy secretion of oestrogen, progesterone, prolactin and placental growth hormones result in lobuloalveolar growth and ductal development to prepare for lactation and breastfeeding (Fig. 5.3).

CLINICAL NOTES

Developmental abnormalities of the breast include:
- Amastia: absence
- Hypoplasia: underdevelopment
- Virginal hypertrophy: excessive pubertal growth
- Accessory nipples: nonfunctioning nipples on the milk line, which extends from the axilla to the groin
- Accessory breast tissue: common in the axilla, grows during pregnancy

---

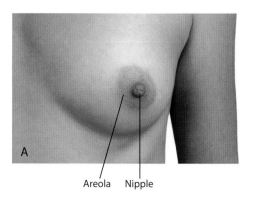

Areola Nipple

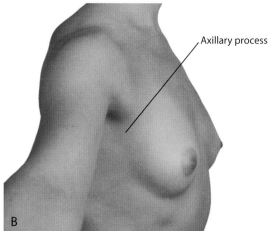

Axillary process

Fig. 5.1 Surface anatomy of the breast. (A) Frontal view of the breast. (B) Lateral view of the breast and axilla. (From Drake RL, Vogl AW, Mitchell AWM. *Gray's Basic Anatomy*. Churchill Livingstone, Elsevier Inc. 2013.)

BREAST SURGERY PRESENTATIONS

History taking

Opening the consultation
Introduce yourself, confirm the patient's details and gain consent to proceed.

Presenting complaint (PC)
Begin with an open question to identify the presenting complaint.

History of presenting complaint (HPC)
Explore the presenting complaint in more detail. Common presentations include:

- Breast lump: a lump or asymmetry may be noticed incidentally or during a regular self-examination, and may represent benign or malignant pathology.

155

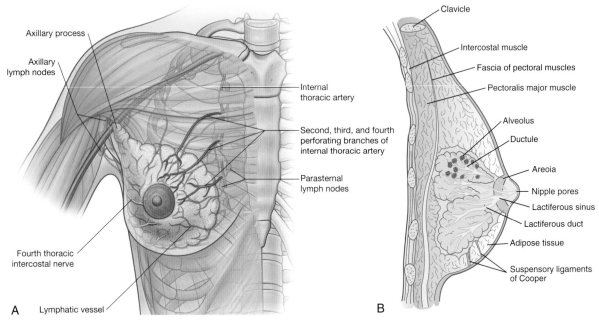

Fig. 5.2 (A) Arterial supply and lymphatic drainage of the breast. (B) Mammary glands, ducts and secretory lobules. (A. From Drake RL, Vogl AW, Mitchell AWM. *Gray's Anatomy for Students, 2nd Edition*. Churchill Livingstone, Elsevier Inc. 2010. B. From Shiland BJ, Zenith. *Medical Assistant: Pediatrics, Geriatrics, Endocrine and Reproductive Systems—Module F*, 2nd Edition. Elsevier; 2015.)

- Breast pain: may be acute, related to infection or cyclical mastalgia.
- Nipple discharge: bloody discharge from a single duct suggests malignancy. Green or grey discharge suggests duct ectasia.
- Skin changes: erythema, ulcerations, dimpling or nipple inversion suggest malignancy.
- Gynaecomastia: the development of breast tissue in males, which may be benign or associated with underlying pathology.

- **T**iming: progressive growth suggests a tumour. Cyclical change suggests benign hormone-related breast mastalgia/lumps
- **E**xacerbating factors: there may have been a specific trigger (i.e., trauma), and symptoms become worse with menstruation
- **S**everity: assess severity of associated pain and impact of symptoms

---

HINTS AND TIPS

Use **SOCRATES** to explore the presenting complaint:
- **S**ite: assess the location of the lump
- **O**nset: preceding trauma suggests fat necrosis. Lumps associated with breastfeeding include galactocele or abscess.
- **C**haracter: soft, firm, smooth, irregular, mobile or tethered
- **R**adiation: there may be multiple lumps or radiation of pain
- **A**ssociated symptoms: erythema, skin change, pain and nipple discharge

Systemic screen
Briefly assess for key symptoms from other body systems.

CLINICAL NOTES

- Constitutional features (fever, lethargy, appetite and weight change, night sweats) or regional lymphadenopathy suggest infective or malignant pathology.
- Gastrointestinal, musculoskeletal or neurological symptoms may suggest metastatic disease associated with a breast lump.

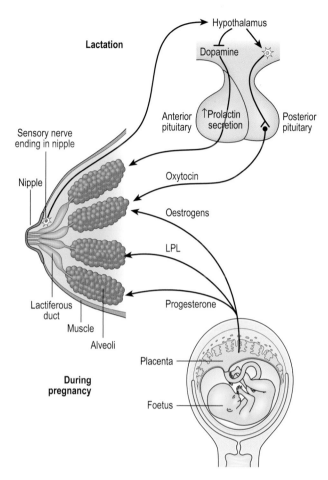

Fig. 5.3 Hormonal control of breast development during pregnancy and lactation. Suckling of the baby at the breast stimulates prolactin release and milk production, and oxytocin release causes alveolar contraction and milk expulsion. (From Hinson J, Raven P, Chew S. *The Endocrine System: Basic Science and Clinical Conditions*, 3rd Edition. Elsevier; 2023.)

Ideas, concerns and expectations

Explore the patient's concerns and identify what they hope to get from the consultation.

COMMUNICATION

Breast lumps can cause significant anxiety. Address concerns early and reassure the patient they have done the right thing seeking medical advice.

Past medical history

Ask about other medical conditions, previous surgeries and recent investigations or procedures. Both previous benign and malignant breast pathology increase the risk of further symptoms.

Menstrual history

A complete menstrual history should be taken:

- Last menstrual period: assess timing of last menstrual period and length of cycle.
- Menarche: determine the age of menarche and menopause, if appropriate.
- Pregnancies: assess gravity and parity, and whether breastfeeding occurred.
- Hormonal contraception: take a full contraception history and identify which hormones have been taken.

Drug history

Obtain a complete drug history, including use of over-the-counter medications, compliance and side-effects. Determine allergy status and type of reaction.

Family history

Enquire about family members with breast pathology, and the age they developed symptoms. Specifically enquire about gynaecological or breast malignancy.

Social history

Assess for risk factors in the social history:

- Functional status: assess independence, type of accommodation and support needs.
- Smoking: a significant risk factor for breast cancer. In those with a current or ex-smoking history, calculate pack-years.
- Alcohol: assess weekly units and type of alcohol consumed. Excess use is a significant risk factor for breast cancer.
- Recreational drugs: anabolic steroid use is an important cause of gynaecomastia in males. Intravenous drug use can predispose to abscess development.
- Occupation: enquire about current occupation, and the impact of symptoms.

Closing the consultation

Summarize the key points of the history back to the patient and thank them for their time.

DIFFERENTIAL DIAGNOSIS

Breast lump

The differential diagnosis of a breast lump includes benign and malignant pathologies (Fig. 5.4).

The age of presentation can offer clues as to the likely diagnosis (Fig. 5.5).

Investigation of a breast lump

Any unexplained breast lump should be referred for a triple diagnostic assessment:

- Clinical assessment: history and examination by a breast specialist.
- Imaging: mammogram for those >35, and ultrasound (US) if <35.
- Breast biopsy: fine-needle aspiration (FNA), core-needle biopsy (CNB) or excisional biopsy, for histological diagnosis.

Breast pain (mastalgia)

The differential diagnosis of breast pain includes hormonal changes and inflammatory disorders (Fig. 5.6).

Investigations for breast pain

1. Bedside
   - Pregnancy test: early pregnancy commonly causes breast pain.
2. Bloods
   - FBC: ↑WBC suggests infection. ↓Hb suggests anaemia, which may be related to chronic disease.
   - Blood cultures: in severe systemic infection, to guide antibiotic therapy.

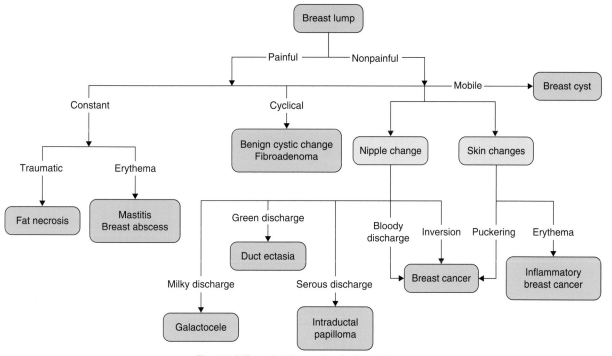

Fig. 5.4 Differential diagnosis of a breast lump.

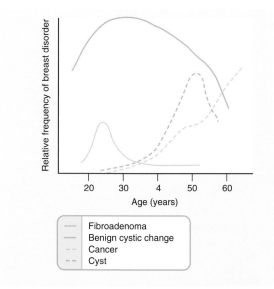

Fig. 5.5 Age distribution of breast lumps. (From Kontoyannis A., Sweetland H. *Crash Course: Surgery*, 3rd Edition, Elsevier; 2008.)

3. Imaging
   • Breast US: to identify underlying abscesses.
   • Mammogram: if there is suspicion for underlying malignancy.

• FNA: cytology and histology can be sent to differentiate between infection or malignancy, and therapeutic drainage performed for abscesses.

HINTS AND TIPS

For simple mastitis, a biopsy is not required. For atypical presentations, recurrent infections or abscesses, biopsy should be taken to exclude malignancy.

Nipple discharge

Nipple discharge is common, and can relate to infective, malignant or endocrinological pathology (Fig. 5.7).

Investigations
1. Bedside
   • Pregnancy test: hormonal changes in pregnancy can cause changes in discharge.
2. Bloods
   • FBC: ↓ Hb indicates anaemia, which may be associated with malignancy. ↑ WBC suggests infection.
   • Prolactin: hyperprolactinemia is the primary cause of galactorrhoea.

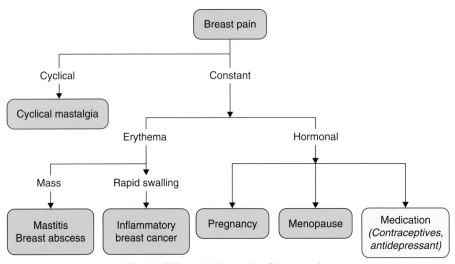

Fig. 5.6 Differential diagnosis of breast pain.

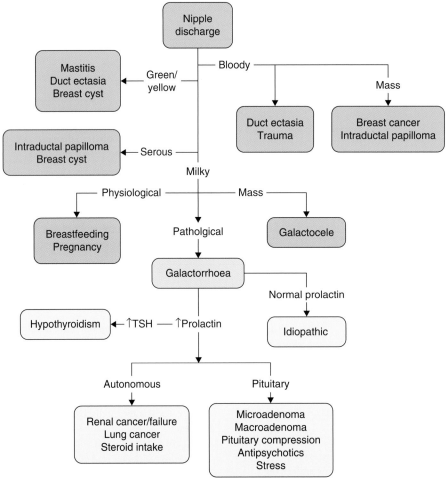

Fig. 5.7 Differential diagnosis of nipple discharge.

- TSH: ↑ hypothalamic TRH release, triggers both ↑ TSH and prolactin release from the pituitary.
- U&Es: indicated to diagnose chronic renal disease.
3. Imaging
   - Mammogram: to help to help characterize and diagnose a mass.
   - CXR: the first line investigation for suspected lung cancer.
   - MRI head: to diagnose pituitary lesions or compression.

Gynaecomastia

Gynaecomastia is the abnormal growth of breast tissue in men. It is common, and often physiological, relating to hormonal fluctuation through life (Fig. 5.8).

HINTS AND TIPS

Examine patients with gynaecomastia carefully, to exclude pseudogynaecomastia, which relates to local fat deposition only.

CLINICAL NOTES

- In chronic liver disease, reduced oestrogen metabolism may cause gynaecomastia.
- Adrenal neoplasms may secrete androgen precursors converted to circulating oestrogen.
- Adipose tissue contains aromatase, a key enzyme in oestrogen synthesis.

Investigations

Both breast and testicular exams are essential to identify masses. Further investigations can be performed if underlying pathology is suspected:

- Hormone assays: to identify hormonal derangement.
- Testicular US: if a mass is identified, US should be performed.
- Mammogram: to aid the diagnosis of any identified masses.
- Adrenal CT: to diagnose underlying adrenal lesions, if suspected.

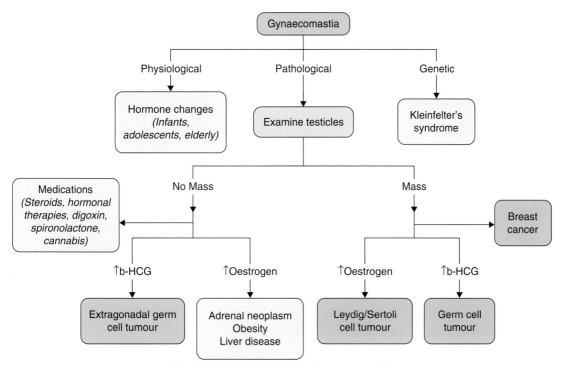

Fig. 5.8 Differential diagnosis of gynaecomastia.

THE BREAST EXAM

Introduce yourself, wash your hands and gain consent to proceed.

Inspection

Ask the patient to sit on the side of the bed with their hands on their lap, then with their hands pushing into their hips and then arms above their head while leaning forward, to accentuate underlying pathology:

- Masses: a mass may be visible on accentuation.
- Asymmetry: while often normal, can underlying pathology.
- Skin changes: erythema, puckering and 'peau d'orange' suggest underlying infection or malignancy.
- Nipple abnormalities: recent inversion suggests malignancy. Discharge is most commonly benign, but can be associated with infection or malignancy.
- Scars: suggestive of previous breast surgery.

Palpation

Palpate the normal breast first, with the patient's ipsilateral hand behind their head. Palpate the breast and axillary tail systematically using the flats of your fingers, and assess for any masses:

- Location: ask the patient to identify the lump first, to make it easier for you to find.
- Size: Small lesions are typically benign. Larger lesions suggest malignancy.
- Shape: irregular masses suggest malignancy. Smooth lumps are typically benign.
- Consistency: masses may be firm, soft or cystic.
- Fluctuance: tethering of abreast mass suggests malignancy.
- Mobility: a very mobile lump suggests fibroadenoma.
- Tenderness: tenderness suggests infective pathology or cyclical breast changes.

Elevate the breast with your hand to inspect for pathology underneath the breast (Fig. 5.9).

Palpate the nipple and areola to assess for any discharge:

- Colour: bloodstained discharge suggests malignancy. Serous discharge may be benign.
- Consistency: thick, offensive discharge suggests infection. Milky discharge may be normal or indicate galactorrhoea.
- Volume: minimal discharge may be normal. Significant discharge suggests pathology.

Palpate the regional lymph nodes on each side, including the axillary, supraclavicular and internal mammary chain:

- Tenderness: suggests reactive lymphadenopathy in infection.
- Consistency: hard, rubbery nodes suggest malignancy.
- Irregularly: irregular nodes suggest malignancy. Smooth nodes are likely benign.
- Tethering: malignant nodes are often tethered to underlying structures.

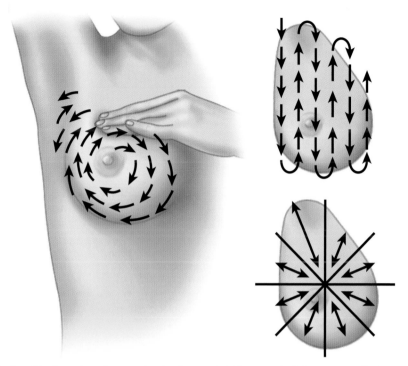

Fig. 5.9 Breast examination. The breast can be examined using a spiral, linear or clock-face approach. Any approach is acceptable if it is systematic and covers all breast tissue. (From Silvestri LA, Silvestri A. *Saunders Comprehensive Review for the NCLEX-RN® Examination*, 9th Edition. Elsevier; 2023.)

Completing the examination

Thank the patient, offer them privacy to get dressed and summarize your findings.

Further tests include:

- Breast imaging: mammography if >35, breast US if <35.
- Biopsy: FNA or CNB can provide a histological diagnosis.

> **RED FLAG**
> Further investigations are required if aspirate is blood stained or a residual lump remains.

BREAST DISORDERS

Benign breast disorders

There are many benign conditions that affect the breast. Most women can be reassured and discharged following the exclusion of significant disease (Table 1, Fig. 5.10).

> **CLINICAL NOTES**
> - A phyllodes tumour is a rare benign breast mass common in older women.
> - It presents with a 4-7 cm smooth nontender breast lump.
> - There is malignant potential.

Mastitis and breast abscess

Mastitis is inflammation of the breast tissue. Puerperal mastitis relates to lactation, affecting up to 10% of breastfeeding mothers. Risk factors include insufficient milk drainage, breast engorgement and nipple fissures. Staphylococcus aureus is the most common cause. Nonlactational mastitis is rare, and may relate to trauma, cigarette smoking (periductal mastitis) and immunosuppression.

Table 5.1 Benign breast conditions

Condition	Aetiology	Clinical features	Management
Cyclical mastalgia	Cyclical hormone fluctuations	Bilateral breast aching, heaviness Premenstrual syndrome – low mood, fatigue, headaches	Supportive bra, NSAIDs/heat packs Avoid caffeine
Fibrocystic change	Most common Cyclical fibrosis of breast tissues Age 20–50	Premenstrual mastalgia Multiple bilateral nodules	Triple assessment Manage as cyclical mastalgia
Breast cyst	Age-related tissue involution Ages 35–50	Sudden appearance of smooth tender lump(s) Mobile, fluctuant	Breast US Aspiration if symptomatic Complicated cysts – biopsy +/– excision
Fibroadenoma	Benign lobular tumour arising during breast development Ages 20–30	Nontender, rubbery, mobile mass (1–2 cm)	Triple assessment Asymptomatic – surveillance Symptomatic/large – excision or ablation
Intraductal papilloma	Benign tumour arising in ducts Ages 30–50	Solitary – palpable areolar lump, bloody/serous discharge Multiple – asymptomatic	Triple assessment Biopsy: No atypia – surveillance Cellular atypia – excision
Duct ectasia	Duct dilation and inflammation Ages 40–50	Unilateral white, green, grey nipple discharge Nipple tenderness, inversion Breast lump	Triple assessment May spontaneously resolve Antibiotics if infected Excision if refractory
Fat necrosis	Traumatic fibrosis/necrosis of fat tissue	Painless, hard, irregular lump Tethering, skin dimpling/nipple inversion	Triple assessment May spontaneously resolve Symptomatic – excision
Galactocele	Blocked lactiferous duct	Typically found after cessation of breastfeeding Firm, painless areolar lump	May spontaneously resolve Symptomatic – aspiration Antibiotics if infected

Symptoms and signs

Symptoms include:

- Unilateral mastalgia, oedema and erythema
- Fever, rigors and malaise
- Pain and difficulty breastfeeding

A breast abscess can complicate mastitis and presents with additional symptoms (Fig. 5.11):

- Purulent unilateral nipple discharge
- Fluctuant mass
- Overlying skin necrosis

> **RED FLAG**
> - Inflammatory breast cancer can present similarly to mastitis.
> - Have a high index of suspicion, and investigate further if there is a poor response to initial treatment.

Investigations

Mastitis is a clinical diagnosis. Investigations are performed in refractory or atypical symptoms:

- Breast milk culture: to guide antibiotic therapy in treatment failure or severe infection.
- Breast US: to diagnose a breast abscess (Fig. 5.12).
- Mammogram: in suspected inflammatory cancer, with confirmatory biopsy if required.

Management

Management includes:

- Supportive measures: warm and cold compresses, NSAIDs, continue breastfeeding.
- Antibiotics: empirical flucloxacillin or IV vancomycin if severe.
- Smoking cessation: in periductal mastitis, to reduce risk of recurrence and complications.
- FNA: to treat breast abscesses. Fluid culture can be sent to guide antibiotic therapy.

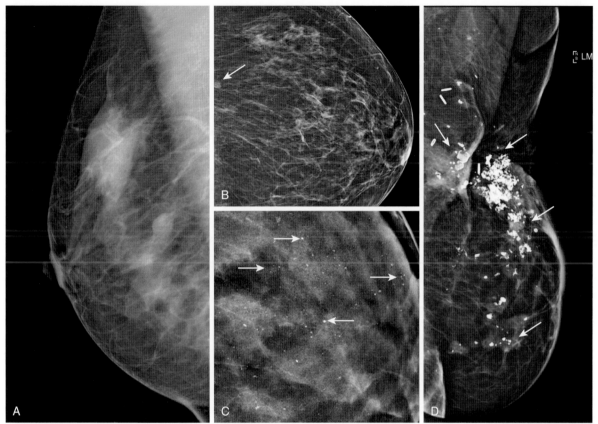

Fig. 5.10 Benign breast conditions. Mammography findings in benign breast conditions. (A) Discrete oval mass suggestive of fibroadenoma. (B) Smooth, round mass indicating breast cyst. (C) Diffuse microcalcifications suggestive of fibrocystic breast change. (D) Diffuse dystrophic calcifications secondary to progressive diffuse fat necrosis. (A. From Deakin PJ, Quick CRG, Biers SM, Arulampalam THA. *Essential Surgery: Problems, Diagnosis and Management*, 6th Edition. Elsevier; 2020. B. From Herring W. *Learning Radiology: Recognizing the Basics*, 5th Edition. Elsevier; 2024. C. From Berg WA, Leung JWT. *Diagnostic Imaging: Breast*, 3rd Edition. Elsevier; 2019. D. From Joe BN, Lee AY. *Breast Imaging: The Core Requisites*, 4th Edition. Elsevier; 2023.)

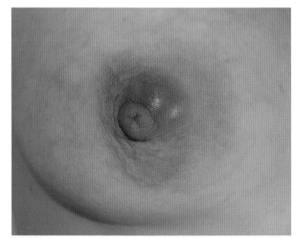

Fig. 5.11 Periductal mastitis with associated periareolar abscess. (From Garden OJ, Parks RW, Wigmore S. *Principles and Practice of Surgery*, 8th Edition. Elsevier; 2023.)

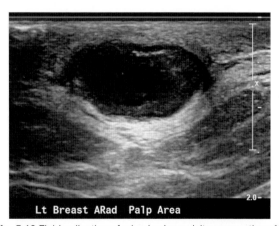

Fig. 5.12 Fluid collection of mixed echogenicity, suggestive of breast abscess. US-guided aspiration can be performed. (From Philpotts LE, Hooley RJ. *Breast Tomosynthesis*. Elsevier; 2017.)

- Incision and drainage: for large necrotic abscesses or those refractory to aspiration.
- Duct excision: for recurrent cases of periductal mastitis.

The prognosis is good, and most cases resolve with antibiotics. Lactational counselling should be offered to breastfeeding mothers to reduce risk of recurrence.

Breast cancer

Breast cancer is the commonest malignancy in the UK. One in eight women are affected in their lifetime. Only 1% of cases occur in men. Risk factors include increased oestrogen exposure, dense breast tissue, obesity, smoking and genetic factors, including the *BRCA1/BRCA2* genes, which account for 5% of cases.

CLINICAL NOTES

In the UK, all women aged 50-70 are invited for mammography screening every 3 years or annually if high risk, to detect asymptomatic cancers early.

Classification

Premalignant disease:

- Ductal carcinoma in situ (DCIS): asymptomatic, often detected on screening. May spread locally or become invasive. Requires full excision and adjuvant treatment.
- Lobular carcinoma in situ (LCIS): asymptomatic, undetectable on mammograms. Typically diagnosed incidentally. Often managed with close surveillance.

  Malignant disease

- Invasive ductal carcinoma (IDC): most common, associated with aggressive metastases.
- Invasive lobular carcinoma (ILC): less common, less aggressive, may be bilateral.
- Inflammatory breast cancer (IBC): rare, advanced, rapidly progressive carcinoma.

Symptoms and signs

Symptoms include (Fig. 5.13):

- Breast lump: nontender, firm, irregular lump, commonly in the upper outer quadrant.
- Skin changes: skin thickening and dimpling (peau d'orange), retractions.
- Nipple changes: inversion, bloodstained discharge.
- Axillary lymphadenopathy: hard, tethered nodes suggest lymphatic spread.

HINTS AND TIPS

- Inflammatory breast cancer presents with rapid onset breast erythema, oedema and skin dimpling (peau d'orange), with bloody nipple discharge.
- There may be signs of metastatic disease, including axillary lymphadenopathy.

Investigations

Suspected breast cancer should undergo triple assessment:

- Clinical examination: history and examination from a breast specialist.
- Imaging: US if <35, and mammogram if >35 (Fig. 5.14).
- Breast biopsy: FNA if low risk, or CNB in suspicious masses. Excisional biopsy can be performed if CNB is inconclusive.

HINTS AND TIPS

In younger women, ultrasound is preferred, as denser breast tissue makes mammogram less sensitive for detecting pathology.

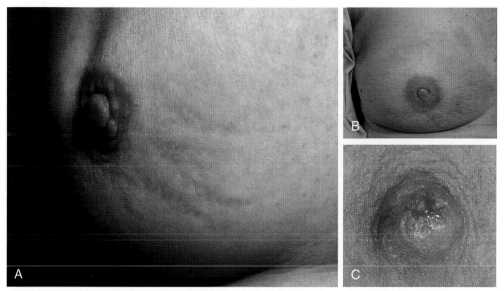

Fig. 5.13 (A) Nipple retraction and skin dimpling in invasive breast cancer. (B) Patchy erythema, flattened nipple and peau d'orange associated with inflammatory breast cancer. (C) Paget's disease of the nipple, with crusty erythema indicating underlying malignant change. (From A. Ball JW, Dains JE, Flynn JA, Solomon BS, Stewart RW. *Seidel's guide to physical examination*, 10th Edition. St. Louis: Elsevier; 2023. B. Dover AR, Innes JA, Fairhurst K. et al. *Macleod's Clinical Examination*, 15th Edition. Elsevier; 2024. C. Habif TP, Dinulos JG, Chapman MS, Zug KA. *Skin Disease: Diagnosis and Treatment*, 4th Edition. Elsevier; 2018.)

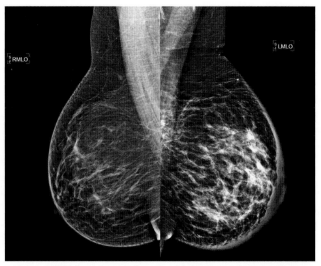

Fig. 5.14 Mammogram in breast cancer. Diffuse skin and trabecular thickening of the left breast, suggestive of cancer. (From Joe BN, Lee AY. *Breast Imaging: The Core Requisites*, 4th Edition. Elsevier; 2023.)

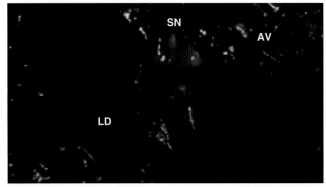

Fig. 5.15 Sentinel lymph node biopsy. Fluorescent dye is injected near the tumour. The first lymph node stained with dye is identified and removed for histopathological examination. If malignant cells are found, radical lymph node dissection is performed. (From Applications of indocyanine green in surgery: a single center case series. *AMSU* 2022.)

Following a diagnosis of breast cancer, further investigations should be performed:

- Receptor status: immunohistochemical staining to assess for oestrogen (ER), progesterone (PR) or human-epidermal growth factor receptor 2 (HER2) receptor status.
- Tumour markers: CA 15-3, CA 27-29 and CEA may be elevated, and can be monitored to assess treatment response.
- Staging: further imaging to assess lymph node status, and metastatic disease.

Management

Management of all malignancies should involve an MDT approach, considering the patient's wishes, cancer stage and goals of treatment.

Surgical management:

- Breast-conserving surgery: removal of cancerous tissue only.
- Mastectomy: with sentinel lymph node biopsy (SLNB) to determine need for radical lymph node dissection (Fig. 5.15).
- Double mastectomy: removal of both breasts, as a prophylactic measure in those at high risk of malignancy, typically used for those with BRCA gene mutations.

CLINICAL NOTES

- SLNB detects malignant lymph node infiltration.
- The sentinel node refers to the first axillary node that drains cancerous breast tissue.
- If the sentinel node is negative, there is a low likelihood of lymphatic spread.

Adjuvant treatment includes:

- Targeted therapy: Trastuzumab (Herceptin), a monoclonal antibody against HER2 receptors. Indicated for all HER2+ve tumours.
- Hormone therapy: indicated for all ER/PR positive tumours, typically tamoxifen if premenopausal or aromatase inhibitors if postmenopausal.
- Radiotherapy: for those at high risk of local recurrence.
- Chemotherapy: neoadjuvant or adjuvant therapy, for triple-negative receptor status or HER-2 positive disease.

Complications

Complications include

- Metastasis: regional lymphatic or distant haematogenous spread.
- Pleural effusions: malignant pleural effusion is common.
- Lymphoedema: axillary surgery or radiation can lead to arm lymphedema.

RED FLAG

Metastatic disease commonly affects the BBLL:
- Bone – bone pain, pathological fractures
- Brain – seizures, headache, focal neurological deficits
- Liver – abdominal pain, distention, jaundice
- Lung – SOB, cough, haemoptysis, chest pain

Prognosis relates to the speed of diagnosis and treatment. Larger, hormone-negative tumours or those associated with metastatic spread have a poorer prognosis.

Chapter Summary

- The triple assessment of a breast lump involves clinical assessment, imaging and breast biopsy.
- Examination features associated with breast cancer include a breast lump, skin puckering, peau d'orange, nipple inversion, retraction and bloody discharge.
- Increased oestrogen exposure including early menarche, late menopause, nulliparity and use of HRT increases the risk of breast cancer.
- BRCA1/2 genes are associated with a significantly increased risk of breast and ovarian cancer.
- Puerperal mastitis is common in breastfeeding mothers and should be treated with warm and cold compresses, NSAIDs and flucloxacillin, if required.
- Mammogram screening every 3 years for breast cancer should be offered to all women between 50 and 70 years of age.
- Breast cancer should be managed with surgical excision, targeted therapies or hormonal therapies in receptor +ve tumours, and adjuvant chemoradiotherapy if high risk.
- Breast cancer commonly metastasises to the BBLL: bone, brain, liver and lung.

UKMLA Conditions

Brain metastases
Breast abscess/mastitis
Breast cancer
Breast cysts
Contraception request/advice
Difficulty with breastfeeding
Disease prevention/screening
Family history of possible genetic disorder
Fever
Fibroadenoma
Fits/seizures
Incidental findings
Menopausal problems
Menopause
Menstrual problems
Metastatic disease
Ovarian cancer
Pathological fracture
Pubertal development

UKMLA Presentations

Amenorrhoea
Bone pain
Breast lump
Breast tenderness/pain
Congenital abnormalities
Contraception request/advice
Fever
Fits/seizures
Menopausal problems
Menopause
Menstrual problems
Nipple discharge
Ovarian cancer
Pleural effusion
Postsurgical care and complications
Pubertal development

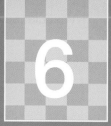

Vascular surgery 6

CLINICAL ANATOMY

The vascular system is the circulatory system of vessels that carry blood and lymph through the body.

The aorta carries oxygenated blood from the heart and branches into arteries, arterioles and capillary beds, to provide oxygenated blood to tissues. The aorta begins at the aortic valve. The aortic arch gives off the brachiocephalic trunk, which divides into the right subclavian and right carotid artery, and the left common carotid and the left subclavian artery. The aorta continues as the thoracic and then abdominal aorta to supply the systemic circulation (Figs 6.1 and 6.2).

Vertebral levels correspond to the major branches of the abdominal aorta supplying the gut (Fig. 6.3).

Veins carry deoxygenated blood from tissues to the heart. Upper limb veins drain into the superior vena cava (SVC), and the inferior vena cava (IVC) drains the lower limb systemic and portal circulation (Fig. 6.4).

The lymphatic system is a vessel network that drains lymph from tissues and circulates it through lymphatic organs, before returning it to the venous circulation via the thoracic duct (Fig. 6.5).

VASCULAR SURGERY PRESENTATIONS

History taking

Opening the consultation
Introduce yourself and confirm the patient's details.

Presenting complaint (PC)
Use open questioning to identify the presenting complaint.

History of presenting complaint (HPC)
Explore the presenting complaint in detail using SOCRATES. Common symptoms of vascular pathology include:

- Calf pain/swelling: claudication is cramping muscle pain in the calves or buttocks, exacerbated by exertion, improved by rest. Acute calf pain may relate to deep vein thrombosis (DVT) or acute limb ischaemia (ALI).
- Ulceration: relating to arterial, venous or neuropathic pathology. May be painful or painless.
- Digital discolouration: red, purple or black discolouration of the toes suggests ischaemia.
- Abdominal pain: aching, poorly localized abdominal pain may represent abdominal aortic aneurysm (AAA).

CLINICAL NOTES

- In intermittent claudication, quantify the distance at which pain occurs, and the time taken to improve with rest.
- Rest pain implies severe arterial disease.

HINTS AND TIPS

- In peripheral arterial disease (PAD), pain is worse walking uphill, with increased muscle demand for oxygenated blood, and the effects of gravity on arterial blood supply.
- Venous claudication improves with leg elevation, as gravity helps return static blood to the heart.
- In neurogenic claudication, leaning forward widens the spinal canal and reduces nerve impingement.

RED FLAG

ALI presents with the **6 P's**:
- **P**ain - sudden and severe
- **P**ulselessness
- **P**aresthesia
- **P**aralysis
- **P**oikilothermia (cold)
- **P**allor

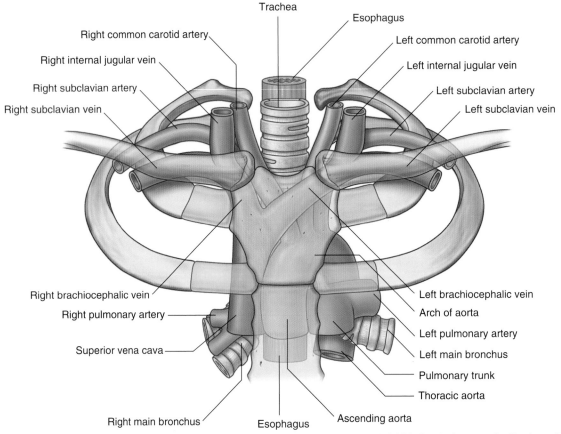

Fig. 6.1 Aortic arch. The great vessels and aortic arch. (From Drake RL, Vogl W, Mitchell AWM. *Gray's Anatomy for Students,* 5th Edition. Elsevier; 2024.)

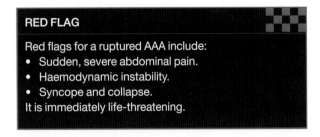

RED FLAG

Red flags for a ruptured AAA include:
- Sudden, severe abdominal pain.
- Haemodynamic instability.
- Syncope and collapse.

It is immediately life-threatening.

CLINICAL NOTES

Systems relevant to vascular surgery include:
- Cardiovascular: PAD is closely associated with coronary artery disease (CAD)
- Respiratory: smoking is a risk factor for respiratory and vascular disease
- Gastrointestinal: to exclude differentials for AAA
- MSK/rheumatology: to screen for traumatic/inflammatory pathology, associated with vasculitidies
- Neurology: to evaluate for neurogenic causes of claudication and sensory loss, or symptoms of TIA/stroke

Systemic screen

Screen for key symptoms from related body areas, and constitutional features including **FLAWS**:

- **F** - Fever
- **L** - Lethargy
- **A** - Anorexia
- **W** - Weight loss
- **N** - Night sweats

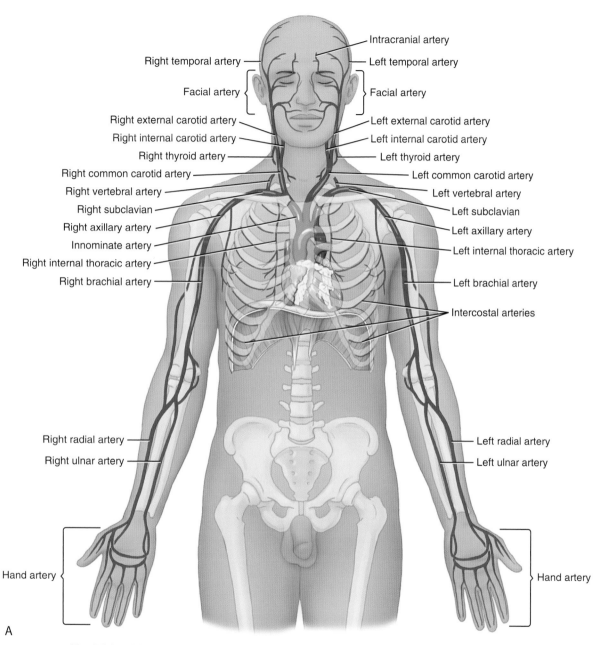

Fig. 6.2 Arterial circulation. (A) Branches of the thoracic aorta supplying the upper limbs and head.

Lower arteries

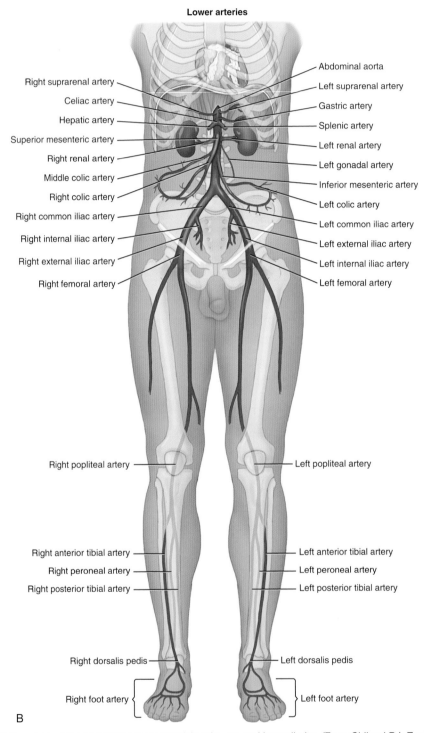

Right suprarenal artery
Celiac artery
Hepatic artery
Superior mesenteric artery
Right renal artery
Middle colic artery
Right colic artery
Right common iliac artery
Right internal iliac artery
Right external iliac artery
Right femoral artery

Abdominal aorta
Left suprarenal artery
Gastric artery
Splenic artery
Left renal artery
Left gonadal artery
Inferior mesenteric artery
Left colic artery
Left common iliac artery
Left external iliac artery
Left internal iliac artery
Left femoral artery

Right popliteal artery

Left popliteal artery

Right anterior tibial artery
Right peroneal artery
Right posterior tibial artery

Left anterior tibial artery
Left peroneal artery
Left posterior tibial artery

Right dorsalis pedis

Left dorsalis pedis

Right foot artery

Left foot artery

B

Fig. 6.2, cont'd (B) Branches of the abdominal aorta supplying the gut and lower limbs. (From Shiland BJ, Zenith. *Medical Assistant: Cardiopulmonary Systems, Vital Signs, Electrocardiography and CPR—Module D,* 2nd Edition. Elsevier; 2015.)

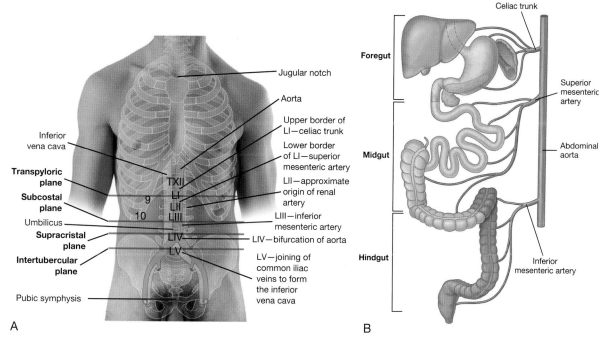

Fig. 6.3 Abdominal aorta. (A) Vertebral level landmarks of the branches of the abdominal aorta. (B) Divisions of the abdominal aorta supplying the foregut, midgut and hindgut. (From Vogl AW, Mitchell AWM, Drake RL. *Gray's Basic Anatomy*. Churchill Livingstone, Elsevier Inc. 2013.)

Past medical history

Other medical conditions, past surgeries and investigations may be related to the diagnosis.

> **HINTS AND TIPS**
>
> - Risk factors for vascular disease include diabetes, hypertension and hyperlipidaemia.
> - A sudden worsening of symptoms in patients with known PAD suggest acute thrombotic ischaemia of a critically stenosed vessel (acute on chronic ischaemia).
> - Be sure to screen for a history of venous thromboembolism (VTE).

Drug history

Document a complete drug history, assessing compliance, recent changes and over-the-counter medications. Document any allergies and the nature of reaction.

> **HINTS AND TIPS**
>
> Statins, antihypertensives or antiplatelets suggest underlying cardiovascular disease, which increase the risk of future vascular events.

Family history

Screen for family members with associated conditions and record the age of diagnosis.

Social history

Screen for risk factors in the social history

- Baseline functional status: to assess independence and symptom impact.
- Smoking: the major risk factor for vascular disease. Record the number of pack years.
- Alcohol use: excess alcohol use is associated with peripheral neuropathy and ulcers.

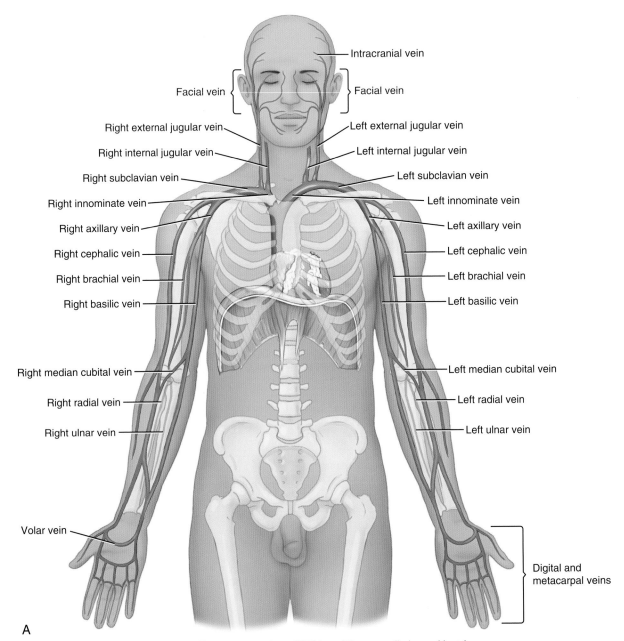

Fig. 6.4 The venous system. (A) Veins of the upper limbs and head.

A

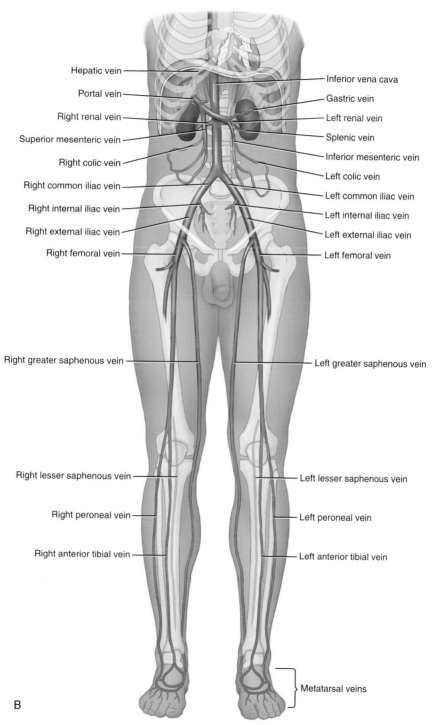

Hepatic vein

Portal vein

Right renal vein

Superior mesenteric vein

Right colic vein

Right common iliac vein

Right internal iliac vein

Right external iliac vein

Right femoral vein

Inferior vena cava

Gastric vein

Left renal vein

Splenic vein

Inferior mesenteric vein

Left colic vein

Left common iliac vein

Left internal iliac vein

Left external iliac vein

Left femoral vein

Right greater saphenous vein

Left greater saphenous vein

Right lesser saphenous vein

Left lesser saphenous vein

Right peroneal vein

Left peroneal vein

Right anterior tibial vein

Left anterior tibial vein

Metatarsal veins

B

Fig. 6.4, cont'd (B) Veins of the abdomen and lower limbs. (From Shiland BJ, Zenith. *Medical Assistant: Cardiopulmonary Systems, Vital Signs, Electrocardiography and CPR—Module D,* 2nd Edition. Elsevier; 2015.)

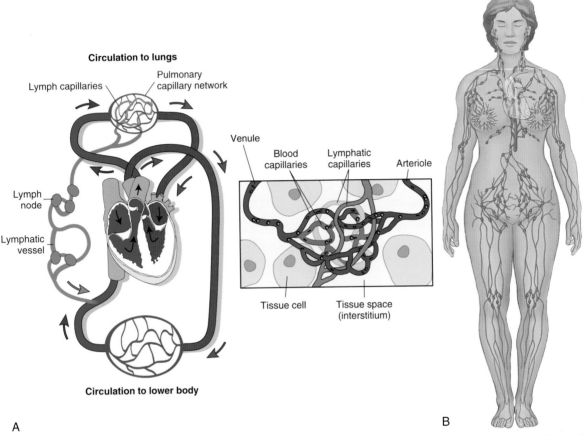

Fig. 6.5 The lymphatic system. (A) The lymphatic system filters lymphatic fluid and returns it to the venous circulation. (B) Lymph nodes and lymphatic vessels are found throughout the body. (From Shiland BJ, Zenith. *Medical Assistant: Cardiopulmonary Systems, Vital Signs, Electrocardiography and CPR—Module D,* 2nd Edition. Elsevier; 2015.)

- Recreational drug use: stimulants can increase cardiovascular risk.
- Diet and weight: obesity and high salt/fat diets increase the risk of vascular disease.

COMMUNICATION

- Smokers must be advised to immediately stop smoking, due to the risk of progressive vascular complications with continued tobacco use.
- Referral to smoking cessation services is advised.

Ideas, concerns and expectations

Explore the patient's ideas, concerns and expectations, to identify what they want from the consultation, and address any concerns.

Closing the consultation

Summarize the history, answer any questions and thank the patient for their time.

DIFFERENTIAL DIAGNOSIS

Calf pain

The differential diagnosis of calf pain includes acute occlusive, infective or traumatic causes, and chronic neurovascular insufficiency (Fig. 6.6).

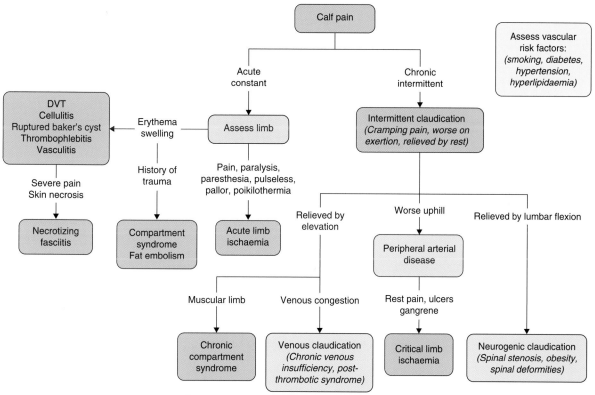

Fig. 6.6 Differential diagnosis of vascular leg pain.

- Referred pain from the joints above and below can mimic vascular calf pain.
- Be sure to examine the joints to exclude joint injury, infection or inflammation.
- In vascular calf pain, the musculoskeletal examination will be normal.

Investigations for calf pain

CLINICAL NOTES

- Determining the neurovascular status of the limb is essential.
- Absence pulses or sensation suggest an acutely limb-threatening diagnosis.

1. Bedside
   - CBG: ↑ >11 mmol/dL suggests diabetes, a significant vascular risk factor.
   - ECG: cardiac assessment is required in those with vascular risk factors.
   - ABPI: compares ankle pressure readings to the arm, as an index of lower limb vessel competency.
   - Compartment pressures: in suspected acute or chronic compartment syndrome.
2. Bloods
   - FBC: ↑ Hb suggests polycythaemia, a significant VTE risk factor.
   - U&Es: long-standing ischaemia may lead to rhabdomyolysis and renal failure.
   - CRP/ESR: ↑ suggests systemic inflammation, associated with vasculitis.
   - Clotting screen: coagulopathies can lead to vascular thrombosis.
   - Lipid profile: ↑ triglycerides/cholesterol increase the risk of atherosclerosis.
   - Thrombophilia screen: in recurrent thrombosis, thrombophilia should be excluded.

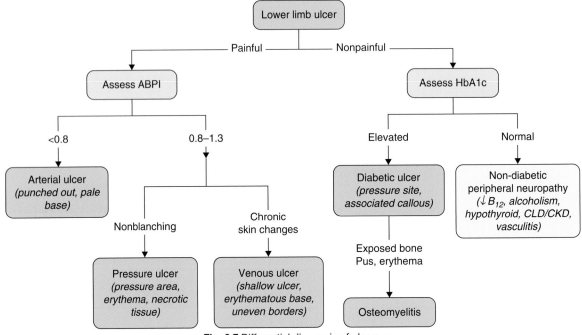

Fig. 6.7 Differential diagnosis of ulcers.

3. Imaging
   - Doppler ultrasound (US): for bedside assessment of vascular disease.
   - MRI/CT angiography: to assess location and extent of stenosis, and plan intervention.
   - CXR: there may be associated features of cardiovascular disease on CXR.
   - Abdominal US: to diagnose asymptomatic aortic aneurysms.

HINTS AND TIPS

ABPI should be 1, indicating comparable pressure readings in the ankle and arm:
- 0.8–1.3 – no evidence of significant arterial disease
- 0.5–0.8 – suggestive of arterial disease
- 0.5 – severe arterial disease
- >1.3 – suggests arterial calcification, common in diabetes

Ulcers

The differential diagnosis of limb ulcers includes vascular, neuropathic or traumatic causes (Fig. 6.7, Table 6.1).

Investigations for a lower limb ulcer

1. Beside
   - Wound swabs: if there is evidence of infection, send swabs for MC&S.
   - ABPI: to assess lower limb vessel competency. <0.5 suggests critical limb ischaemia (CLI), associated with ulcers.
   - CBG: >11 mmol/dL with osmotic symptoms is diagnostic of diabetes.
   - ECG: to assess for associated cardiovascular disease.
2. Bloods
   - FBC: ↑WBC suggests infection.
   - U&Es: there may be end-organ damage relating to diabetic nephropathy.
   - HbA1c: >48 mmol/mol confirms a diagnosis of diabetes.
   - CRP/ESR: ↑ suggests osteomyelitis, associated with neuropathic ulcers.
   - Blood cultures: if there is evidence of severe systemic infection.
   - Lipid profile: hyperlipidaemia increases vascular risk.
   - Thrombophilia screen: in patients with recurrent thrombosis.

Table 6.1 Differential diagnosis of leg ulcers

	Arterial	Venous	Neuropathic (diabetic)
Location	Lower limb pressure points	Medial malleoli	Plantar pressure points
Aetiology	Vessel occlusion Tissue ischaemia	Chronic venous hypertension Tissue ischaemia	Microvascular/neuropathic disease Impaired wound healing
Features	Punched out No exudate Well-defined borders	Shallow, superficial exudative Irregular borders	Deep Hyperkeratotic borders Surrounding callous
Pain	Severe	Mild/moderate	Absent
Associated symptoms	Varicose veins Oedema Venous eczema	Cold, pale limbs Hair loss Absent pulses	Sensory loss Charcot deformities

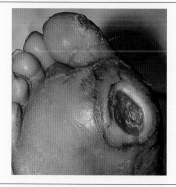 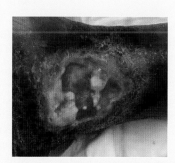 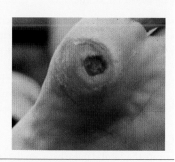

Neuropathic ulcers commonly relate to diabetes.
Source: Arterial –Viik J, Min M, Kekonen A, Annus P. Bioimpedance and Spectroscopy. *Elsevier; 2021; venous –Gohel M, Shortell.* Venous Ulcers, *2nd Edition. Elsevier; 2023. Neuropathic – Gordon CJ, Craft JA, Brashers VL, McCance KL, Turton J, Huether SE.* Understanding Pathophysiology, *4th Edition. Elsevier; 2023.*

3. Imaging
   - Doppler US: elevated peak systolic velocity suggests increased vascular resistance and vascular stenosis, and for chronic venous insufficiency (CVI).
   - X-ray: for evaluation of bony injuries in peripheral neuropathy.
   - Probe-to-bone test: to evaluate for osteomyelitis in chronic diabetic ulcers.
   - Tissue biopsy: to guide antibiotic therapy in infection and exclude malignancy.
   - MRI/CT angiography: to assess vascular stenosis and occlusions.

HINTS AND TIPS

The acronym **WIPER** can be used to prepare for the exam:

- **W** - **W**ash your hands
- **I** - **I**ntroduce yourself
- **P** - **P**atient details
- **E** - **E**xplain the procedure and **E**xpose appropriately
- **R** - **R**eposition patient

VASCULAR EXAMINATIONS

Peripheral arterial exam

Wash your hands, introduce yourself and confirm the patient's details.

General inspection

Inspect the patient from the end of the bed for evidence of vascular pathology:

- Peripheral cyanosis: discolouration of the tissues suggesting poor limb perfusion.

- Scars: suggestive of previous operations, including bypass surgery.
- Missing limbs/digits: severe PAD can result in gangrene and limb loss.
- Equipment: medications, mobility aids and monitoring devices may suggest underlying pathology.

Upper limbs

Inspect the upper limbs:

- Pallor: pale limbs are associated with PAD.
- Tar staining: evidence of smoking, a significant vascular risk factor.
- Xanthomata: lipid deposits in the hand, suggestive of hypercholesterolaemia.

Palpate the upper limbs:

- Temperature: PAD is associated with cool, pale extremities.
- CRT: >2s suggests inadequate peripheral perfusion.
- Pulses: palpate radial and brachial pulses, assessing rate and rhythm, radio–radio delay.
- Blood pressure (BP): measure the BP in both arms to assess for hypertension. A wide pulse pressure or difference between arms suggests aortic dissection (Fig. 6.8).

Carotids

Locate the carotid pulse between the larynx and anterior border of the sternocleidomastoid

- Auscultation: auscultate for bruit, suggestive of severe carotid stenosis.
- Palpation: if there are no bruits, palpate the pulse and assess volume and character.

Abdomen

Examine the abdomen:

- Inspection: inspect for obvious midline pulsation, suggestive of AAA.
- Palpation: the aorta should be pulsatile but not expansile.
- Auscultation: auscultate the aorta and renal arteries to detect bruits.

Lower limbs

Inspect the lower limbs:

- Pallor: pale extremities suggest poor peripheral perfusion
- Discolouration: pallor/cyanosis with elevation and reddening (dependant rubor) when lowered suggests PAD.
- Hair loss: poor arterial supply results in hair loss.

- Ulcers: arterial ulcers are small, well-defined, deep and painful, and venous ulcers large and shallow, with irregular borders.
- Gangrene: tissue necrosis associated with CLI, with black discolouration and skin breakdown.
- Muscle weakness: CLI can result in muscle loss, paralysis and paraesthesia.

Palpate the lower limbs:

- Temperature: cold limbs suggest PAD.
- CRT: >2s suggests inadequate limb perfusion.
- Pulses: palpate the femoral, popliteal, posterior tibial and dorsalis pedis pulses, and assess for radio-femoral delay.
- Sensation: grossly assess light touch. Glove and stocking sensory loss suggests peripheral neuropathy (Figs 6.9 and 6.10).

Buergers test

Buergers test assesses lower limb arterial supply:

- Lay the patient supine and raise both legs to 45 degree for 1 minute.
- Observe limb colour. Pallor suggests inadequate perfusion. Note the angle this occurs.
- Assess for venous guttering, collapsing of the veins into the subcutaneous tissue suggestive of limb ischaemia.
- Sit the patient up and hang their legs over the bed. Reperfusion of the limb with gravity will result in blue, then red discoloration of the limb (reactive hyperaemia) (Fig. 6.11).

CLINICAL NOTES

In healthy individuals, the limb should remain pink. An angle <20° suggests CLI.

Completing the examination

Wash your hands, thank the patient and summarize your findings.

Further tests include:

- Cardiovascular exam: a complete cardiovascular examination should be performed.
- ABPI: to assess the extent of lower limb arterial insufficiency.
- Doppler US: to assess the extent of vascular resistance and vessel stenosis.
- Peripheral venous exam: arterial and venous pathology is often comorbid.
- Diabetic foot exam: in patients with diabetes, it is essential to examine the feet regularly.

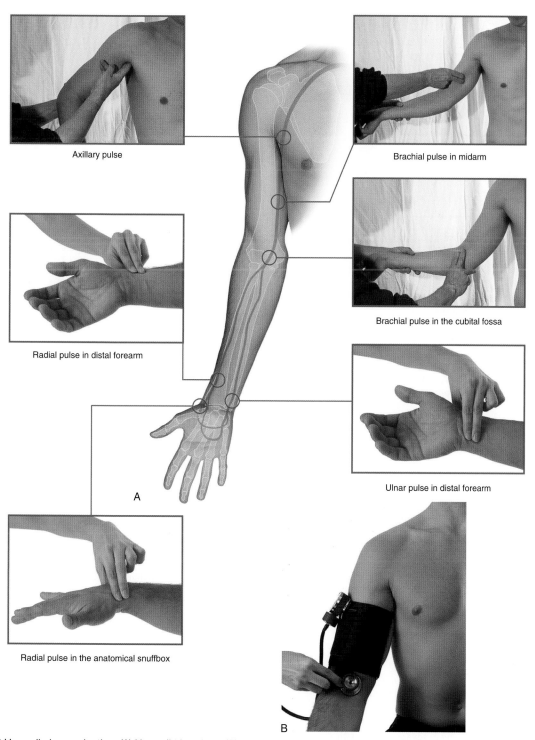

Axillary pulse

Brachial pulse in midarm

Brachial pulse in the cubital fossa

Radial pulse in distal forearm

Ulnar pulse in distal forearm

A

Radial pulse in the anatomical snuffbox

B

Fig. 6.8 Upper limb examination. (A) Upper limb pulses. (B) Assessment of blood pressure. (From Drake RL, Mitchell AWM, Vogl AW. *Gray's Anatomy for Students,* 5th Edition. Elsevier; 2024.)

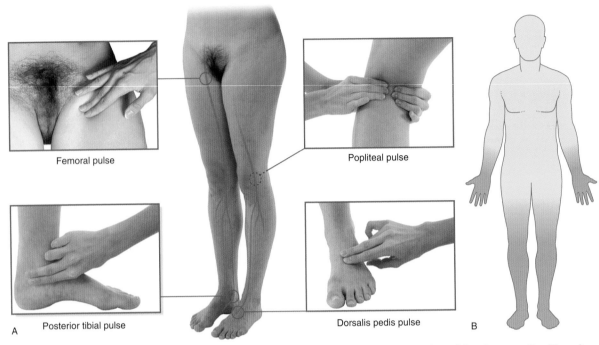

Fig. 6.9 Lower limb examination. (A) Lower limb pulses. (B) Glove and stocking sensory loss in peripheral neuropathy. (From A. Drake RL, Mitchell AWM, Vogl AW. *Gray's Anatomy for Students,* 5th Edition. Elsevier; 2024. B. Gruener G, Mtui E, Dockery P. *Fitzgerald's Clinical Neuroanatomy and Neuroscience,* 8th Edition. Elsevier; 2021.)

Peripheral venous exam

Introduce yourself and confirm the patient's details.

> **HINTS AND TIPS**
>
> - Prepare for the examination using the WIPER structure.
> - Assess for any bedside adjuncts including mobility aids, medications and monitoring devices.

Inspection

Inspect the lower limbs:

- Venous eczema: red, itchy, crusted skin, resulting from fluid stasis and inflammation.
- Lipodermatosclerosis: panniculitis, with skin induration, swelling and thickening in advanced CVI, with a characteristic inverted champagne bottle appearance.
- Haemosiderin deposition: hyperpigmentation of the legs resulting from red blood cell breakdown and iron release, and staining due to poor venous return.
- Ulcers: venous ulcers are shallow, irregular and large, and may be painful.
- Varicose veins: dilated tortuous superficial veins, typically affecting the medial leg (great saphenous vein insufficiency) or posterior leg (small saphenous vein insufficiency).
- Saphena varix: dilation of the saphenous vein, with a small, blue, soft groin lump that disappears on lying flat.
- Arterial disease: pale, cool, hairless legs with arterial ulcers or gangrene suggests PAD.
- Scars: may relate to vein harvesting or stripping of varicosities (Fig. 6.12).

> **HINTS AND TIPS**
>
> Scars may not be visible due to increasing use of minimally invasive treatments for venous disease.

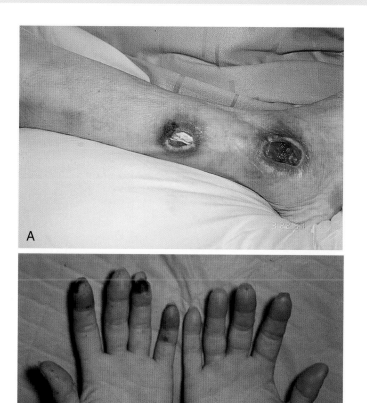

Fig. 6.10 Arterial disease. (A) Arterial ulcers, small, with well-defined borders, and a 'punched-out' appearance. (B) Digital gangrene in severe PAD. (From A. Kumagai CK, deWit SC. *Medical-Surgical Nursing: Concepts & Practice,* 2nd Edition. Elsevier; 2013. B. Sidawy AN, Landry GJ, Repella TL, Perler BA. *Rutherford's Vascular Surgery and Endovascular Therapy,* 10th Edition. Elsevier; 2023.)

CLINICAL NOTES

- Assess varicosities for phlebitis, which presents with vein erythema and pain.
- A tender, hard varicosity suggests underlying thrombus (thrombophlebitis).

Palpation

Palpate the lower limbs:

- Pitting oedema: suggestive of CVI. Move up the leg to establish the level of oedema.

- Pulses: assess the femoral, popliteal, posterior tibial and dorsalis pedis pulses.

Completing the examination

Wash your hands, thank the patient and summarize your findings.

Further tests include:

- Doppler US: to confirm the location of incompetence and suitability for treatment.
- Peripheral arterial exam: arterial and venous pathology is often comorbid.
- ABPI: to assess for PAD or neuropathic calcification.
- Diabetic foot exam: in comorbid diabetes, it is essential to examine the feet thoroughly.

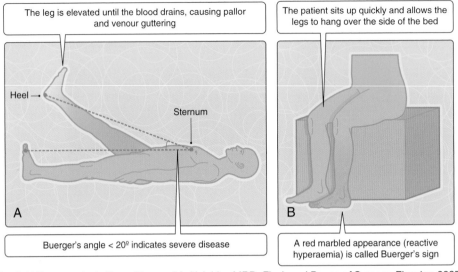

The leg is elevated until the blood drains, causing pallor and venour guttering

The patient sits up quickly and allows the legs to hang over the side of the bed

Heel →

Sternum

A

B

Buerger's angle < 20º indicates severe disease

A red marbled appearance (reactive hyperaemia) is called Buerger's sign

Fig. 6.11 Buergers test. (From Bhangu AA, Keighley MRB. *Flesh and Bones of Surgery*. Elsevier; 2007.)

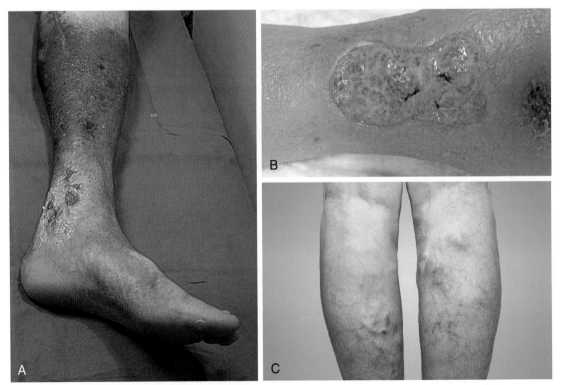

Fig. 6.12 Venous disease. (A) Lipodermatosclerosis, hemosiderin staining and venous eczema are evident, with large venous ulcer over the medial malleolus. (B) Large venous ulcer, with irregular border and shallow, sloughy appearance. (C) Bilateral varicose veins in the small saphenous vein territory. (From A. Kinross J, Rasheed S, Chaudry MA. *Clinical Surgery*, 4th Edition. Elsevier; 2023. B. Gosnell K, Cooper K. *Foundations and Adult Health Nursing*, 9th Edition. Elsevier; 2023. C. Brashers VL, Zettel S, Power-Kean K, El-Hussein MT. *Huether and McCance's Understanding Pathophysiology*, Second Canadian Edition. Elsevier; 2023.)

- Abdominal exam: to exclude abdominal pathology obstructing venous return.

Diabetic foot exam

Wash your hands, introduce yourself and confirm the patient details.

Inspection

Inspect the lower limbs and toes:

- Discolouration: pallor and cyanosis suggest poor perfusion. Black skin suggests gangrene, associated with chronic ischaemia, tissue necrosis and skin breakdown.
- Ulcers: diabetic ulcers are common in diabetic polyneuropathy, occurring over pressure areas, relating to sensory loss, chronic trauma and hyperglycaemia. Venous or arterial ulcers may also be present.
- Missing digits: CLI or complicated diabetic ulcers can result in digit/limb loss.
- Calluses: loss of sensation and ill-fitting footwear result in callus formation.
- Deformities: chronic bony injuries may result in deformities including Charcot foot, with associated effusion and loss of function.
- Footwear: note the pattern of wear on the soles, check they are the correct size, and for foreign objects causing foot trauma (Fig. 6.13).

Palpation

Palpate the lower limbs:

- Temperature: cool extremities suggest poor perfusion.
- Pulses: palpate the posterior tibial and dorsalis pedis pulses.
- Sensation: using a monofilament, assess foot sensation with the patient's eyes closed. Sensory loss suggests neuropathy.

Gait

Assess the patient's gait by asking them to walk to the end of the room and back. Findings associated with peripheral neuropathy include:

- Slow speed: reduced walking speed may suggest impaired sensation.
- Broad-based gait: indicative of an unstable gait.
- High stepping gait: suggestive of foot drop, associated with peroneal nerve damage.
- Difficulty turning: impaired sensation and proprioception can cause difficulties turning.

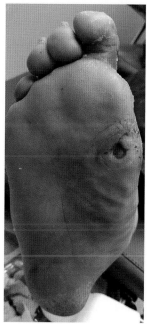

Fig. 6.13 Diabetic foot. Diabetic foot, with ulceration, calluses, a significant Charcot deformity. (From Robertson RP. *DeGroot's Endocrinology: Basic Science and Clinical Practice,* 8th Edition. Elsevier; 2023.)

CLINICAL NOTES

- Assess vibration sensation using a 128 Hz tuning fork.
- Reduced proprioception sensation and reflexes suggest severe disease.

Completing the examination

Wash your hands, thank the patient and summarize your findings.

Further tests include:

- CBG/HbA1c: to assess glycaemic control. Treatment is required if elevated.
- Lower limb neurological exam: for complete assessment of neurological impairment.
- Peripheral vascular exams: both arterial and venous pathology may be comorbid.

VASCULAR DISORDERS

Peripheral arterial disease

Peripheral arterial disease (PAD) describes the atherosclerotic stenosis of the peripheral arteries. It typically affects the lower limbs. Risk factors include smoking, hypertension, hypercholesterolaemia, diabetes, obesity and cardiovascular disease. PAD commonly coexists with coronary artery disease (CAD).

Symptoms and signs

PAD may be asymptomatic or manifest with:

- Intermittent claudication (IC): muscle ischaemia on exertion due to insufficient blood supply.
- Critical limb ischaemia (CLI): severe PAD resulting in ischaemia at rest.
- Acute limb ischaemia (ALI): acute occlusion of a peripheral vessel, due to thrombotic occlusion in severe PAD or acute embolism, due to AF or myocardial infarction (Table 6.2).

> **DIFFERENTIALS**
> - Leriche syndrome describes severe aortoiliac vasculo occlusive disease.
> - Symptoms include bilateral buttock/thigh claudication, erectile dysfunction and absent femoral pulses.

HINTS AND TIPS

Causes of ALI include:
- Thromboembolism
- Traumatic vessel injury
- Compartment syndrome
- Aortic dissection
- Acute arterial vasoconstriction

Investigations

Investigations are only performed if they do not delay urgent revascularization:

- Doppler US: elevated peak systolic velocities suggest vascular stenosis.
- MRI/CT angiography: the gold standard imaging to detail site and extent of occlusion.

Management

ALI is a surgical emergency, requiring urgent vascular consult and revascularization (Fig. 6.14).

RED FLAG

- Compartment syndrome is both a cause and consequence of ALI.
- Acute swelling in the closed limb compartments following trauma or reperfusion injury increases compartmental pressures, resulting in limb ischaemia.
- Management is with urgent fasciotomy.

Table 6.2 Manifestations of peripheral arterial disease

	IC	CLI	ALI
Symptoms	Cramping muscle pain distal to occlusion Worse on exertion, relieved by rest	Rest pain Nonhealing ulcers Tissue loss	Thrombotic – subacute, history of IC Embolic – acute onset, 6 P's: Pain, pulseless, pallor, paralysis, paraesthesia, poikilothermia
Signs	Cool, pale, limbs Hair and muscle loss Reduced pulses Buergers angle <90 degrees	As IC + arterial ulcers, gangrene, necrosis Buergers angle <20 degrees	
Ix	ABPI <0.9	ABPI <0.3	Arterial/venous Doppler – reduced/absent flow
Mx	Structured exercise program Reduce cardiovascular risk	As IC + consideration of revascularization Manage complications	Urgent vascular consult and revascularization

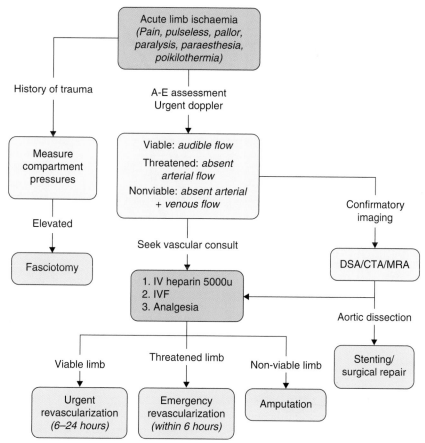

Fig. 6.14 Approach to management of acute limb ischaemia. *CTA*, CT angiography; *DSA*, digital subtraction angiography; *MRA*, MRI angiography.

Management of chronic PAD includes:

- Structured exercise therapy: walking until claudication occurs, then resting until pain subsides, 3 times a week for 12 weeks, to improve blood flow and exercise tolerance.
- Lifestyle changes: to reduce cardiovascular risk, including smoking cessation, weight loss, improved diet and exercise, and management of comorbidities.
- Medical management: secondary prevention of cardiovascular disease, including antiplatelet therapy (aspirin or clopidogrel) and high-dose statins.
- Foot care: regular foot examinations and foot care are essential to detect ulcers.
- Analgesia: pain may be complex, and require referral to pain management services.

Revascularization is performed for ALI, and considered for complicated CLI:

- Endovascular: balloon angioplasty +/− stent placement and atherectomy, for short stenosis or aortoiliac disease.

- Surgical: bypass surgery or endarterectomy, for extensive or multifocal disease.
- Amputation: for unsalvageable, gangrenous limbs. May be performed following revascularization attempts or as the primary treatment modality in severe CLI (Fig. 6.15).

Complications

Complications include:

- Amputation: in severe ALI/CLI, irreversible ischaemia may result in amputation.
- Neurological injury: ischaemia may result in sensory loss, and paralysis.
- Reperfusion syndrome: significant endothelial inflammation following reperfusion can cause acidaemia, hyperkalaemia and oedema, and result in compartment syndrome.
- Arterial ulcers: impaired peripheral blood flow results in painful ulceration.

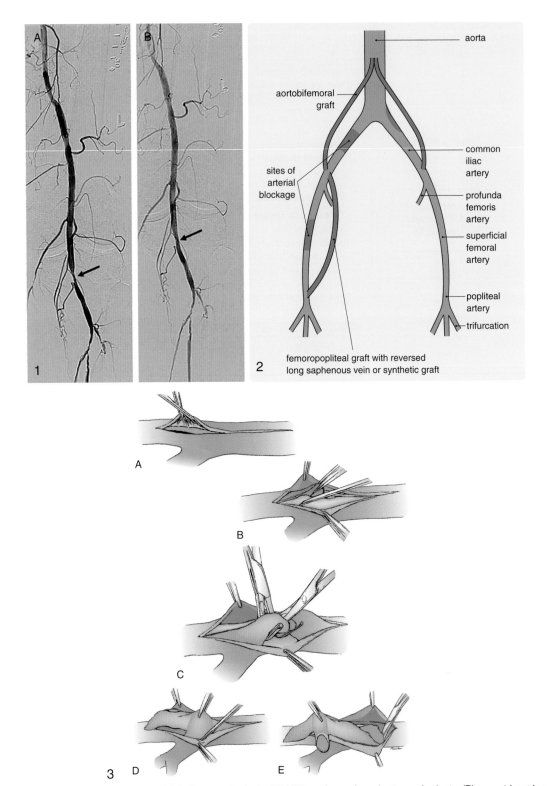

Fig. 6.15 Revascularization techniques. (1) Balloon angioplasty. (A) MRI angiography prior to angioplasty, (B) repeat imaging following successful dilation of stenosis. (2) Common arterial bypass grafts. (3) Open endarterectomy. Steps A–E outline the removal of atherosclerotic plaques. (From A. Stacy MR, Suri JS, El-Baz AS. *Diabetes and Cardiovascular Disease*. Elsevier; 2021. B. Kontoyannis A. *Crash Course: Surgery,* 3rd Edition. Elsevier; 2008. C. Sidawy AN, et al. *Rutherford's Vascular Surgery and Endovascular Therapy,* 10th Edition. Elsevier; 2023.)

- Dry gangrene: necrosis resulting from severe chronic ischaemia, with black discolouration of necrotic tissue and possible autoamputation. Revascularization can be attempted prior to amputation.
- Wet gangrene: bacterial superinfection of gangrene, presenting with oedema, blistering and discharge. Urgent antibiotics and debridement required due to the risk of sepsis. Revascularization +/− amputation are performed following management of acute infection (Fig. 6.16).

DIFFERENTIALS

- Raynaud's phenomenon is a vasoconstrictive response of digital arteries to cold or emotional stress.
- It is idiopathic (Raynaud disease) or related to underlying autoimmune pathology.
- Symptoms include digital discolouration from white (ischaemia), to blue (hypoxia), then red (reactive hyperaemia).
- Prolonged ischaemia can result in ulcers and gangrene.
- Management is with trigger avoidance, and vasodilators (nifedipine).

Chronic venous insufficiency

Chronic venous insufficiency (CVI) describes chronic venous dysfunction and impaired peripheral venous return. It typically affects the great and short saphenous veins in the legs. Elevated venous pressures result in valve incompetence, vein dilation and blood stasis, manifesting with fluid extravasation, oedema, inflammation and tissue hypoperfusion. Risk factors include increasing age, females, smoking, previous VTE or raised intraabdominal pressure (obesity/pregnancy).

Symptoms and signs

Symptoms include:

- Limb pain: leg cramping or discomfort, worse when standing and with heat.
- Oedema: ascending from the ankle to the calf as disease progresses.
- Varicose veins: dilated, tortuous superficial veins in lower limbs.
- Pruritus: with associated with paraesthesia and numbness.

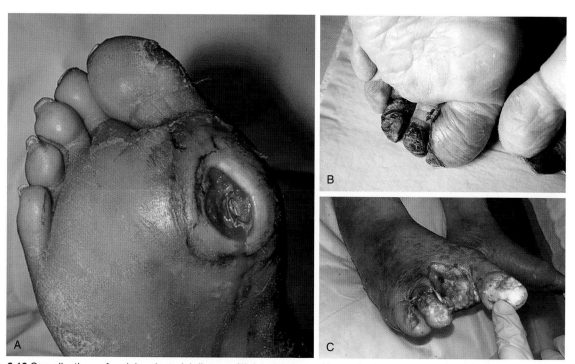

Fig. 6.16 Complications of peripheral arterial disease. (A) Arterial ulcer, with punched out appearance, well defined borders, occurring over a pressure area. (B) Dry gangrene of the toes. (C) Wet gangrene, with evidence of local infection and autoamputation. (From A. Viik J, Min M, Kekonen A, Annus P. *Bioimpedance and Spectroscopy*. Elsevier; 2021; B. Craft JA, et al. *Understanding Pathophysiology,* 4th Edition. Elsevier; 2023. C. Ramachandran M, Gladman MA. *Clinical Cases and OSCEs in Surgery: The Definitive Guide to Passing Examinations,* 3rd Edition. Elsevier; 2018.)

- Skin changes: telangiectasis, hemosiderin standing, lipodermatosclerosis.
- Ulcers: resulting from severe CVI, due to chronic tissue ischaemia.
- Venous eczema: fluid stasis results in skin inflammation, crusting and itch (Fig. 6.17).

Investigations

Investigations include:

- Venous US: will demonstrate venous reflux, or features of acute/chronic DVT.
- ABPI: to diagnose comorbid arterial disease.

Management

Management includes:

- Management of commodities: treatment of associated VTE and PAD.
- Lifestyle changes: including leg elevation, exercise, emollients, smoking cessation, weight loss and avoiding prolonged standing and heat.

- Compression therapy: to improve venous return, using compression stockings or bandages. Contraindicated in PAD.

HINTS AND TIPS

- Compression therapy is not contraindicated in active ucleration.
- Wounds should be managed appropriately while compression therapy is used.
- Improved venous return will prompt healing and reduce wound complications.

For refractory symptoms or complications, interventional approaches include:

- Vein ablation: minimally invasive thermal ablation of varicosities.
- Vein resection: ligation with vein stripping, with removal of the saphenous veins.
- Vein valvuloplasty: reconstruction of deep veins in legs.

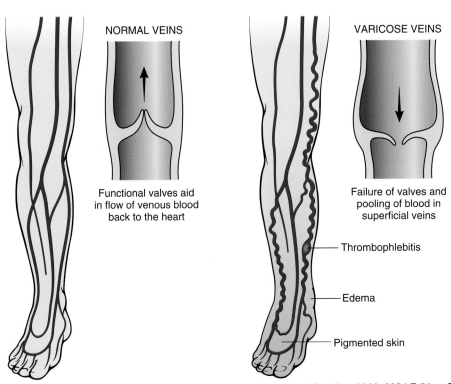

NORMAL VEINS

Functional valves aid in flow of venous blood back to the heart

VARICOSE VEINS

Failure of valves and pooling of blood in superficial veins

Thrombophlebitis

Edema

Pigmented skin

Fig. 6.17 Formation of varicosities. (From *ICD-10-CM/PCS Coding: Theory and Practice,* 2023–2024 Edition. Elsevier; 2023.)

Complications

Complications include:

- Cellulitis: chronic venous eczema predisposes to superimposed infection.
- Superficial thrombophlebitis: inflammation and thrombosis of superficial veins, presenting with pain, erythema and induration.
- DVT: venous status predisposes to thrombosis formation.
- Venous ulcers: chronic skin lesions occurring above the ankles, associated with pain, pruritus, and risk of infection. Difficult to heal with high recurrence rates.

DIFFERENTIALS

Thrombophlebitis migrans is a migratory superficial thrombophlebitis, relating to malignancy (Trousseau syndrome), thromboangiitis obliterans or Behçet disease.

Diabetic foot

Neuropathic diabetic foot describes the clinical manifestation of peripheral polyneuropathy related to chronic hyperglycaemia. Ischaemic diabetic foot can also occur, related to hyperglycaemia-induced microangiopathy and PAD. There is often a mixed picture.

Symptoms and signs

Features of diabetic feet include:

- Symmetrical sensory loss: glove and stocking distribution.
- Painless neuropathic ulcers: on plantar pressures areas, typically metatarsals/heel.
- Recurrent skin infections: including athlete's foot and cellulitis.
- Painless cutaneous lesions: callus and corns relating to recurrent skin trauma.
- Deformities: including hallux valgus, hammer toes and Charcot deformities.

HINTS AND TIPS

- A neuropathic diabetic foot will be warm, with palpable pedal pulses.
- An ischaemic diabetic foot is cold and pulseless.

Investigations

A thorough clinical examination should be performed including diabetic foot exam, neurological exam and arterial and venous exam.

Further investigations include:

- ABPI: to evaluate arterial insufficiency.
- Foot X-rays: to diagnose associated traumatic bony injury.
- Lower limb MRI: to diagnose for osteomyelitis and soft tissue injury.
- Doppler US: to assess arterial and venous circulation.

Management

Supportive management includes:

- Wound dressings: to protect chronic ulcers and promote healing.
- Mechanical offloading: therapeutic footwear or casts to reduce pressure.
- Antibiotics: for superimposed wound infection or osteomyelitis.
- Tight glycaemic control: essential to reduce risk of complications.

Surgical management includes:

- Debridement: removal of necrotic skin to aid healing.
- Revascularization: for associated PAD.
- Amputation: in severe ulcers or life-threatening complications (osteomyelitis, gangrene). The level of amputation required depends on the extent of infection (Fig. 6.18).

CLINICAL NOTES

- Following amputation active rehabilitation is required to encourage prosthesis use and resumption of a normal lifestyle.
- Many patients experience severe phantom limb pain and psychological complications following amputation.

Complications

Complications include:

- Osteomyelitis: deep tissue infection resulting in severe bone pain and systemic infection.
- Charcot deformities: recurrent foot trauma may result in deformity and loss of function (Fig. 6.19).

Abdominal aortic aneurysms

An aneurysm is an abnormal vessel dilation due to vessel wall weakening. Abdominal aortic aneurysms (AAA) are the dilation of the abdominal aorta to >1.5× its normal diameter. They are common, particularly in older males. Smoking, hypertension and atherosclerosis are significant risk factors (Fig. 6.20).

Symptoms and signs

Aneurysms are often asymptomatic and picked up incidentally. Symptoms may include:

- Nonspecific back/abdominal pain
- Pulsatile abdominal mass
- Audible vascular bruit
- Peripheral thrombosis (DVT)

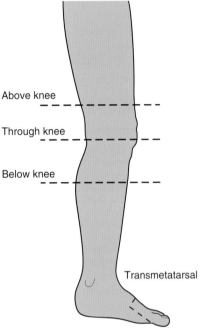

Fig. 6.18 Levels of amputation. (From Tambyraja AL, Parks RW, Garden OJ, Wigmore S. *Principles and Practice of Surgery,* 8th Edition. Elsevier; 2023.)

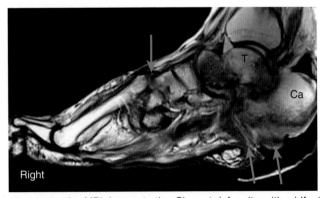

Fig. 6.19 Complications of diabetic neuropathy. MRI demonstrating Charcot deformity, with midfoot osteolysis and collapse, tarso-metatarsal dislocation (*short arrow*). There is a large infected plantar ulcer under the calcaneus (*long arrows*) and reduced signal within the talus/calcaneus, indicating osteomyelitis. (From Pierre-Jerome C. *The Essentials of Charcot Neuroarthropathy: Biomechanics, Pathophysiology, and MRI Findings.* Elsevier; 2022.)

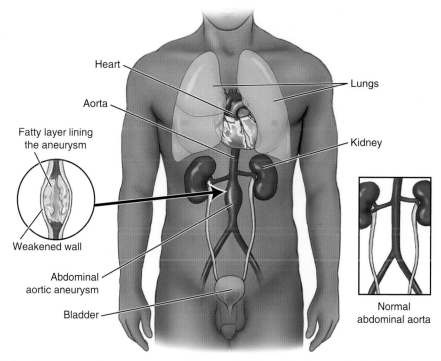

Fig. 6.20 Abdominal aortic aneurysm. Aneurysms are most commonly infrarenal and may extend to the iliac arteries. (From LaFleur Brooks M, Levinsky D, LaFleur Brooks D. *Basic Medical Language,* 7th Edition. Elsevier; 2024.)

RED FLAG

- A ruptured AAA is a surgical emergency.
- Symptoms include sudden, severe, tearing abdominal/back pain, hypotension and a painful pulsatile mass.
- Emergency vascular consult and operative repair within 90 minutes are required due to the risk of profound blood loss and death.
- The mortality rate is over >80%.

CLINICAL NOTES

- One-off US screening for AAA is offered for males aged 65-75 with a smoking history.
- Frequent surveillance is indicated for larger aortic diameters:
  - 3.0-4.4 cm — repeat scan offered in 12 months
  - 4.5-5.4 cm — repeat scan offered in 3 months
- At diameters >5.5cm, repair is required due to the risk of rupture.

Investigations

Investigations include:

- Abdominal US: for asymptomatic patients, to detect and locate aneurysm.
- CTAP: to confirm the diagnosis and plan surgical intervention (Fig. 6.21).

Management

A ruptured AAA is a surgical emergency, requiring urgent vascular consult and surgical repair (Fig. 6.22).

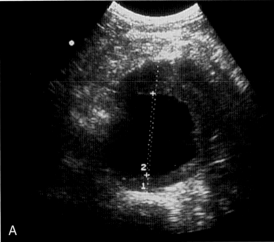

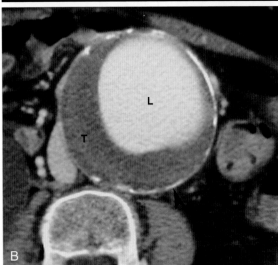

Fig. 6.21 Imaging findings in AAA. AAA is diagnosed when aortic dilation exceeds 3 cm. (A) US showing transverse section through an AAA. Measurement 1 demonstrates the diameter of the aneurysm, and measurement 2 the aortic lumen within the aneurysmal sac. (B) CT demonstrating AAA, with dilation of the aorta >5 cm. A large thrombus (T) surrounds the aortic lumen (L). (From A. Garden OJ, Harunarashid H, Parks RW. *Principles and Practice of Surgery,* 7th Edition. Elsevier; 2018. B. Ferri FF. *Ferri's Clinical Advisor 2023.* Elsevier; 2023.)

For stable patients, management involves:

- Conservative measures: reduction of cardiovascular risk, including smoking cessation, weight loss and management of comorbidities (hypertension, diabetes, hyperlipidaemia).
- AAA surveillance: for aneurysms <5.5 cm, interval US surveillance is appropriate, to identify expansion rate and need for operative intervention.

Elective repair is indicated for aneurysms >5.5 cm or expanding >1 cm per year. Options include:

- Endovascular aneurysm repair (EVAR): minimally invasive placement of expandable stent graft via femoral arteries. Indicated for most patients.
- Open surgical repair (OSR): replacement of dilated aortic segment with prosthetic graft. Typically used if EVAR failed or was associated with complications (Fig. 6.23).

Complications

Complications include:

- AAA rupture: presenting with profound blood loss and haemodynamic instability.
- Embolism: aneurysmal thrombosis secondary to blood stasis can cause emboli.
- Aortic dissection: the weak aneurysmal wall is prone is intimal injury and dissection, which can result in visceral and limb ischaemia and haemodynamic instability.
- Surgical complications: organ ischaemia due to thrombus migration, graft infection.
- EVAR complications: endoleaks, aneurysmal regrowth, device migration/failure.

CLINICAL NOTES

Complications following EVAR are common, hence CTA at 1 month, 12 months, then annually is required.

Venous thromboembolism

Venous thromboembolism (VTE) includes deep vein thrombosis (DVT), formation of a clot in the deep venous system and pulmonary embolism (PE) which typically resulting from embolus of a DVT to the pulmonary circulation. The aetiology of thrombus formation involves Virchow's triad (Fig. 6.24 and Table 3.3).

Symptoms and signs

DVTs commonly affect deep veins in the lower extremities, presenting with:

- Leg swelling, warmth and erythema
- Dull, aching pain along venous system
- Superficial vein dilation (Fig. 6.25)

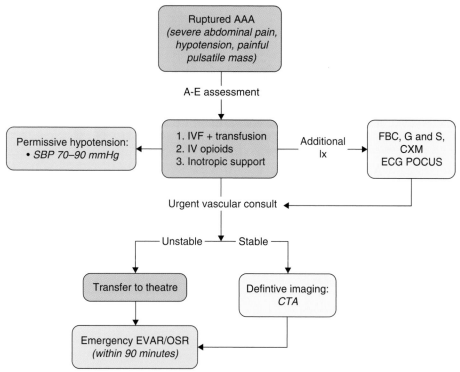

Fig. 6.22 Approach to the management of ruptured AAA. *AAA*, Abdominal aortic aneurysm; *CTA*, CT angiogram; *EVAR*, endovascular aneurysm repair; *OSR*, open surgical repair; *POCUS*, point of care ultrasound.

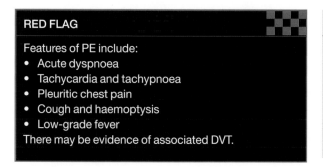

RED FLAG

Features of PE include:
- Acute dyspnoea
- Tachycardia and tachypnoea
- Pleuritic chest pain
- Cough and haemoptysis
- Low-grade fever

There may be evidence of associated DVT.

HINTS AND TIPS

- D-dimer is a sensitive but not specific markers to screen for VTE in low-risk patients
- It is raised in many inflammatory states including infection, pregnancy, malignancy and surgery
- In high-risk patients, definitive imaging should be prioritized.

Investigations

The Wells criteria is used to calculate the probability of VTE (Table 6.4).

To confirm the diagnosis, investigations include

- D dimer: to exclude DVT in low-risk patients (wells = 0).
- Doppler US: to diagnose DVT in intermediate-high risk patients (wells >1).
- CTPA: contrast-enhanced CT chest. Intraluminal filling defects indicate PE (Fig. 6.26).

Management

Acute VTE is a medical emergency, and should be managed with urgent assessment, treatment initiation, and resuscitation and haemodynamic support as required (Fig. 6.27).

HINTS AND TIPS

Be cautious with fluid resuscitation in massive PE, due to the risk of fluid overload on worsening ventricular function, decreasing cardiac output and precipitating cardiac arrest.

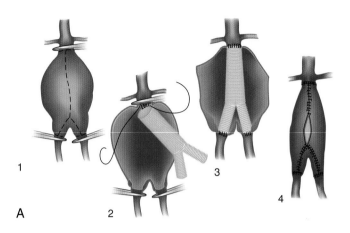

A

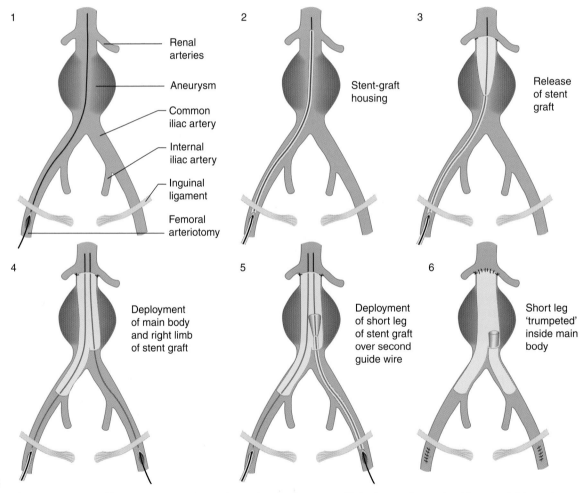

B

Fig. 6.23 AAA repair (A) OSR, with aneurysm dissection and stent placement. (B) Endovascular repair, with expandable aortic graft and iliac limbs placed via the femoral arteries. (From A. Kent KC, et al. *Surgical principles for operative treatment of aortic aneurysms.* In Lindsay J. Jr, editor: *Diseases of the aorta.* Philadelphia. 1994; Lea & Febiger. B. Garden OJ, et al. *Principles and Practice of Surgery*, 8th Edition, Elsevier; 2023.)

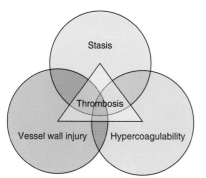

Fig. 6.24 Virchow's triad. (Professional illustration by Kenneth X. Probst.)

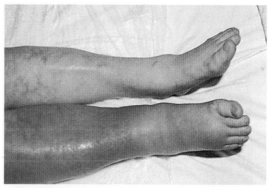

Fig. 6.25 Clinical features of DVT. (From Shiland BJ, Zenith. *Medical Assistant: Cardiopulmonary Systems, Vital Signs, Electrocardiography and CPR—Module D,* 2nd Edition. Elsevier; 2015.)

Table 6.3 Risk factors for VTE

Venous stasis	Endothelial injury	Hypercoagulability
Immobility – illness, long haul travel, limb injury, age Chronic venous insufficiency Surgery Obesity	Smoking Hypertension Atherosclerosis IVDU Indwelling devices	Malignancy ↑ Oestrogen – pregnancy, OCP, HRT Autoimmune disorders Inherited thrombophilia

HRT, Hormone replacement therapy; OCP, oral contraceptive pill.

Table 6.4 Wells criteria

Wells criteria for DVT	Score	Wells criteria for PE	Score
Active cancer	1	Clinical symptoms of DVT	3
Previous DVT	1	PE is most likely diagnosis	3
Paralysis, paresis or recent immobilization of lower limb	1	Previous PE/DVT	1.5
Recently bedridden >3 days Major surgery within past 12 weeks	1	Tachycardia >100 bpm	1.5
Localized deep venous tenderness	1	Surgery/immobilization past 4 weeks	1.5
Entire leg swelling	1	Haemoptysis	1
Swelling >3 cm versus other leg	1	Malignancy	1
Pitting oedema in symptomatic leg	1		
Distended superficial veins	1		
Alternative diagnosis as/more likely	−2		
Pretest probability • 0: low • 1-2: intermediate • >3: high		Pretest probability • <4: PE unlikely • >4 PE likely	

Calf swelling is measured 10 cm below the tibial tuberosity. DVT, Deep vein thrombosis; PE, pulmonary embolism

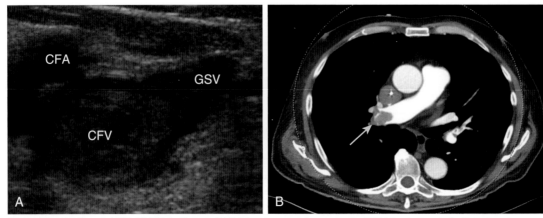

Fig. 6.26 Imaging findings in VTE. (A) US findings in DVT. The common femoral vein (CFV) is obstructed, dilated and noncompressible, with an intraluminal hyperechoic mass, suggesting thrombosis. (B) CTPA demonstrating right main pulmonary artery PE. (From A. Courtesy Gregory Piazza, MD, MS. B. Kabrhel C, Walls RM. *Rosen's Emergency Medicine: Concepts and Clinical Practice, 2-Volume Set,* 10th Edition. Elsevier; 2023.)

Long-term management of VTE includes:

- Provoked VTE (>1 risk factor in history): anticoagulation for 3 months.
- Unprovoked VTE (no risk factor in history): anticoagulation for 6 months.
- Recurrent VTE/underlying risk factors: indefinite anticoagulation, with treatment of underlying risk factors if possible.

CLINICAL NOTES

Anticoagulation options include:
- Bridging with low molecular-weight heparin (LMWH) for 5-10 days and subsequent direct oral anticoagulants (apixaban/dabigatran).
- Specific indications (i.e., mechanical heart valves) require warfarin.
- VTE prophylaxis is used to prevent VTE in high-risk situations (i.e., inpatient admissions), typically LMWH +/– compression stockings.

Complications

Complications of DVT include

- Venous gangrene: severe ischaemic necrosis of distal extremity following large DVT.

- Post thrombotic syndrome: chronic venous insufficiency following DVT.
- Pulmonary embolism: acute embolus of thrombus causes PE.

Complications of PE include:

- Respiratory complications: atelectasis, pleural effusion, pulmonary infarction.
- Cardiac arrest: massive PE can result in haemodynamic instability and cardiac arrest.
- Right ventricular failure: submassive/massive PE can result in ventricular failure, with ECG signs of right heart strain (S1Q3T3, new right bundle branch block, ST elevation) – elevated troponins, and RV dysfunction on echocardiography.

Carotid artery stenosis

Carotid artery stenosis (CAS) is the atherosclerotic occlusion of the common and internal carotid arteries. It is common in older adults with comorbid cardiovascular disease. Smoking, hypertension and diabetes are significant risk factors.

Symptoms and signs

CAS may be asymptomatic. More extensive stenosis presents with cerebral ischaemia:

- Transient ischaemic attack (TIA): transient loss of sensory or motor function or amaurosis fugax, lasting <24 hours.
- Ischaemic stroke: contralateral motor/sensory loss, lasting >24 hours.

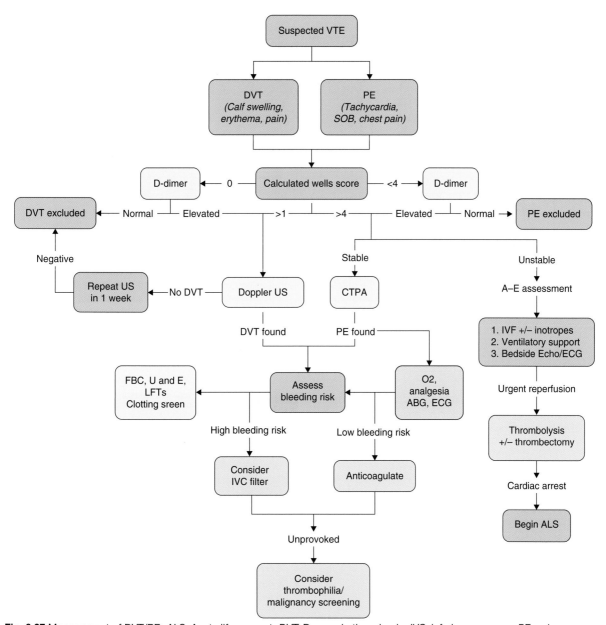

Fig. 6.27 Management of DVT/PE. *ALS,* Acute life support; *DVT,* Deep vein thrombosis; *IVC,* inferior vena cava; *PE,* pulmonary embolism.

HINTS AND TIPS

There may be audible carotid artery bruits due to turbulent blood flow through stenosis.

Investigations

Investigations include:

- Carotid Doppler US: increased peak systolic flow velocity suggests stenosis. Absence suggests total occlusion.

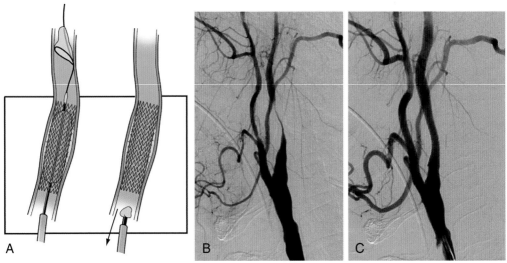

Fig. 6.28 Carotid artery stenting. (A) Stenting of the carotid bifurcation to treat internal carotid artery stenosis. (B) DSA showing severe stenosis in the proximal internal carotid artery. (C) DSA after stent placement of a stent across the carotid bifurcation, demonstrating correction of stenosis. (From Winn HR. *Youmans and Winn Neurological Surgery*, 8th Edition. Elsevier Inc.; 2023.)

- CTA/Digital subtraction angiography (DSA): to confirm location and extent of stenosis.
- CT/MRI head: to exclude ischaemic stroke/TIA.

CLINICAL NOTES

Stenosis is graded by severity:
- Clinically significant (>50%)
- Moderate (50%–69%)
- Severe (70%–99%)

Management

Management relates to the extent of stenosis and presence of symptoms:

- Lifestyle modifications: smoking cessation, improved diet and exercise, weight loss.
- Medical management: antiplatelet therapy, statins and optimization of comorbidities (hypertension, diabetes).
- Revascularization: for symptomatic patients, severe stenosis, or bilateral disease, with endarterectomy or angioplasty and stenting (Fig. 6.28).

RED FLAG

Evidence of ischemic stroke or TIA is an urgent indication for CT head and consideration of thrombolysis +/– thrombectomy and antiplatelet therapy based on the findings.

Complications

Complications include:

- Cerebrovascular accident: stroke, myocardial infarction.
- Compilations of surgery: injury to adjacent structures, haemorrhage, embolic stroke.

Lymphoedema

Lymphoedema relates to lymphatic obstruction and impaired lymphatic clearance, resulting in collection of lipid and protein-rich fluid in the interstitial space. Primary lymphoedema is rare, relating to genetic abnormalities. Secondary lymphoedema relates to infection, or injury/obstruction to lymphatic flow due to tumours, inflammation, radiation or following surgery.

Symptoms and signs

Symptoms include:

- Aching, heavy legs
- Difficulty moving legs
- Recurrent skin infections
- Skin hardening and tightening
- Warty growths and fluid leakage

Lymphoedema is progressive, with gradual worsening of symptoms. Stages include:

- Reversible limb oedema (pitting)
- Irreversible limb oedema with skin fibrosis (nonpitting)
- Progressive limb enlargement and fibrosis (irreversible elephantiasis) (Fig. 6.29)

Management

Management involves:

- Conservative: lymphatic massage and compression garments, limb elevation, exercise and management of the underlying cause.
- Surgical: lymphatic vessel resection, grafting or lymph node transfer.
- Management of complications: antibiotics for skin infections and psychological support.

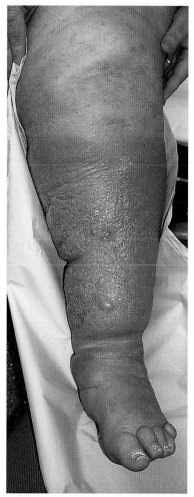

Fig. 6.29 Lymphoedema. Massive lymphoedema, with leg swelling, skin blistering, fluid leakage and skin fibrosis. (From Parks RW, Wigmore S, Tambyraja AL, Garden OJ. *Principles and Practice of Surgery,* 8th Edition. Elsevier; 2023.)

Chapter Summary

- PAD presents with intermittent claudication, cramping muscle pain on exertion that relieves with rest, and an ABPI <0.8.
- CLI presents with rest pain, arterial ulcers and gangrene, and an ABPI <0.5.
- ALI presents with the 6P's – pain, pulselessness, paralysis, pallor, paraesthesia and poikilothermia (perishingly cold). It typically relates to PAD or AF.
- Smoking cessation is essential in PAD, to reduce the risk of CLI and limb loss.
- Neuropathic ulcers result from peripheral neuropathy, chronic limb trauma and poor wound healing. There is a risk of osteomyelitis and limb loss.
- A ruptured AAA presents with sudden, severe tearing abdominal/back pain, hypotension and a painful pulsatile mass. The mortality is >80%.
- The Wells criteria is used to assess VTE risk and guide diagnostic investigations.
- Carotid artery stenosis can be asymptomatic, or present with symptoms of cerebral hypoperfusion (stroke/TIA). Surgery is indicated if there are symptoms or severe (>70%) stenosis.

UKMLA Conditions

Acute coronary syndromes
Adverse drug effects
Aneurysms
Aortic aneurysm
Aortic dissection
Aortic valve disease
Arrhythmias
Arterial thrombosis
Arterial ulcers
Cardiac arrest
Cardiac failure
Cellulitis
Compartment syndrome
Decreased/loss of consciousness
Deep vein thrombosis
Deteriorating patient
Diabetes mellitus type 1 and 2
Diabetic neuropathy
Disease prevention/screening
Essential or secondary hypertension
Gangrene
Hyperlipidaemia
Incidental findings
Intestinal ischaemia
Ischaemic limb and occlusions
Limp
Loss of libido

UKMLA Presentations

Abdominal distension
Acute abdominal pain
Acute and chronic pain management
Acute change in or loss of vision
Acute joint pain/swelling
Altered sensation, numbness and tingling
Back pain
Blackouts and faints
Breathlessness
Cardiorespiratory arrest
Chest pain
Chronic abdominal pain
Cold
Cough
Cyanosis
Decreased/loss of consciousness
Deteriorating patient
Diabetes mellitus type 1 and 2
Erectile dysfunction
Fever
Flashes and floaters in visual fields
Haemoptysis
Hypertension
Immobility
Limb claudication
Limb weakness
Limp

● **Chapter Summary—cont'd**

UKMLA Conditions
Lower limb soft tissue injury
Musculoskeletal deformities
Myocardial infarction
Necrotizing fasciitis
Obesity
Osteomyelitis
Pallor
Patient on anticoagulant therapy
Patient on antiplatelet therapy
Peripheral nerve injuries/palsies
Peripheral vascular disease
Polycythaemia
Pressure sores
Pulmonary embolism
Respiratory arrest
Respiratory failure
Sepsis
Shock
Stroke
Subarachnoid haemorrhage
Transient ischaemic attacks
Venous ulcers

UKMLA Presentations
Loss of libido
Low blood pressure
Massive haemorrhage
Muscle pain/myalgia
Musculoskeletal deformities
Neuromuscular weakness
Pain on inspiration
Painful
Painful swollen leg
Pale
Pallor
Peripheral oedema and ankle swelling
Pleural effusion
Postsurgical care and complications
Pruritus
Pulseless leg/foot
Scarring
Sepsis
Shock
Skin ulcers
Soft tissue injury
Weight gain

CLINICAL ANATOMY

The kidneys are retroperitoneal organs that regulate fluid balance and homeostasis, and filter and remove waste products of metabolism from the blood (Figs. 7.1–7.2).

Production of urine by the kidneys is known as diuresis. The nephron is the functional unit of the kidney, and contains millions of glomeruli, which filter blood to remove waste products, regulate electrolyte homeostasis and reabsorb water. Urine is the end product which drains into the renal calyces and pelvis before travelling to the bladder via the ureters (Fig. 7.3).

The bladder lies within the anterior pelvic cavity. The ureters drain into the bladder at the ureterovesical junctions. The urethra exits the bladder inferiorly via the internal urethral orifice at the bladder neck. The detrusor muscle in the bladder wall relaxes to store between 500 and 1000 mL of urine, and contracts to expel urine during micturition (Fig. 7.4).

The urethra drains urine from the bladder. In females, the urethra is approximately 4 cm long, and travels inferiorly through the deep perineal pouch, before forming the external urethral orifice between the labia minora, anterior to the vaginal opening. In males, the urethra is approximately 20 cm long,

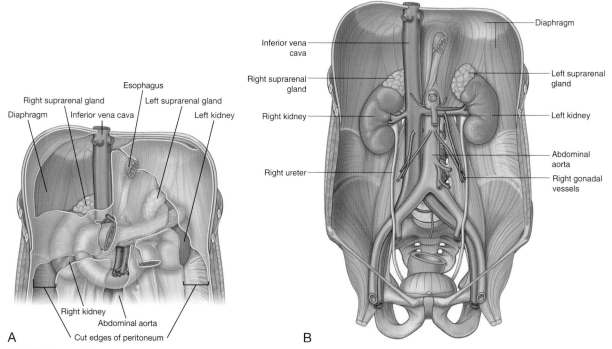

Fig. 7.1 Anatomical relations of the kidney. (A) Abdominal location of the kidney. (B) Abdominal relations of the kidney, ureters and bladder. (From A. Vogl AW, Mitchell AWM, Drake RL. *Gray's Basic Anatomy*. Churchill Livingstone, Elsevier Inc. 2013. B. Mitchell AWM, Drake RL, Vogl AW. *Gray's Anatomy for Students Flash Cards,* 5th Edition. Elsevier; 2024.)

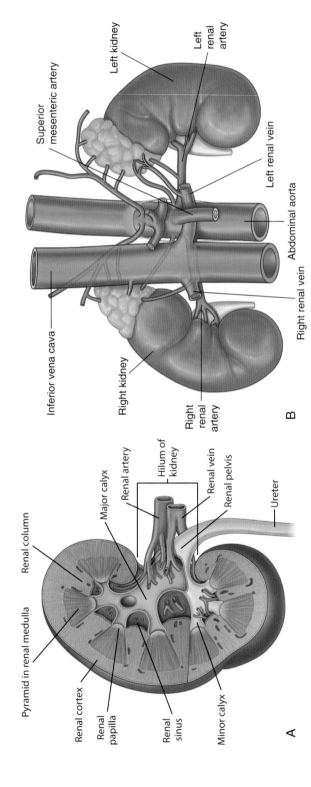

Fig. 7.2 (A) Cross-sectional anatomy of the kidney. (B) Vascular anatomy of the kidney. The renal arteries branch from the aorta at L2 to supply the kidneys. The left renal vein crosses under the superior mesenteric artery (SMA) to join the IVC, making it vulnerable to compression by an aortic or SMA aneurysm. (From A. Vogl AW, Mitchell AWM, Drake RL. *Gray's Basic Anatomy*. Churchill Livingstone, Elsevier Inc. 2013. B. Mitchell AWM, Vogl AW, Drake RL. *Gray's Anatomy for Students*, 4th Edition. Elsevier; 2020.)

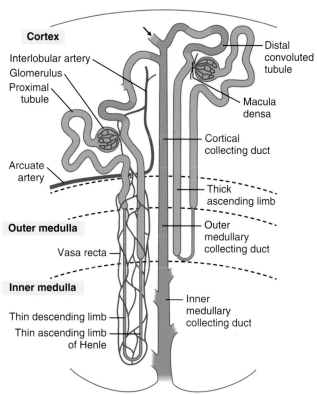

Fig. 7.3 Two nephrons situated in the cortex and medulla of the kidney. Several nephrons converge and empty into a collecting duct. (From Gilbert SF, Weiner DE. *National Kidney Foundation Primer on Kidney Diseases,* 8th Edition. Elsevier; 2023.)

exiting the bladder and passing inferiorly through the prostate, before bending anteriorly to enter the base of the penis. The urethra bends inferiorly as it courses through the penis before forming the external urethral orifice (Fig. 7.5).

The prostate is an accessory structure of male reproduction that surrounds the urethra. It is composed of glandular and muscular tissue. It secretes prostatic fluid, which contains proteolytic enzymes such as prostate-specific antigen (PSA) that liquefy and maintain semen fluidity and drains into the urethra and is expelled as part of the male ejaculate. The peripheral zone contains most of the glandular tissue. The central zone surrounds the ejaculatory ducts, and the transitional zone surrounds the urethra (Fig. 7.6).

The testes are the primary male reproductive organ. The testes develop in the retroperitoneal space and descend through the inguinal ring into the scrotum, typically at week 33 of pregnancy. The testes are composed of multiple seminiferous tubules, which are the site of spermatogenesis. Leydig cells in between the tubules secrete testosterone and testosterone

precursors in response to pituitary LH release. The epididymis stores maturing sperm, which is propelled into the ductus deferens, spermatic cord, ejaculatory duct and finally urethra during ejaculation. The prostatic ducts and seminal vesicles drain into the ejaculatory duct as it courses through the prostate (Fig. 7.7).

UROLOGY PRESENTATIONS

History taking

COMMUNICATION

- Urological symptoms are highly personal.
- Take time to build rapport to ensure you identify all relevant symptoms.

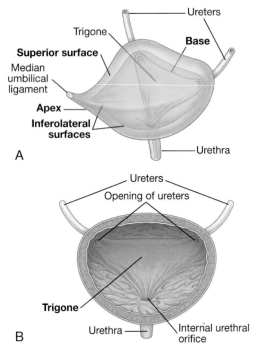

A

B

Fig. 7.4 Internal and external anatomy of the bladder. (A) Superior surface of the bladder. (B) Internal view of the bladder showing the connections of the ureters and urethra. Note the smooth detrusor muscle in the wall of the bladder, which controls urine storage and expulsion. (From Vogl AW, Mitchell AWM, Drake RL. *Gray's Basic Anatomy*. Churchill Livingstone, Elsevier Inc. 2013.)

Opening the consultation
Introduce yourself and confirm the patient details.

Presenting complaint (PC)
Ask an open question to identify the patient's presenting complaint.

History of presenting complaint (HPC)
Explore the presenting complaint further using SOCRATES and obtain a timeline of symptoms.

CLINICAL NOTES

- SOCRATES is a useful structure to explore many symptoms, not only pain.
- Any nonrelevant parts can simply be skipped.

Common symptoms of urological pathology are:

- Dysuria: discomfort, burning or stinging when passing urine.
- Lower urinary tract symptoms (LUTS): issues with storing urine or urination.
- Haematuria: blood in the urine, which may be microscopic or macroscopic.
- Loin pain: may be described as flank or back pain. May radiate to the groin.
- Lump in groin: a lump or swelling in the groin or scrotum.
- Male sexual dysfunction: erectile dysfunction, loss of libido or infertility.

HINTS AND TIPS

LUTS describes both storage and voiding symptoms:
- Storage – frequency, urgency, nocturia, incontinence
- Voiding – hesitancy, poor stream, terminal dribbling, difficulty passing urine

---

RED FLAG

Red flags in urology include:
- Severe loin pain, fever, and vomiting
- A complete inability to pass urine
- Unexplained micro/macroscopic haematuria
- New LUTS and erectile dysfunction
- Sudden, severe scrotal pain
- Painless growth or change in testes shape/texture

Associated features include:

- Fevers and rigors: may indicate infective pathology.
- Nausea and vomiting: common in infective, traumatic or malignant pathology.
- Abdominal pain: typically suprapubic tenderness or unilateral back pain.
- Weight loss: unintentional weight loss is red flag feature for malignancy.

Ideas, concerns and expectations
Elicit ideas, concerns and expectations early in the consultation, to ensure any concerns are addressed, and you understand what the patient hopes to achieve with the consultation.

Systemic enquiry
A brief systemic enquiry may highlight other relevant features to the presenting complaint, or prompt further relevant questions before you move on to the rest of the history.

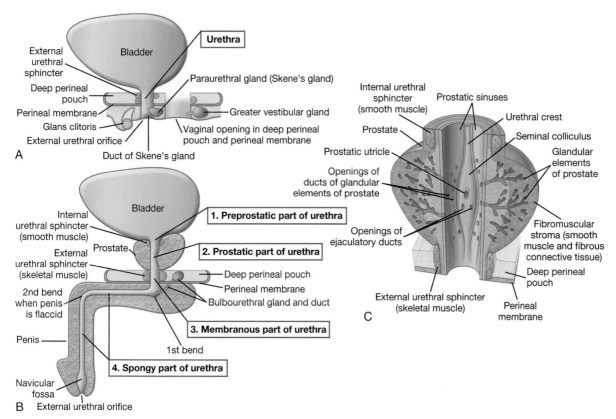

Fig. 7.5 Urethral anatomy in men and women. (A) Female urethra. (B) Male urethra. (C) Prostatic relations of the male urethra. (From Vogl AW, Mitchell AWM, Drake RL. *Gray's Basic Anatomy*. Churchill Livingstone, Elsevier Inc. 2013.)

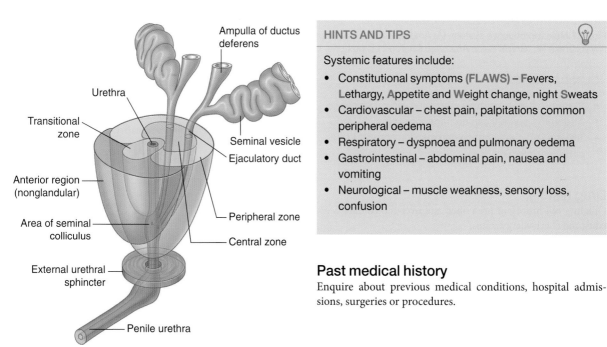

Fig. 7.6 Zonal anatomy of the prostate. (From Drake RL, Mitchell AWM, Vogl AW. *Gray's Anatomy for Students,* 5th Edition. Elsevier; 2024.)

Past medical history

Enquire about previous medical conditions, hospital admissions, surgeries or procedures.

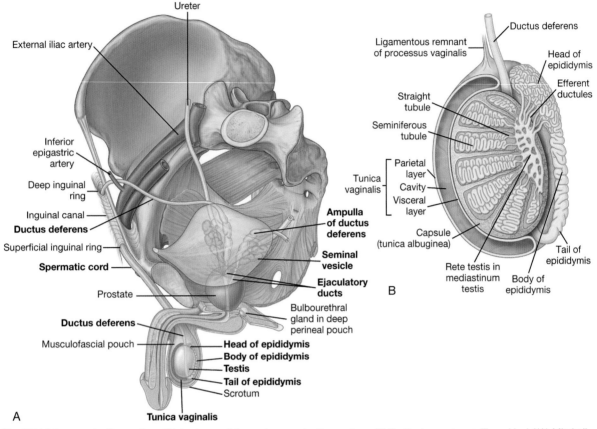

Ureter

External iliac artery

Inferior
epigastric
artery

Deep inguinal
ring

Inguinal canal

Ductus deferens

Superficial inguinal ring

Spermatic cord

Prostate

Ductus deferens

Musculofascial pouch

Ligamentous remnant
of processus vaginalis

Straight
tubule

Seminiferous
tubule

Parietal
layer
Tunica   Cavity
vaginalis Visceral
layer

**Ampulla
of ductus
deferens**

Capsule
(tunica albuginea)

**Seminal
vesicle**

**Ejaculatory
ducts**

B

Bulbourethral
gland in deep
perineal pouch

Head of epididymis
Body of epididymis
Testis
Tail of epididymis
Scrotum

Ductus deferens

Head of
epididymis

Efferent
ductules

Rete testis in
mediastinum
testis

Body of
epididymis

Tail of
epididymis

A

Tunica vaginalis

Fig. 7.7 Male reproductive system. (A) Anatomy of the male reproductive system. (B) Testicular anatomy. (From Vogl AW, Mitchell AWM, Drake RL. *Gray's Basic Anatomy*. Churchill Livingstone, Elsevier Inc. 2013.)

CLINICAL NOTES

- Systemic disease may have associated urinary symptoms.
- Abdominal surgery can damage the urological tract.
- Traumatic catheterisation can result in chronic LUTS or urinary infection.

Drug history

Obtain a full history of prescribed and over-the-counter remedies and check allergy status.

HINTS AND TIPS

- Diuretics can cause LUTS.
- Psychotropic medications can cause sexual dysfunction
- Medications may alter the colour of urine.
- Check medication compliance, recent changes and any new side effects.

Sexual history

A brief sexual history includes last sexual partner, recent unprotected sexual intercourse and previous sexually transmitted infections (STIs). In women, take a menstrual history, including last menstrual period, gravity and parity, and any postcoital or intermenstrual bleeding.

Family history

Screen for close family members with a history of urological symptoms.

Social history

The general social context of the patient should be explored:

- Baseline functional status: assess independence with activities of daily living (ADLs), including personal hygiene. Patients with reduced mobility may have difficulties managing continence.
- Smoking: assess smoking status and calculate the number of pack-years. Smoking is associated with urological malignancy.

- Alcohol: record the quantity and type of alcohol consumed each week.
- Recreational drugs: recreational drugs can be associated with LUTS.
- Diet and fluids: determine daily fluid intake, including quantity and type of fluids.
- Occupation: specific risk factors in occupational histories can highlight potential differential diagnoses.

CLINICAL NOTES

Occupational exposure to rubber, plastics or dyes increases the risk of transitional cell carcinoma of the bladder.

HINTS AND TIPS

- Chronic dehydration and continence issues increases the risk of UTIs.
- Caffeinated or alcoholic beverages cause urinary frequency and dehydration.
- Excessive fluid intake can lead to frequency and nocturia.

Closing the consultation

Summarize the history, thank the patient and answer any questions.

DIFFERENTIAL DIAGNOSIS

Dysuria

Dysuria is discomfort, pain or a burning sensation when passing urine. It may be associated with LUTS, suprapubic or loin pain, and nausea and vomiting. The differential diagnosis of dysuria includes a range of inflammatory and infectious disorders of the urinary tract (Fig. 7.8).

HINTS AND TIPS

Noninfective cystitis may relate to inappropriate use of topical hygiene products.

Investigations for dysuria

1. Bedside
   - Observations: changes in temperature, blood pressure, heart rate and respiratory rate can identify systemic compromise.
   - Urine dipstick: leukocytes, nitrates and red blood cells suggest infection.
   - Urine MC&S: to confirm a diagnosis of infection and guide antibiotic therapy.
   - Pregnancy test: females of childbearing age should have a pregnancy test. Pregnancy is associated with LUTS, and UTIs are significant in pregnancy.
   - STI testing: STIs commonly present with dysuria.
2. Bloods
   - FBC: ↑ WBC is suggestive of bacterial infection.
   - CRP: ↑ in infective or inflammatory pathology.
   - U&Es: ↑ creatinine and urea indicate acute kidney injury (AKI) or chronic kidney disease (CKD). Creatinine clearance can be calculated to approximate GFR.
   - PSA: ↑ in prostatic pathology.
   - Autoantibodies: if glomerulonephritis is suspected.
3. Imaging
   - Ultrasound (US) KUB: to detect structural abnormalities of the urinary tract that increase infection risk or suggest malignancy.
   - CT Kidneys, Ureters, Bladder: first line to formally assess structural urological pathology.
   - Cystoscopy: a flexible or rigid cystoscopy can be used to diagnose and treat urinary obstruction and take tissue biopsies for histology.
   - Renal biopsy: to diagnose the underlying pathology in nephritic syndrome or diagnose renal AKI.
   - Multiparametric MRI +/- prostate biopsy: to diagnose prostate malignancy.
   - Urodynamic studies: measures bladder pressure and flow rates. Abnormal pressures or voiding can occur in obstructive conditions.
   - Micturating cystourethrogram (MCUG): commonly used in paediatrics to assess for structural abnormalities associated with recurrent UTIs.

COMMON PITFALLS

- Simple dysuria without red flag features is likely to be a lower urinary tract infection, which can be diagnosed clinically or on a bedside urine dipstick.
- Be sure to consider the most common diagnoses before investigating further.

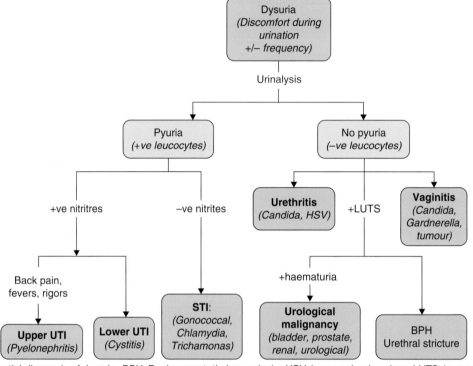

Fig. 7.8 Differential diagnosis of dysuria. *BPH*, Benign prostatic hyperplasia; *HSV*, herpes simplex virus; *LUTS*, lower urinary tract symptoms; *STI*, sexually transmitted infection; *UTI*, urinary tract infection.

CLINICAL NOTES

- Urea and creatinine are filtered and excreted by the kidneys.
- Elevation is associated with kidney injury but creatinine levels will not start rising until GFR has reduced by 50%.
- Urea/creatinine ratio can suggest the underlying cause in AKI:
  - >20:1 indicates a prerenal cause
  - <15:1 indicates a renal cause
  - 10:1–20:1 indicates a postrenal cause

Lower urinary tract symptoms

Lower urinary tract symptoms (LUTS) include storage and voiding symptoms:

- Storage: frequency, urgency, nocturia, incontinence
- Voiding: hesitancy, poor stream, terminal dribbling, straining and a sensation of incomplete voiding

Most urinary pathologies will present with elements of LUTS, with or without other symptoms. Storage symptoms are common in infections or detrusor muscle hyperactivity. Voiding symptoms occur in obstructive conditions or impaired detrusor muscle contractility. However, there is significant overlap between the two, and many conditions present with a mixed picture (Fig. 7.9).

Investigations for LUTS

1. Bedside
   - Bladder diary: assess frequency of urination, voiding volume and fluid intake.
   - Urine dipstick: dip the urine to detect infection, glucose or blood. Send MC&S if there is evidence of infection.
   - Digital rectal exam (DRE): an essential first step in suspected prostate pathology.
2. Bloods
   - FBC: anaemia may suggest underlying bleeding or malignancy. ↑WCC is associated with urinary tract infection.
   - CRP: ↑ in inflammatory states including infection and malignancy.
   - U&Es: ↑ urea and creatinine indicate AKI or CKD.
   - LFTs: ↑ALP is associated with bony metastasis, common in prostate cancer.

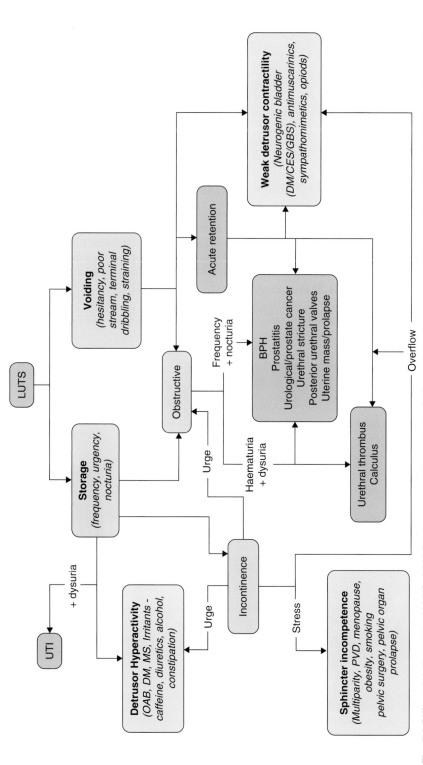

Fig. 7.9 Differential diagnosis of LUTS. *BPH*, Benign prostatic hyperplasia; *CES*, cauda equina syndrome; *DM*, diabetes mellitus; *GBS*, Guillain-Barre syndrome; *LUTS*, lower urinary tract symptoms; *MS*, multiple sclerosis; *OAB*, overactive bladder; *PVD*, previous vaginal delivery; *UTI*, urinary tract infection.

- PSA: ↑PSA suggests prostate pathology including BPH, prostatitis and cancer.
3. Imaging
    - US bladder: a postvoid residual scan may indicate obstructive pathology.
    - US prostate: to assess prostate size and shape following an abnormal DRE.
    - AXR: urinary calculi may be radiopaque and visible on a plain abdominal film.
    - CTKUB: used to visualize lesions, calculi, strictures or masses.
    - CT urogram: to visualize filling defects or obstructions to urinary flow (Fig. 7.10).
    - Multiparametric MRI: the gold standard for suspected prostate cancer.
    - Urodynamic studies: to measure bladder pressure and flow rates. Useful in the investigation of detrusor instability and overactive bladder (OAB), or in obstructive pathology.
    - Cystoscopy: to accurately assess obstructive lesions of the urethra, prostate and bladder neck, and take tissue samples for histology.
    - Nerve conduction studies: if neurogenic bladder is suspected.

CLINICAL NOTES

- Target your investigations to the demographics and clinical history.
- Older males are more likely to have underlying prostate or bladder pathology.
- Older women with several children are more likely to have pelvic pathology.

Haematuria

Haematuria is defined as the presence of RBCs in the urine. Microscopic haematuria is not visible to the naked eye. Macroscopic haematuria presents with visible urine colour change. Microscopic haematuria suggests glomerular damage. Macroscopic haematuria may indicate damage anywhere in the urinary tract (Fig. 7.11).

Investigations for haematuria

1. Bedside

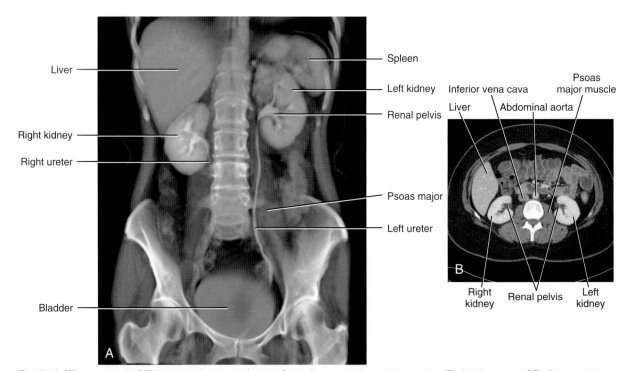

Fig. 7.10 CT urogram. (A) CT Urogram demonstrating the flow of contrast through the ureter. (B) Axial contrast CT of the renal pelvis. CT image with contrast in the axial plane. (From A. Drake RL, Mitchell AWM, Vogl AW. *Gray's Anatomy for Students Flash Cards,* 5th Edition. Elsevier; 2024. B. Vogl AW, Mitchell AWM, Drake RL. *Gray's Basic Anatomy.* Churchill Livingstone, Elsevier Inc. 2013.)

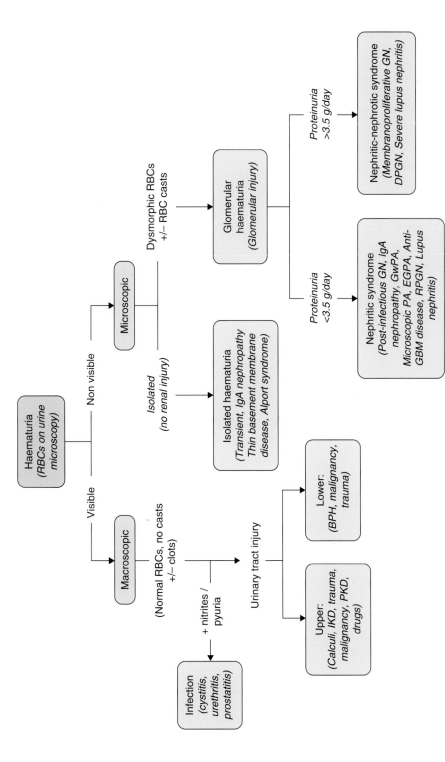

Fig. 7.11 Differential diagnosis of haematuria. Haematuria refers to red blood cells (RBCs) in the urine. Myoglobinuria, ingestion of beetroot, menstrual blood and several medications including rifampicin, phenytoin and nitrofurantoin, can darken the urine and cause false positive results. *anti-GBM*, Anti-glomerular basement membrane disease; *BPH*, benign prostatic hyperplasia; *DPGN*, diffuse proliferative glomerulonephritis; *EGPA*, eosinophilic granulomatosis with polyangiitis; *GN*, Glomerulonephritis; *GwPA*, Granulomatosis with polyangiitis; *IKD*, interstitial kidney disease; microscopic *PA*, microscopic polyangiitis; *PKD*, polycystic kidney disease; *RPGN*, rapidly progressive glomerulonephritis; *UTI*, urinary tract infection.

- Urine dipstick: to detect blood and protein.
- Urinalysis: MC&S can confirm the presence of haemoglobin, evaluate for RBC casts and proteinuria in glomerular disease, and culture infective organisms.

2. Bloods
   - FBC: ↓Hb indicates anaemia, associated with malignancy or chronic bleeding. ↑WCC suggests infection.
   - CRP/ESR: ↑ in systemic inflammatory disorders.
   - U&Es: ↑ urea/creatinine indicate AKI.
   - PSA: if prostatic pathology is suspected.

3. Imaging
   - US KUB: to screen for structural abnormalities of the urinary tract.
   - CT urogram: to identify filling defects, renal parenchymal changes, and assess the collecting system.
   - Cystoscopy: the gold standard for evaluating suspected urological malignancy.

HINTS AND TIPS

Consider nonurological causes that may present with haematuria, including vaginal bleeding, haematological pathology or vasculitis.

Loin pain

Loin pain, sometimes referred to as flank pain, has a wide differential diagnosis. Common and significant causes include renal colic (associated with ureteric calculi) and upper urinary tract infection, however, there are several nonurological causes that should be considered (Fig. 7.12).

Investigations for loin pain

1. Bedside
   - Urine dip: nitrites and leukocytes indicate infective pathology, and haematuria may indicate inflammatory pathology or renal stones.
   - Urinalysis: acidic or alkaline urine may suggest calculi and the likely composition of stones. Urine MC&S should be performed in infective pathology.
   - Pregnancy test: ectopic pregnancy is a life-threatening differential diagnosis in females of childbearing age and should be excluded.

2. Bloods
   - FBC: ↓Hb indicates anaemia, and ↑WCC is associated with infection.
   - U&Es: to screen for renal impairment.
   - LFTs: if hepatic or cholestatic pathology is suspected.
   - Amylase: a sensitive marker for pancreatitis.

3. Imaging
   - US KUB: to detect obstructive defects and nephrolithiasis.
   - AXR: radiopaque calculi may be visible on a plain X-ray film.
   - CT urogram: to characterize obstructive lesions and filling defects.
   - CT abdomen/pelvis: to identify kidney stones and detect abdominal or renal masses. Angiography can be used if

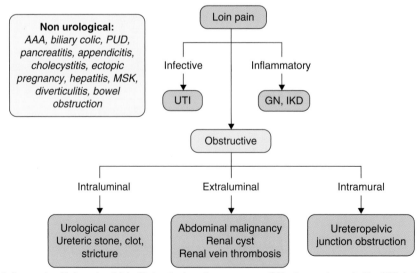

Fig. 7.12 Differential diagnosis of loin pain. *AAA*, Abdominal aortic aneurysm; *GN*, glomerulonephritis; *IKD*, interstitial kidney disease; *MSK*, musculoskeletal; *PUD*, peptic ulcer disease; *UTI*, urinary tract infection.

renal vein thrombosis is suspected.
- Cystoscopy: if urological malignancy is suspected.

Groin lump

Groin lump or swelling is a common surgical presentation. While it may be benign, there are several significant pathologies that can present with a groin lump (Fig. 7.13).

CLINICAL NOTES

A thorough examination of the lump, a hernia exam, a testicular exam, external genitalia, digital rectal and abdominal exam, is an essential first step.

Investigations for a groin lump

1. Bedside
   - Urinalysis: MC&S should be sent in infective pathology to confirm the diagnosis and guide antibiotic therapy.
   - STI testing: if an STI is suspected as the cause of groin swelling.
2. Bloods
   - FBC: ↓Hb is associated with anaemia in malignancy. ↑ WCC indicates infective pathology.

- Tumour markers: ↑ AFP, b-HCG and LDH may indicate testicular malignancy.
- HIV test: HIV infection may cause painful inguinal lymphadenitis.
3. Imaging
   - US abdomen/groin/testes: to differentiate between solid or cystic masses, or those containing intestinal contents.
   - CTCAP: for staging in malignancy, or to detect hernias not visible on ultrasound.
   - Excisional biopsy: for histological diagnosis in suspected malignancy.

RED FLAG

Testicular torsion presents with:
- Sudden testicular swelling and pain
- Lower abdominal pain
- Hemiscrotal elevation with a transverse testes
It is a urological emergency. Urgent scrotal exploration in high clinical suspicion is indicated, without waiting for confirmatory investigations.

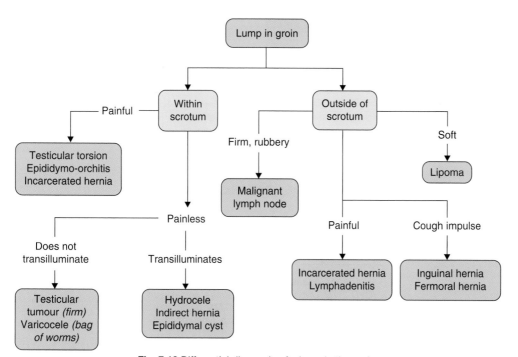

Fig. 7.13 Differential diagnosis of a lump in the groin.

Male reproductive dysfunction

While there is a range of urological pathologies that can manifest with male reproductive dysfunction, the differential diagnosis remains broad and includes a range of psychiatric, cardiovascular, endocrine and neurological causes (Fig. 7.14).

COMMUNICATION

- Psychogenic sexual dysfunction is typically acute in onset, and manifests during sexual intercourse, not independently. There may be a background of relationship issues.
- Organic sexual dysfunction is typically gradual in onset, occurs in all sexual scenarios, and follows a constant course.

Investigations for male reproductive dysfunction

1. Bedside
   - Semen analysis: the first-line test in the assessment of infertility.
   - Capillary blood glucose (CBG): to screen for diabetes.
   - Urine dip: haematuria may indicate urological trauma or malignancy.
2. Bloods
   - U&Es: to screen for acute or chronic renal impairment.
   - PSA: if prostate pathology is suspected.
   - HbA1c: to accurately assess long-term blood glucose control.
   - Fasting lipids: ↑ in cardiovascular disease.
   - Hormone assays: to screen for underlying endocrine disturbance if there are relevant associated symptoms.
   - Autoimmune screen: autoantibodies can detect underlying connective tissue disease.
3. Imaging
   - US bladder/prostate/testes: if urological, prostate or scrotal pathology is suspected.

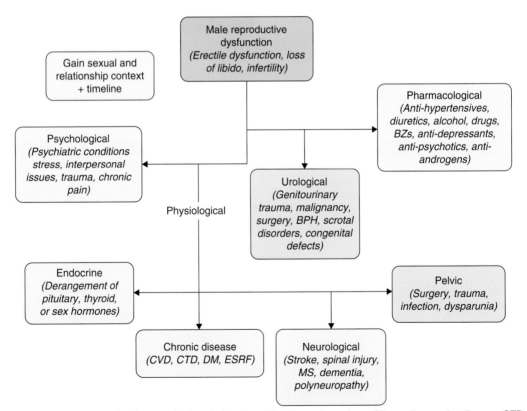

Fig. 7.14 Differential diagnosis of male reproductive dysfunction. *BZs*, Benzodiazepines; *CD*, cardiovascular disease; *CTD*, connective tissue disease; *DM*, diabetes mellitus; *ESRF*, end-stage renal failure; *MS*, multiple sclerosis.

- CT pelvis: to characterize obstructive or malignant pathology.
- Cystoscopy: to accurately visualize lesions of the urinary tract and take tissue biopsies for histology.

UROLOGICAL EXAMINATION

HINTS AND TIPS

The acronym **WIPER** can be used to prepare for the exam:

- **W** – **W**ash your hands
- **I** – **I**ntroduce yourself
- **P** – **P**atient details
- **E** – **E**xplain the procedure and **E**xpose appropriately
- **R** – **R**eposition patient

General inspection

Inspect the patient from the end of the bed:

- Pallor: may suggest anaemia, associated with bleeding and malignancy.
- Cachexia: significant muscle wasting associated with malignancy.
- Peripheral oedema: lower limb or abdominal swelling is associated with renal, hepatic and cardiovascular pathology.

Fluid status assessment

It is important to assess fluid status in renal or urological pathology to identify dehydration or fluid overload.

- Capillary refill time: delayed if hypovolaemic.

- Observations: tachycardia and hypotension may indicate dehydration or hypovolemia.
- Mucous membranes: dry mucous membranes indicate dehydration.
- Skin turgor: well-hydrated skin should spring back when pinched. A slow return to normal (reduced skin turgor) indicates dehydration.
- Oedema: pedal, sacral or abdominal oedema (ascites).
- JVP: a raised JVP indicates fluid overload.

Abdominal examination

Examination of the abdomen should be performed:

- Loin pain: loin-to-groin pain is a key feature of infective or inflammatory pathology.
- Suprapubic pain: common in lower urinary tract pathology including infections or retention, and radiation of scrotal pathology.
- Renal angle tenderness: pain elicited on percussion of the 12th rib on the back, that suggests renal pathology including pyelonephritis or ureteric calculi.
- Distention: lower abdominal distention may suggest urinary retention or malignancy.
- Masses: balloting the kidneys may indicate enlargement or a mass. A transplanted kidney will be palpable in the right iliac fossa.
- Scars: associated with previous abdominal surgery.
- Shifting dullness: indicates free fluid in the abdomen (ascites).

Completing the examination

Wash your hands, thank the patient and perform further examinations if required:

- Testicular exam: essential in the assessment of a male with scrotal or groin symptoms.
- Vaginal exam: may reveal pelvic organ prolapse, a pelvic mass or vaginal bleed.
- Digital rectal examination: to identify prostate pathology (Fig. 7.15).

HINTS AND TIPS

- A vaginal and rectal examination is essential.
- The close anatomical relations of the genitourinary and intestinal organs often result overlapping clinical syndromes.

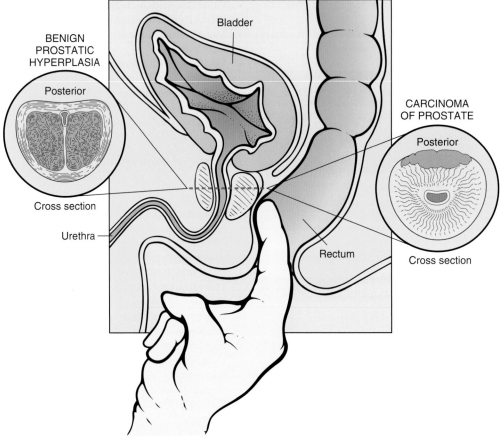

Fig. 7.15 Prostate pathology on digital rectal examination. (A) The normal prostate should be smooth, the size of a walnut, with a palpable central sulcus. (B) BPH, with an asymmetrically enlarged prostate. The central sulcus may be lost. (C) An asymmetrical nodular prostate, likely representing malignancy. (From ICD-10-CM/PCS. *Coding: Theory and Practice,* 1st Edition. Elsevier; 2023.)

Testicular exam

Introduction

Wash your hands, introduce yourself and gain consent to proceed.

COMMUNICATION

Gaining informed consent for an intimate examination is essential. Explain what the examination will involve and that a chaperone will be present, and ensure the patient is happy before proceeding.

General inspection

General inspection can indicate signs of underlying pathology:

- Pain: pain or discomfort may be evident from the end of the bed.
- Abdominal distension: may be present in urinary retention or mass.
- Cachexia: muscle wasting is associated with underlying malignancy.
- Pallor: anaemia of chronic disease can occur in malignancy.
- Equipment: note any medications, monitoring devices or mobility aids, that may suggest underlying comorbidities and baseline functional status.

Groin inspection

Inspect the external genitalia, perineum and lower abdomen.

- Swelling: oedema, masses or hernias may present as a visible lump or swelling.
- Skin changes: note any erythema, ulcers, lesions or scars. A red itchy rash may suggest fungal infection, and scars from previous abdominal or scrotal surgery.

- Scrotal position: one testis typically hangs marginally lower than the other.
- Cremasteric reflex: stroking the skin of the inner thigh causes cremaster muscle contraction and elevation of the ipsilateral testicle toward the inguinal canal.

> **COMMUNICATION**
>
> - Ask the patient to lift their penis out of the way, rather than doing so yourself.
> - It will make the patient feel more comfortable and frees up both of your hands to examine the scrotum.

Palpation

Penis

Retract the foreskin (if uncircumcised), and inspect the glans penis:

- Skin: assess for penile ulcers, warts, discharge or erythema.
- Foreskin: should be easily retracted and replaced. A tight unretractable foreskin suggests phimosis.

Testicles

If there is pain or pathology, inspect the normal testicle first.

- Anchor the scrotum and contralateral testis with your other hand.
- Place your thumb and index finger around the testicle and immobilize the testicle with your remaining fingers.
- Roll the testicle between your thumb and index finger to examine the whole surface systematically.

> **CLINICAL NOTES**
>
> - If you cannot locate the testes they may be undescended.
> - Palpate along the path of the inguinal ligament to locate the testes.

If a mass is identified:

- Characteristics: assess the site, size, shape, consistency, fluctuance and tenderness.
- Transillumination: A transilluminable mass suggests fluid.
- Cough impulse: exacerbation of the lump with coughing suggests hernia or varicocele.
- Reducibility: a reducible lump suggests hernia.

- Palpate above the lump: an ability to palpate above the lump suggests scrotal mass, rather than hernia.

> **HINTS AND TIPS**
>
> - A varicocele feels like a 'bag of worms'. The testis is palpable through it.
> - A hydrocele transilluminates and the testes are not usually palpable.
> - An incarcerated hernia will not be reducible nor exacerbated with coughing and will be painful.

> **CLINICAL NOTES**
>
> - Ask the patient to lay flat to assess for spontaneous reduction.
> - If the lump is still present, ask the patient to manually reduce it.
> - Hernias may reappear upon cessation of pressure, standing or coughing.

Further palpation includes:

- Epididymis: tenderness suggests epididymitis. A palpable lump separate from the testes is likely to represent an epididymal cyst.
- Spermatic cord: palpable from the superior aspect of the testicle. Assess for masses and tenderness.

Completing the examination

Thank the patient and offer them privacy to get dressed. Further assessments include:

- Abdominal examination: a complete abdominal examination should be performed.
- Digital rectal examination: to assess for associated prostate pathology.
- Ultrasound abdomen/testis: for assessment of any masses identified.

UROLOGICAL DISORDERS

Urinary tract infection

Urinary tract infections (UTIs) are infections of the urinary system. Lower UTIs describe infection of the bladder and urethra, known as cystitis, and upper UTIs involve the kidneys and ureters, known as pyelonephritis. They are very common, particularly in females, and may be recurrent. E.coli is the most common cause (Table 7.1).

Symptoms and signs

Features of lower UTIs include:

- Dysuria
- Increased urinary frequency and urgency
- Malodorous, concentrated urine
- Haematuria
- Suprapubic tenderness

Pyelonephritis (upper UTI) presents with:

- Fever
- Loin pain/renal angle tenderness
- Lethargy and malaise
- Nausea and vomiting

RED FLAG

- Pyelonephritis is a medical emergency, due to the risk of urosepsis.
- Vulnerable groups may present atypically and are at high risk of mortality.
- Suspect urinary infection in elderly patients with acute delirium or altered mental status.

Table 7.1 Risk factors for the development of UTIs

Pathophysiology	Aetiology
Obstructed urinary flow	BPH, renal stones, ureteric stricture Constipation, pelvic/abdominal mass
Urinary stasis	VUR, urinary retention, neurogenic bladder Dehydration
Introduction of bacteria	Poor hygiene, sexual intercourse, catheters Female anatomy (shorter urethra)
Susceptibility to infection	Immunosuppression (HIV, steroids, diabetes, age, malnutrition)
Hormonal changes	Pregnancy, postmenopause, contraception changes

BPH, *Benign prostatic hyperplasia*; VUR, *vesicoureteric reflux*.

Investigations

Symptomatic, uncomplicated UTIs are a clinical diagnosis and can be empirically treated.

Further investigations include:

- Urine dipstick: nitrites, leucocytes and RBCs indicate likely infection.
- Urine MC&S: for complicated UTIs, atypical symptoms or unclear diagnoses.
- Urinary tract imaging: if there is evidence of complications or underlying pathology (Figs. 7.16–7.17).

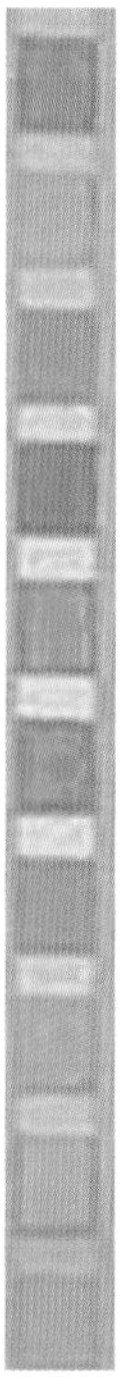

Glucose mmol/L	N	5.5	17	55		
Bilirubin	N	+	++	+++		
Ketones mg/dL	N	0.5	1.5	5	15	
Specific gravity	1	1.05	1.01	1.02	1.025	1.03
RBCs ery/µL	N	5-10	10	25	50	250
pH	5.0	6.0	6.5	7.0	8.0	9.0
Protein mg/dL	N	15	30	100	300	1000
Urobilin mg/dL	N	1	4	8	12	
Nitrites	N	+	++			
leuko leuko/µL	N	15	75	125	500	

Fig. 7.16 Urine dipstick findings

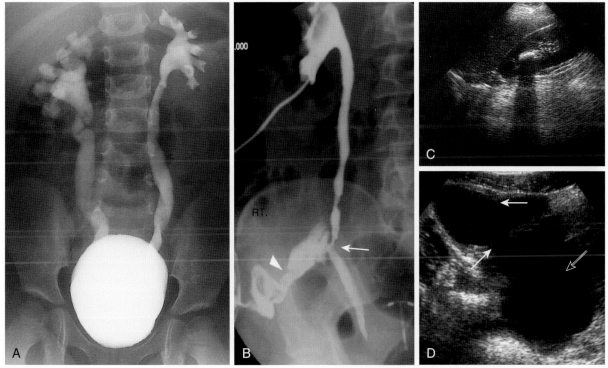

Fig. 7.17 Imaging findings in urinary pathology predisposing to UTIs. (A) Micturating cystourethrogram showing bilateral vesicoureteric reflux. (B) Antegrade pyelogram of a renal TB patient showing a ureteric stricture (*arrow*) and a fistulous tract to the skin (*arrowhead*). Renal TB is associated with HIV infection, which is another cause of recurrent UTIs. (C) Ultrasound demonstrating large renal calculus. (D) Transabdominal ultrasound shows a large diverticulum with a wide neck arising from the urinary bladder. (From A. Carroll W, Lissauer T. *Illustrated Textbook of Paediatrics,* 6th Edition. Elsevier; 2022. B. Multimodality imaging of genitourinary tuberculosis. Radwan A, Menias CO, El-Diasty MT, Etchison AR, Elshikh M, Consul N, Nassar S, Elsayes KM. Multimodality Imaging of Genitourinary Tuberculosis. *Curr Probl Diagn Radiol.* 2021;50(6):867-883. https://doi.10.1067/j.cpradiol.2020.10.005. Epub 2020 Nov 15. PMID: 33272721. C. Kowalczyk N. *Radiographic Pathology for Technologists,* 8th Edition. Elsevier; 2022. D. Kamaya A, Wong-You-Cheong J. *Diagnostic Ultrasound: Abdomen & Pelvis,* 2nd Edition. Elsevier; 2022.)

COMMON PITFALLS

- Asymptomatic bacteriuria is common in elderly and catheterized patients.
- It represents colonization rather than infection and does not typically require treatment, unless there are specific vulnerabilities or immunocompromise.

Management

Conservative management includes avoiding dehydration, good genital hygiene, timing bladder emptying and postcoital voiding.

Medical management includes:

- Uncomplicated lower UTIs: empirical antibiotic therapy according to local guidelines (typically nitrofurantoin/trimethoprim for 3 days).
- Complicated lower UTIs: broad-spectrum antibiotics for 7 to 14 days.
- Recurrent UTIs: prophylactic antibiotics taken daily for up to 1 year.

- Catheter-associated UTI (CAUTI): catheter removal/replacement, and antibiotics.

mechanical obstruction or functional voiding impairment (Table 7.2, Fig. 7.19).

Urinary incontinence

Urinary incontinence is the involuntary leakage of urine. It is relatively common, particularly in older females. There are several underlying risk factors and aetiologies. Adequate and timely management is essential due to the negative psychological and social effects (Table 7.3).

Complications

- Pyelonephritis: infection of the renal parenchyma from ascending urinary infection (Fig. 7.18).
- Acute urinary retention: severe ascending infection can result in retention.
- Perinephric/renal abscess: collections can develop as a complication of pyelonephritis.
- Urosepsis: systemic inflammatory response can result in sepsis.
- Renal papillary necrosis: AKI with necrosis of the renal parenchyma typically relating to pyelonephritis or obstruction.
- Fournier's gangrene: necrotizing fasciitis of the external genitalia, which can occur as a complication of UTIs in older males or immunocompromised hosts.

Urinary retention

Urinary retention describes an inability to voluntarily empty the bladder. It can develop acutely, or chronically, relating to

Management

Benign transient causes including UTI and constipation should be identified and treated to rapidly alleviate symptoms.

Conservative management is trialled initially.

- Treatment of cause: treatment of associated UTI or constipation if identified.

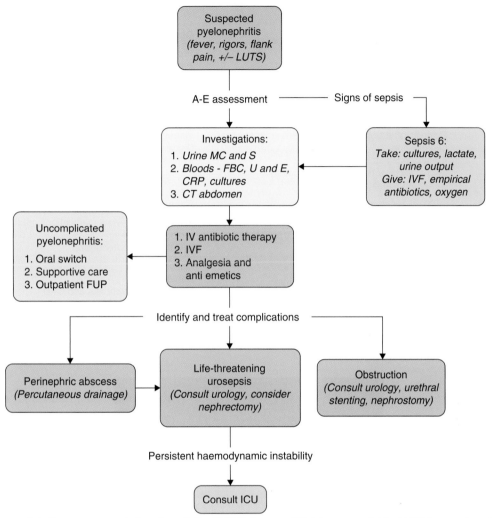

Fig. 7.18 Approach to the management of pyelonephritis. *FUP*, Follow-up; *IVF*, intravenous fluids; *LUTS*, lower urinary tract symptoms; *MC&S*, microscopy culture and sensitivity.

- Lifestyle changes: weight loss, smoking cessation, reducing alcohol and caffeine, reducing excess fluid intake.
- Manage comorbidities: uncontrolled diabetes or chronic cough can worsen symptoms.
- Medication review: to evaluate and consider removal of triggering medications.
- Pelvic floor exercises: pelvic floor weakness often occurs postpartum and manifests as stress incontinence.
- Bladder training: timed voiding to increase intervals, relaxation techniques.

CLINICAL NOTES

- Nocturnal enuresis (bedwetting) is the involuntary release of urine at night.
- It is common and typically resolves spontaneously before 5 years of age.
- Bedwetting persisting beyond this can be managed with fluid restriction, behavioural modification, and in refractory cases, desmopressin or an enuresis alarm.

Table 7.2 Acute versus chronic urinary retention

	Acute	Chronic
Clinical features	Sudden, painful inability to void Suprapubic pain Palpable bladder Agitation	Progressive painless difficulty emptying the bladder Palpable bladder Overflow incontinence/ nocturnal enuresis
Aetiology	Intrinsic obstruction – BPH, malignancy, calculi, stricture, clot Extrinsic obstruction – pelvic organ prolapse/mass, constipation Postoperative retention Medication – anticholinergics, opioids, sympathomimetics	Mechanical obstruction – BPH, cancer Neurogenic bladder- SCC/CES, stroke, MS, PD, diabetic neuropathy, splanchnic nerve trauma Medication – anticholinergics, opioids, sympathomimetics
US findings	>400 mL residual volume	PV residual volume >300 mL
Management	Urgent catheterization Treat cause – review medications, treat obstruction	Treat cause – review medications, treat obstruction, urological stenting LTC if refractory/recurrent
Complications	Obstructive nephropathy AKI and acute renal failure Postobstructive diuresis	Recurrent UTIs Renal stones Hydroureteronephrosis and CKD Overflow incontinence

BPH, *Benign prostate hyperplasia;* CES, *cauda equina syndrome;* CCBs, *calcium channel blockers;* LTC, *long-term catheter;* MS, *multiple sclerosis;* PD, *Parkinson disease;* PV, *postvoid;* SCC, *spinal cord compression;* TCAs, *tricyclic antidepressants.*

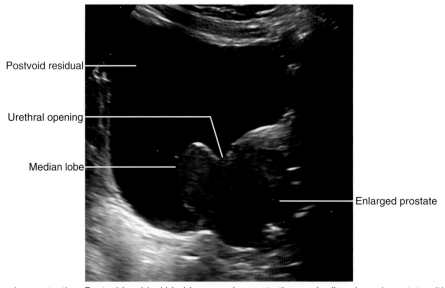

Postvoid residual

Urethral opening

Median lobe

Enlarged prostate

Fig. 7.19 Chronic urinary retention. Postvoid residual bladder scan demonstrating markedly enlarged prostate with a hypertrophied median lobe projecting into the bladder, and significant postvoid residual volume. (From Kamaya A, Wong-You-Cheong J, Woodward PJ. *Diagnostic Ultrasound for Sonographers*. Elsevier; 2019.)

Table 7.3 Types of urinary incontinence

	Stress	Urge	Overflow
Clinical features	Involuntary urinary leakage upon ↑ intraabdominal pressure (coughing, sneezing, exercising)	Sudden urgency, involuntary urine leakage	Involuntary dribbling of urine when bladder full, no urinary urge Postvoid residual volume
Aetiology	Urethral dysfunction – weak pelvic floor muscles, sphincter weakness (ageing, obesity, trauma)	Detrusor overactivity OAB Neurogenic bladder	Impaired detrusor contractility Neurogenic bladder Medications Bladder outlet obstruction
Urinary stress test	Leakage with Valsalva	Delayed leakage	No leakage
Postvoid residual volume	<50 mL	<50 mL	>200 mL

The urinary stress test involves introduction of water into the bladder via catheter. The catheter is removed, and the patient performed a Valsalva manoeuvre. If involuntary leakage of urine occurs, the type of incontinence can be diagnosed. BPH, Benign prostate hypertrophy; CTD, connective tissue disease; OAB, overactive bladder.

Type-specific management is initiated if conservative measures have failed after 6 to 8 weeks:

- Stress incontinence: vaginal pessaries, urethral slings, colposuspension.
- Urge incontinence: muscarinic antagonists (oxybutynin), sympathomimetics (mirabegron).
- Botox injections.
- Overflow incontinence: Intermittent catheterization, treat obstruction, muscarinic agonists (bethanechol).

COMMON PITFALLS

- Medical options for incontinence have several side effects.
- Oxybutynin and mirabegron can cause urinary retention, and bethanechol can lead to urinary urgency.
- All should be used with caution, with close monitoring for side effects.

RED FLAG

Red flags in incontinence which are indications for urological referral include:
- Pain
- Haematuria or proteinuria
- Significant postvoid residual volume
- Obstructive symptoms
- Pelvic organ prolapse
- Recurrent UTIs

Urinary tract calculi

Urinary tract calculi, also known as nephrolithiasis or renal/ureteric stones, is the formation of calculi along the urogenital tract. They have a range of compositions, relating to underlying risk factors. Risk factors include dehydration, loop diuretics and high-sodium diets (Table 7.4, Fig. 7.20).

HINTS AND TIPS

Uric acid stones are radiolUcent, and cannot be seen on X-ray

Signs and symptoms

Small stones may be asymptomatic and diagnosed incidentally on abdominal imaging. Larger stones produce symptoms, related to urinary obstruction and local inflammation:

- Renal colic: severe, paroxysmal, unilateral loin to groin pain.
- LUTS: dysuria, frequency or urgency.
- Agitation: extreme restlessness and inability to lie still.
- Haematuria: micro or macroscopic relating to the size of stones.
- Nausea and vomiting: due to severe pain.

Investigations

Investigations include:

- Urinalysis: to confirm haematuria. Urinary pH can indicate the likely stone composition.
- FBC: ↑ WBC suggests associated infection.
- U&Es: ↑urea/creatinine indicates development of obstructive AKI.

Table 7.4 Urinary calculi composition

Stone type	Aetiology	Investigations	Management
Calcium oxalate (75%)	Hypercalciuria Hyperoxaluria Antifreeze poisoning Malabsorptive conditions – IBD	Radiopaque ↓ Urine pH	Hydration Low sodium, protein and oxalate diet Thiazide diuretics Urine alkalinization
Uric acid (10%)	Gout, hyperuricemia High cell turnover – leukaemia, chemotherapy	Radiolucent ↓ Urine pH	Hydration Low purine diet Allopurinol Urine alkalinization
Struvite (5%–10%)	UTI with urease-producing bacteria Indwelling catheters	Weakly radiopaque ↑Urine pH	Treat UTI Hydration Urine acidification Surgical removal
Calcium phosphate (<5%)	Hyperparathyroidism Type 1 RTA	Radiopaque ↑Urine pH	Hydration Low sodium diet Thiazide diuretics Urine acidification
Cystine (<5%)	Hereditary – cystinuria	Weakly radiopaque ↓ Urine pH	Hydration Low sodium diet Urine alkalinization
Xanthine (<5%)	Hereditary – xanthinuria	Radiolucent	Low purine diet

IBD, *Inflammatory bowel disease;* RTA, *renal tubular acidosis.*

- CTAP: to confirm the diagnosis, locate the stone and exclude other pathology.

Management

Symptomatic renal stones or those associated with complications should be managed with an A–E approach with approach resuscitation before definitive interventions are performed (Table 7.5, Fig. 7.21).

HINTS AND TIPS

- NSAIDs (typically PR diclofenac) are the preferred analgesia in renal colic.
- They decrease ureteric peristalsis, oedema and renal pressure via reducing GFR.

Complications

Complications include:

- Infection: pyelonephritis, urosepsis and renal parenchymal/perinephric abscesses.

- AKI: obstructive nephropathy can result in AKI.
- Hydronephrosis: obstruction can result in hydronephrosis, which without treatment, can result in permanent glomerular injury and CKD.
- CKD: recurrent obstructed stones and AKIs can predispose to the development of CKD.

RED FLAG

- Obstructed infected stones are a surgical emergency, risking permanent glomerular injury, urosepsis and death.
- Urgent surgical extraction is required.

Urinary tract cancer

Urinary tract cancer most commonly develops in the bladder. Rarely, it can develop in the renal pelvis, ureters or urethra. The most common histological subtype is transitional cell carcinoma (TCC), although squamous cell carcinoma and adenocarcinoma can also occur. Risk factors include smoking, amine exposure (dyes and rubber), recurrent UTIs/renal stones and long-term catheters.

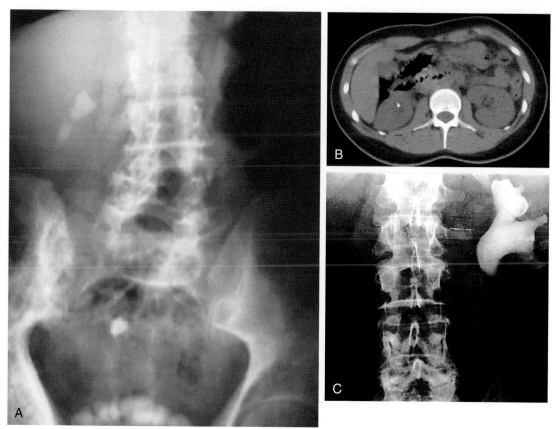

Fig. 7.20 Nephrolithiasis. (A) Right-sided renal stones on plain X-ray film. (B) CTKUB with a large stone in the renal pelvis of the right kidney. (C) A large staghorn calculus in the calyces of the left renal pelvis. (From A. Used with permission from Melmed S, et al. *Williams Textbook of Endocrinology*. 14th Edition: South Asia Edition, 2 Vol SET. Elsevier; 2020. B. Dighe M, Grajo JR, Lee L. *Abdominal Imaging*. Elsevier; 2022. C. Talley N, O'Connor S. *Talley and O'Connor's Clinical Examination – 2-Volume Set,* 9th Edition. Elsevier; 2022.)

Table 7.5 Surgical management options for renal stones

Intervention	Description	Indication
Extracorporeal shock wave lithotripsy (ESWL)	Noninvasive acoustic shockwave therapy to fragment stones and encourage passage	Ureteral stones Renal stones <20 mm Lower renal pole stones <10 mm
Ureterorenoscopy (URS)	Transurethral flexible/rigid cystoscopy with stone extraction and intraurethral lithotripsy	
Percutaneous nephrostomy (PCN)	Percutaneous insertion of a catheter into renal pelvis to drain obstruction	Temporizing drainage in infected/obstructed kidney
Percutaneous nephrolithotomy (PCNL)	Percutaneous nephroscopy and stone removal +/– lithotripsy	Renal stones <20 mm Lower renal pole stones >10 mm
Ureterolithotomy	Ureteral incision and manual stone removal	Failure of other interventions

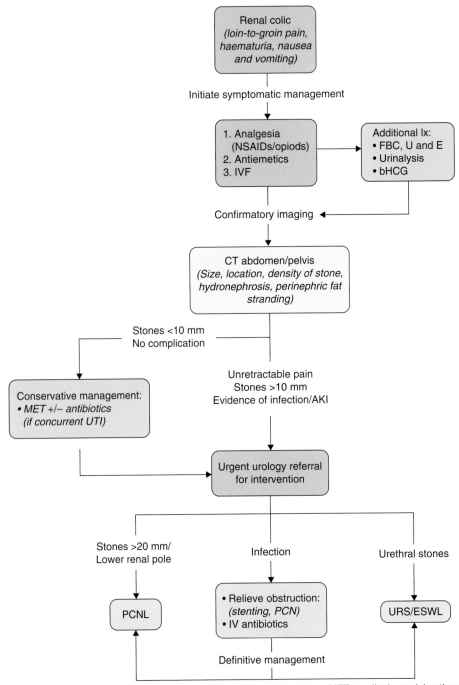

Fig. 7.21 Management of renal stones. *ESWL*, extracorporeal shock wave lithotripsy; *MET*, medical expulsive therapy, typically with tamsulosin or nifedipine; *PCN*, percutaneous nephrostomy; *PCNL*, percutaneous nephrolithotomy; *URS*, ureterorenoscopy.

Symptoms and signs

Urinary tract cancer initially presents with painless visible haematuria. Other features include:

- LUTS: dysuria, frequency, urgency and nocturia.
- Urinary retention: acute or chronic retention secondary to bladder outlet obstruction.
- Abdominal pain: suprapubic, perineal or loin pain.
- Palpable mass: relating to the location of the lesion.
- Constitutional features: fevers, lethargy, appetite and weight loss, night sweats.

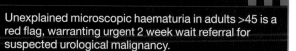

RED FLAG

Unexplained microscopic haematuria in adults >45 is a red flag, warranting urgent 2 week wait referral for suspected urological malignancy.

Investigations

Investigations include:

- Urinalysis: to confirm haematuria and exclude infective/inflammatory pathology.
- Bloods: FBC, U&Es, LFTs and bone profile.
- Urological imaging studies: CT or MR urography, or urinary US.
- Cystoscopy and biopsy: to confirm the diagnosis and take samples for histology.
- CT TAP: for staging and detection of metastasis, most common in the liver, lung or bone (Figs. 7.22–7.23).

Management

The management of all cancer should follow an MDT approach, prioritizing the patient's wishes and considering realistic goals of treatment.

Surgical management includes:

- Radical cystectomy with pelvic lymph node dissection: urinary diversion is required typically via stoma or bladder reconstruction.
- Transurethral resection of the bladder tumour (TURBT): bladder preserving.
- Neoadjuvant platinum-based chemotherapy: used alongside all surgical management.

Metastatic disease is managed with platinum-based palliative chemotherapy, with immunotherapy, radiation therapy and surgery considered for symptomatic management.

Recurrence is common, and patients should be followed up regularly to assess for new urinary symptoms.

Renal cell carcinoma

Renal cell carcinoma (RCC) is the most common renal malignancy. It arises sporadically, relating to risk factors including smoking, obesity, hypertension, chronic nephrolithiasis and long-term heavy paracetamol use. Predisposing genetic conditions account for a small minority of cases, including Von-Hippel-Lindau syndrome, tuberous sclerosis and hereditary renal cell carcinoma.

Symptoms and signs

RCC is typically asymptomatic. Symptomatic patients present with a classic triad:

- Haematuria
- Loin pain
- Palpable abdominal mass

DIFFERENTIALS

- A nephroblastoma (Wilms tumour) is the most common renal malignancy in children.
- Symptoms include abdominal mass, failure to thrive and haematuria.
- There is a 90% cure rate with surgery and chemoradiotherapy.

CLINICAL NOTES

An unexplained left varicocele may represent malignant obstruction of the left rein vein, into which the left gonadal vein drains.

Investigations

Most RCCs are detected incidentally on unrelated abdominal imaging (Fig. 7.24).

Further investigations include:

- Urinalysis: may demonstrate haematuria and proteinuria.
- Bloods: FBC, U&Es, LFTs, bone profile and hormone assays to screen for renal impairment, paraneoplastic phenomena and metastatic disease.
- Imaging: further imaging of the liver, lungs and bone to diagnose metastasis (Fig. 7.25).

Management

Management relates to the extent of disease:

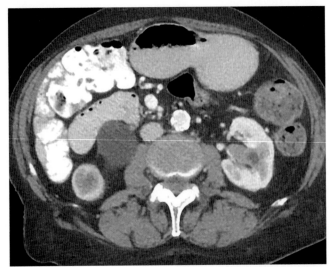

Fig. 7.22 Transitional cell carcinoma (TCC) on CT urography. Large TCC in the urinary bladder on CT urography. A mass extends into the lower left pelvis, with significant filling defect and mural thickening. (From Grajo JR, Lee LK, Dighe MK. *Abdominal Imaging: Case Review Series*. Elsevier; 2022.)

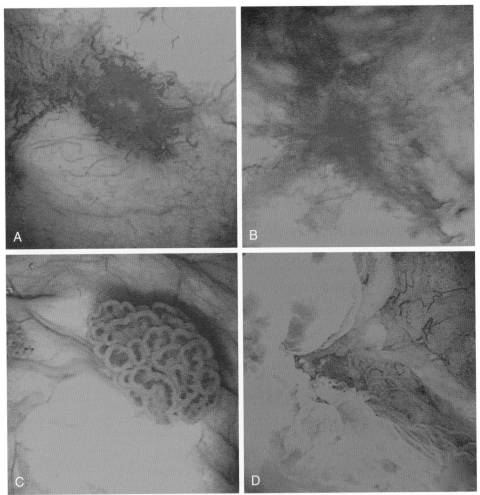

Fig. 7.23 Cystoscopy findings in transitional cell carcinoma. Cystoscopy may demonstrate single or multiple lesions, with a papillary or nodular appearance. (A) Radiation cystitis following high-dose pelvic radiation. (B) A flat erythematous area may indicate carcinoma in situ. (C) Low-grade papillary bladder tumour. (D) Muscle-invasive bladder tumour. (From Frank SJ, Cox JD, Ang KK. *Radiation Oncology: Rationale, Technique, Results,* 9th Edition. Elsevier; 2010.)

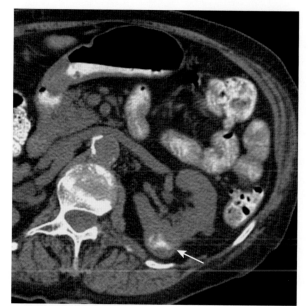

Fig. 7.24 RCC on CT abdomen. Dystrophic calcification is seen in a left kidney, with distortion of the renal outline and thickened irregular walls, diagnosed as a renal cell carcinoma. (From Silverman PM. *Oncologic Imaging: A Multidisciplinary Approach,* 2nd Edition. Saunders, Elsevier Inc. 2022.)

- Local disease: radical nephrectomy, which may be curative.
- Metastatic disease: palliation, with targeted immunotherapies and surgical debulking for symptomatic management.

CLINICAL NOTES

- A radical nephrectomy includes removal of the kidney, adrenal glands and surrounding perinephric fat, +/– locoregional lymph node dissection.
- Radiochemotherapy is not typically used, as most RCCs are radio- and chemo-resistant.

There are several paraneoplastic syndromes related to RCC, which manifest with symptoms related to the underlying hormonal derangement. The management is symptomatic until definitive nephrectomy is performed.

HINTS AND TIPS

Paraneoplastic syndromes associated with RCC include:

- P – secondary Polycythaemia (EPO)
- R – Renin (hypertension)
- C – hyperCalcaemia (PTHrP)
- C – hyperCortisolism (ACTH)

Renal transplant

Renal transplant may be indicated for patients with end-stage renal failure (ESRF) (GFR <15 mL/min or on dialysis). The donor kidney is typically transplanted into the right iliac fossa, with vascular anastomoses to the inguinal vessels (Figs. 7.26–7.27).

CLINICAL NOTES

- Living donors must have two healthy kidneys before donation.
- Any comorbidities that may damage the kidneys (i.e., diabetes, hypertension) are absolute contraindications.

There are several potential complications of a transplant:

- Acute tubular necrosis
- Renal artery thrombosis or stenosis
- Urological leakage or obstruction
- Graft complications: graft rejection and graft versus host disease
- Complications of immunosuppression: infection, posttransplant malignancy (Tables 7.6–7.7)

HINTS AND TIPS

Renal transplant has a better prognosis than dialysis in ESRF.

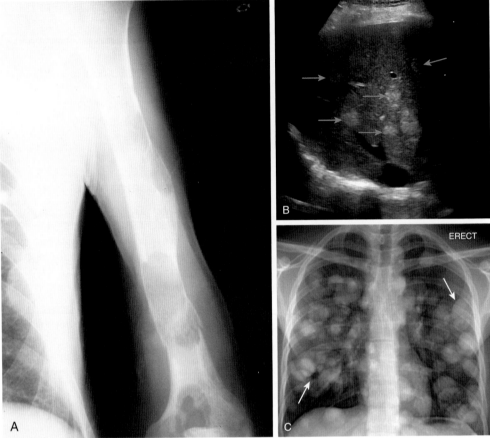

Fig. 7.25 Metastatic RCC. (A) Several lytic lesions are present throughout the humerus. (B) Liver US showing numerous hyperechoic, rounded metastases. (C) Multifocal lung nodules and masses. Note the well-circumscribed, round, 'cannonball' metastases. (From A. Washington CM, et al. *Washington and Leaver's Principles and Practice of Radiation Therapy,* 5th Edition. Elsevier; 2021. B. Kamaya A, Wong-You-Cheong J. *Diagnostic Ultrasound: Abdomen & Pelvis,* 2nd Edition. Elsevier; 2022. C. Uncommon thoracic manifestations from extrapulmonary tumors: Computed tomography evaluation – Pictorial review. Franquet T, Rosado-de-Christenson ML, Marchiori E, Abbott GF, Martínez-Jiménez S, López L. Uncommon thoracic manifestations from extrapulmonary tumors: Computed tomography evaluation - Pictorial review. *Respir Med.* 2020;168:105986. https://doi.10.1016/j.rmed.2020.105986. Epub 2020 Apr 28. PMID: 32469707.)

PROSTATE DISORDERS

Benign prostatic hyperplasia

Benign prostatic hyperplasia (BPH) is the benign growth of the transitional zone of the prostate. It is common, affecting nearly half the male population in older adulthood. It is thought to relate to declining testosterone levels and an increased oestrogen/testosterone ratio.

Symptoms and signs

The key features of BPH include LUTS:

- Storage: frequency, urgency, urge incontinence, nocturia (+/– dysuria).
- Voiding: hesitancy, straining, poor stream, terminal dribbling, incomplete emptying.

HINTS AND TIPS

- Recurrent gross haematuria can develop due to increased vascularity of the hyperplastic gland.
- Appropriate investigations to exclude underlying malignancy should be arranged, even if BPH is suspected as the underlying diagnosis.

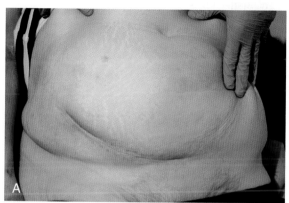

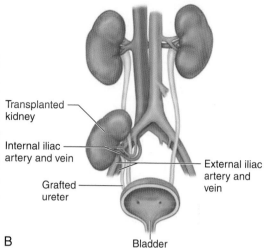

Fig. 7.26 Renal transplant. (A) Surgical scar from a renal transplant. (B) Surgical placement of transplanted kidney. (From A. Dover AR, et al. *Macleod's Clinical Examination*, 15th Edition. Elsevier; 2024. B. Dennison HA, Harding MM. *Lewis's Medical-Surgical Nursing: Assessment and Management of Clinical Problems*, 12th Edition. Elsevier; 2023.)

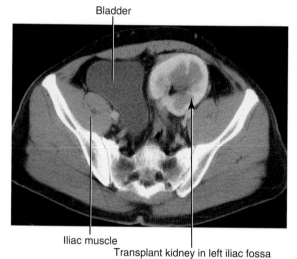

Fig. 7.27 Kidney transplant on CT scan. (From Vogl AW, Mitchell AWM, Drake RL. *Gray's Basic Anatomy*. Churchill Livingstone, Elsevier Inc. 2013.)

A DRE will demonstrate an asymmetrically enlarged, smooth, nontender prostate, with a firm, rubbery texture.

Investigations

Investigations include:

- Urinalysis: to rule out other causes of LUTS.
- Voiding diary: including urinary frequency-volume chart, fluid intake, sleep disturbance and episodes of incontinence.
- Multiparametric MRI: as part of a preoperative assessment.

Management

Management should be based on symptom severity (IPSS score).

- Mild symptoms: watchful waiting.
- Moderate/severe symptoms: medical therapy with alpha-blockers, 5-alpha reductase inhibitors or antimuscarinics.

Table 7.6 Graft complications

	Graft rejection		
	Hyperacute	**Acute**	**Chronic**
Onset	**<48 hours**	**<6 months**	**>6 months**
Aetiology	ABO incompatibility Type 2 hypersensitivity reaction	HLA incompatibility Inadequate immunosuppression Type 2/4 hypersensitivity reaction	Previous acute rejection Poor HLA match Inadequate immunosuppression Type 2/4 hypersensitivity reaction
Clinical features	Intraoperative swelling once perfusion is restored	Pain in the graft Graft oedema Fever and malaise ↑BP, urea and creatinine ↓Urine output	Slow, progressive worsening of kidney function
Mx	Graft removal	Immunosuppression	Graft removal

Table 7.7 Graft versus host disease

	Acute	**Chronic**
Onset	<100 days	>100 days
Aetiology	Donor T lymphocytes mount type 4 hypersensitivity reaction to the host leading to severe organ damage	Unclear ?T lymphocyte and humoral immunity mediated
Clinical features	Skin – painful maculopapular rash Intestines – vomiting, diarrhoea, abdo pain Liver – jaundice, anaemia	Skin – scleroderma skin changes Intestines – bloody diarrhoea, abdo pain, weight loss Liver – jaundice Lung – cough, wheeze, SOB Muscle – myasthenic symptoms, polymyositis
Mx	Optimize prophylaxis (cyclosporine) Systemic +/– topical steroids	Steroids cyclosporin

CLINICAL NOTES

Alpha-blockers act immediately to improve LUTS, whereas 5-alpha reductase inhibitors act over several months to gradually reduce prostate size. Antimuscarinics can aid symptoms, however, there is a risk of falls and urinary retention, particularly in older adults.

Nonpharmacological measures include:

- Medication review: opioids, TCAs and antihistamines can worsen LUTS.
- Dietary advice: reduce alcohol, caffeine and evening fluid intake.

- Bladder retraining: increasing intervals between voiding to increase bladder capacity.

Surgery can be considered if pharmacological and nonpharmacological measures fail to control symptoms:

- Transurethral resection of the prostate (TURP): cystoscopic resection of hyperplastic prostatic tissue surrounding the urethra.
- Prostatectomy: for significantly enlarged prostates.
- Transurethral incision of the prostate: minimally invasive, for moderately enlarged prostates or for patients with significant comorbidities (Fig. 7.28).

Complications

Complications include:

- Chronic urinary retention (may precipitate acute retention)

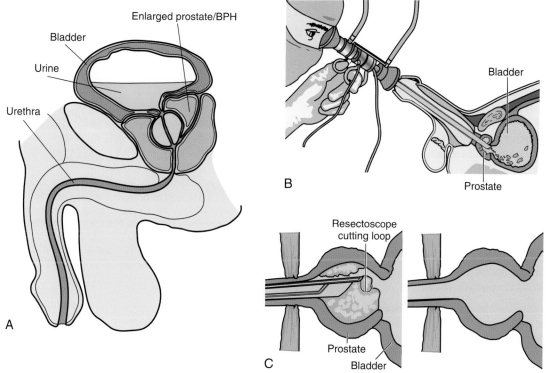

Fig. 7.28 Transurethral resection of the prostate. (A) Enlarged prostate. (B) Transurethral resection of enlarged prostate with resectoscope (TURP). (C) The obstructing prostate is removed with a cutting loop. (From Phillips N, Hornacky A. *Berry & Kohn's Operating Room Technique,* 14th Edition. Elsevier; 2022.)

- Recurrent UTIs, prostatitis
- Bladder calculi
- Hydronephrosis
- Renal impairment and CKD

Complications of surgery include:

- Sexual dysfunction: erectile dysfunction and retrograde ejaculation.
- TURP syndrome: dilutional hyponatremia due to irrigant absorption via prostatic vessels.
- Postoperative urinary retention: relating to transient bladder muscle damage.
- Recurrence: a small percentage of patients may need another procedure in later life.

HINTS AND TIPS

- BPH is not a risk factor for prostate cancer.
- The individual risk of cancer remains the same after TURP, as the peripheral zone remains intact, which is the most common site of malignancy.

CLINICAL NOTES

- Acute bacterial prostatitis typically relates to E.coli infection.
- Symptoms include fever, acute dysuria, severe back and perineal pain and a tender, boggy warm prostate.
- Complications include prostatic abscess, pyelonephritis and severe sepsis.
- Management includes antibiotic treatment for up to 6 weeks.
- Chronic prostatitis can be related to infection or noninfectious inflammation, described as chronic pelvic pain syndrome (CPPS).
- It presents as a milder form of acute prostatitis.
- Cases related to infection are treated with extended courses of antibiotics.
- CPPS is treated with alpha blockers, 5-alpha reductase inhibitors and psychological support for chronic pain.

Prostate cancer

Prostate cancer is one of the most common cancers affecting older men. A family history of prostate cancer significantly increases the risk. Predisposing genes include BRCA2 and Lynch syndrome, which are associated with earlier onset and a more aggressive course.

99% are adenocarcinomas.

Symptoms and signs

Prostate cancer is commonly asymptomatic, detected on screening or found incidentally. Symptoms indicate local spread of disease:

- Urinary retention
- Haematuria
- Urinary incontinence
- Loin pain

Advanced disease presents with constitutional symptoms and features of metastatic disease:

- Constitutional features: fevers, lethargy, anorexia, weight loss, night sweats.
- Bone pain: lumbosacral sclerotic bony metastasis are most common.
- Neurological defects: spinal cord compression related to vertebral fractures.
- Rectal symptoms: constipation, pain, bleeding, obstruction.
- Lymphoedema: metastases may obstruct lymph nodes (Fig. 7.29).

DRE findings include:

- Lobar asymmetry
- Prostatomegaly with an obliterated sulcus
- Hard, nontender nodules on an otherwise smooth surface

COMMON PITFALLS

- DRE may be normal, as most malignancies are confined to the peripheral zones.
- If there is high clinical suspicion, patients should be investigated further even if DRE is normal.

Investigations

Diagnosis is made using a combination of:

- PSA testing: to support a diagnosis and monitor response to treatment.
- Multiparametric MRI (mpMRI): to assess local tumour extent and guide staging.

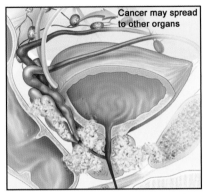

Fig. 7.29 Local spread of prostate cancer. Depiction of prostate cancer originating in the peripheral zone and spreading locally to invade neighbouring organs including the bladder, ureters, urinary sphinc'ters and bowel. (From El-Hussein MT, Zettel S, Power-Kean K, Rodway GW. *Huether and McCance's Understanding Pathophysiology,* Second Canadian Edition. Elsevier; 2023.)

- Prostate biopsy: to confirm the diagnosis and calculate the Gleason score.

PSA level:

- PSA <2.5 ng/mL: prostate cancer unlikely
- PSA <2.5–4 ng/mL: prostate cancer possible if symptomatic
- PSA 4–10 ng/mL: 25% chance of prostate cancer
- PSA >10 ng/ml: >50% chance of prostate cancer

ETHICS

- There is a range of nonmalignant conditions including BPH, prostatitis, increasing age and recent sexual activity that can raise PSA.
- 25% of men diagnosed with prostate cancer have a normal PSA.
- PSA testing may result in significant anxiety and lead to unnecessary invasive investigations.
- Patients should be counselled about this before testing.

The Gleason score is used to grade the metastatic potential of the tumour

- Grade: the degree of differentiation of the tumour cells – (1 = well differentiated, 5 = poorly differentiated).
- Score: the sum of the two most prevalent grades (Fig. 7.30).

Further imaging can detect metastatic disease, typically sclerotic bony lesions (Fig. 7.31).

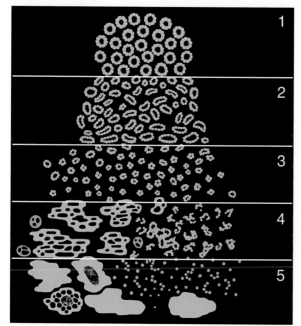

Fig. 7.30 Gleason scoring for prostate adenocarcinoma. 1 – well-differentiated cancer cells that look similar to normal cells, with slow growth. 5 – poorly differentiated cancer cells that are high risk, and likely to grow and spread quickly. (From Amin MB, Tickoo SK. *Diagnostic Pathology: Genitourinary,* 3rd Edition. Elsevier; 2022.)

Management

Management of prostate cancer depends on the tumour stage, patient life expectancy and wishes, and realistic goals of treatment.

- Low risk, limited life expectancy: watchful waiting (regular DRE/PSA).
- Low risk, good life expectancy: active surveillance (regular DRE/PSA/biopsy/mpMRI).
- Intermediate/high risk: radical prostatectomy/radiotherapy + androgen deprivation therapy (ADT).
- Locally advanced disease: ADT + antiandrogen therapy + radiotherapy.
- Metastatic disease: ADT + antiandrogen therapy + radiotherapy.

Options for radiotherapy include brachytherapy (implantable radioactive seeds) or external beam radiation (Fig. 7.32).

Complications

Complications related to local and metastatic spread or treatment side effects:

- Pathological fractures/osteoporosis: bony metastasis, or secondary to ADT.
- Sexual dysfunction: erectile dysfunction/infertility can occur after radical prostatectomy.
- Radiation proctitis: local radiotherapy increases the risk of rectal cancer.

MALE REPRODUCTIVE DISORDERS

Epididymitis

Epididymitis is the inflammation of the epididymis. Orchitis is the inflammation of the testis and can occur as a complication of epididymitis, known as epididymo-orchitis. Acute epididymitis most commonly occurs due to UTIs (typically E.coli) or STIs (typically Chlamydia trachomatis or Neisseria gonorrhoea).

Symptoms and signs

Acute epididymitis presents with:

- Unilateral scrotal pain: develops over days and can radiate to the flank.
- Skin changes: erythema and oedema.
- Fever and rigors: a low-grade fever and chills are common.
- Irritative LUTS: dysuria, frequency, urgency and urethral discharge.
- Positive Prehn sign: reduction in pain when the affected hemiscrotum is elevated (Fig. 7.33).

CLINICAL NOTES

- Chronic epididymitis can develop following multiple or incompletely treated acute epididymitis.
- Symptoms include chronic scrotal discomfort, mild swelling and a thickened epididymis.

Investigations

Epididymitis is a clinical diagnosis. Investigations are used only to guide treatment and exclude differentials:

- Urinalysis + MC&S: to identify the causative organism and tailor antibiotic therapy.
- STI testing: Nucleic acid amplification testing (NAAT) for chlamydia and gonorrhoea, VDRL testing for syphilis and blood tests for HIV.
- Testicular ultrasound: to rule out testicular torsion or scrotal abscess.

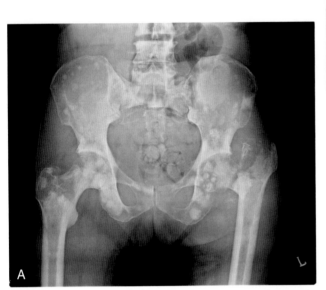

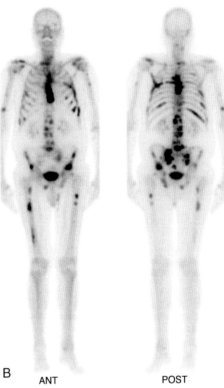

ANT   POST

Fig. 7.31 Sclerotic metastasis in prostate adenocarcinoma. (A) Sclerotic lesions in the pelvis relating to prostate cancer. (B) PET scan showing enhancing sclerotic lesions in the vertebral bodies and pelvis. (From A. Ramya Krishna, Gayathri Devi, Thanigaimani, Indhu Kannan, Rajeswari Kathiah. *Textbook of Pathology*. Elsevier; 2022. B. Thrall JH, O'Malley JP, Ziessman HA. *Nuclear Medicine and Molecular Imaging: The Requisites,* 5th Edition. Elsevier; 2020.)

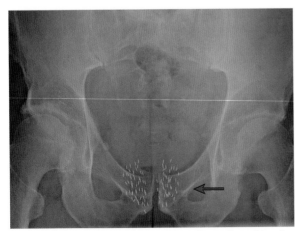

Fig. 7.32 Brachytherapy pellets on X-ray. (https://en.wikipedia. org/wiki/Brachytherapy.)

Management

Management includes:

- Empirical antibiotics: for UTI or STI, depending on the likely aetiology.
- Supportive measures: analgesia, cold packs and scrotal elevation.

Complications

Complications include:

- Epididymo-orchitis: the spread of infection from the epididymis to the testis.
- Epididymal abscess: an enclosed collection of pus in the testicular tissue.
- Chronic epididymitis: recurrent or untreated acute epididymitis can result in chronic inflammation, defined as symptoms >6 weeks.

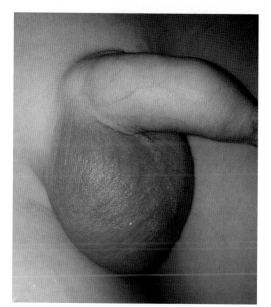

Fig. 7.33 Clinical appearance of epididymitis. The right testis is swollen and erythematous compared to the right. (From Stenzl A, Rausch S. *Elsevier Essentials. Männermedizin: Das Wichtigste für Ärztinnen und Ärzte aller Fachrichtungen.* Elsevier; 2022.)

- Sepsis: severe infection can develop in older or immunocompromised patients.
- Infertility: severe or poorly managed epididymitis can result in epididymal destruction and infertility.

Testicular torsion

Testicular torsion is the twisting of the spermatic cord. It is a urological emergency and can result in testis ischaemia and infarction without urgent identification and treatment. Risk factors include younger age, abdominal surgery, cryptorchidism, malignancy or undiagnosed bell clapper deformity (Fig. 7.34).

Symptoms and signs

Features of testicular torsion include:

- Testicular pain: sudden onset, severe, unilateral scrotal pain, radiating to the lower abdomen.
- Nausea and vomiting.
- Abnormal testis position: high-riding, transverse lie.
- Absent cremasteric reflex.
- Negative Prehn sign: no reduction in pain with elevation of the affected hemiscrotum (Fig. 7.35).

Management

Testicular torsion is a urological emergency. Urgent scrotal exploration is required to save the testis (Fig. 7.36).

Imaging should only be performed if there are atypical clinical features or diagnostic uncertainty (Fig. 7.37).

There is a >90% chance of testicular salvage if surgical exploration is performed within 6 hours. The savage rate significantly decreases after this. Late (>24 hours) or absent surgical intervention increases the risk of testicular ischaemia, necrosis and infertility.

Testicular tumours

Testicular tumours are the most common solid malignancy in males aged 20 to 35. Risk factors include cryptorchidism,

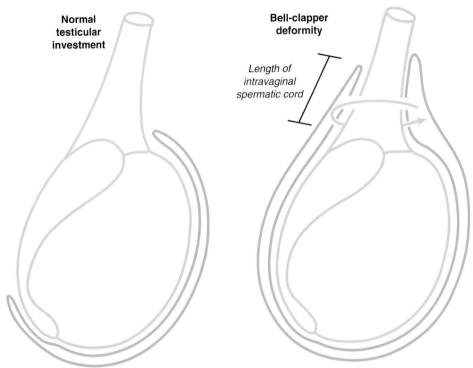

Fig. 7.34 The bell-clapper deformity. The bell-clapper deformity is an abnormally high attachment of the tunica vaginalis, and significantly increases the risk of torsion. (Taghavi K, Dumble C, Hutson JM, Mushtaq I, Mirjalili SA. The bell-clapper deformity of the testis: The definitive pathological anatomy. *J Pediatr Surg.* 2021;56(8):1405-1410. https://doi.10.1016/j.jpedsurg.2020.06.023. Epub 2020 Jun 25. PMID: 32762939.)

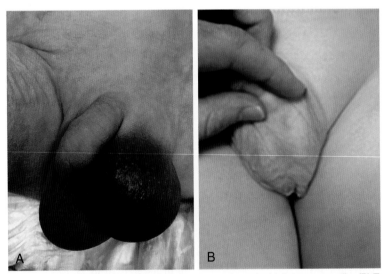

Fig. 7.35 Testicular torsion. (A) A torted left testicle with erythema, necrosis and a high transverse lie. (B) Torsion of the testicular appendage presents similarly to testicular torsion. The blue dot sign indicates infarction of the appendage, which can be seen through the scrotal skin. (From A. Zarit JS, Balest AL, Riley MM, et al. *Zitelli and Davis' Atlas of Pediatric Physical Diagnosis,* 8th Edition. Elsevier; 2023. B. Copp HL, Selekman R, Partin AW, Peters CA, Kavoussi LR, Dmochowski RR. *Campbell-Walsh-Wein Urology: 3-Volume Set,* 12th Edition. Elsevier; 2020.)

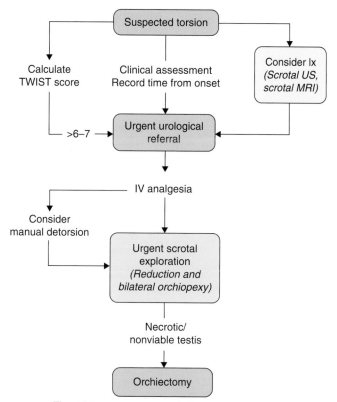

Fig. 7.36 Acute management of testicular torsion.

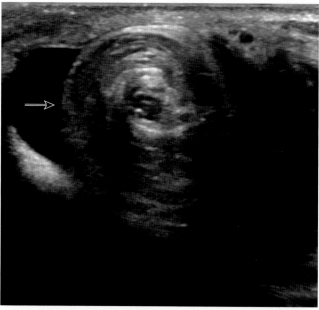

Fig. 7.37 Scrotal US in testicular torsion. US may show enlarged testis, twisting of the spermatic cord (whirlpool sign) and reduced or absent blood flow to the affected testis. (From Fananapazir G, Foster BR. *Diagnostic Imaging: Genitourinary,* 4th Edition. Elsevier; 2022.)

malignancy of the contralateral testicle, family history, chromosomal abnormalities and infertility. There are a range of histopathological subtypes, with varying malignant potential, disease course and clinical features (Table 7.8).

CLINICAL NOTES

- Cryptorchidism can be unilateral or bilateral.
- It is common and typically resolves spontaneously by 6 months.
- Persistent cases are treated with orchidopexy or orchiectomy.
- There is a risk of malignancy in the affected testis.

Symptoms and signs

Symptoms include:

- Unilateral painless testicular nodule/swelling
- Scrotal discomfort/lower abdominal pain
- Negative transillumination
- Gynaecomastia (secondary to ↑bHCG)
- Constitutional features (FLAWS)
- Symptoms of metastasis

RED FLAG

A firm testicular nodule is malignancy until proven otherwise.

Investigations

Investigations include:

- Tumour markers: AFP, bHCG, and LDH may be raised.
- Ultrasound: to characterize the mass and confirm the diagnosis.
- CTCAP: to look for evidence of regional lymph node metastasis.
- X-rays: testicular tumours commonly metastasize to the lungs or bone (Fig. 7.38).

HINTS AND TIPS

- Masses should not be biopsied, due to the risk of seeding and the spread of cancer cells.
- Histopathological diagnosis takes place following orchiectomy.

CLINICAL NOTES

Both testicular cancer and RCC can present with cannonball lung metastasis.

Management

Management options include:

- Surgical resection: radical inguinal orchiectomy and radical lymph node dissection.

Table 7.8 Testicular tumours

Histology	Germ cell (seminoma)	Germ cell (nonseminoma)	Nongerm cell
Features	Most common (40%) Malignant tumour Slow growth, late metastases Better prognosis	Includes embryonal carcinoma, teratoma, choriocarcinoma and yolk sac tumours, and mixed tumours. High malignant potential and early metastases	Rare (5%) Includes Leydig and Sertoli cell Hormone producing Rarely malignant
AFP	Negative	↑↑ in yolk sac tumours May be ↑ in teratoma or mixed	Negative
bHCG	May be ↑	↑↑ in choriocarcinoma May be ↑ in embryonal or mixed	Negative
US findings	Hypoechoic, homogenous, clear margins May have calcifications	Variable in echogenicity, nonhomogenous, poorly defined May be calcified or cystic	

AFP, *Alpha fetoprotein;* bHCG, *beta-human chorionic gonadotropin;* US, *ultrasound.*

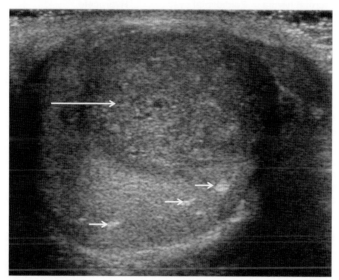

Fig. 7.38 Ultrasound findings. Seminoma (*long arrow*) with focal areas of macrocalcification lying outside the tumour margins (*small arrows*). (From Sidhu PS, Allan PL, Weston MJ, Baxter GM. *Clinical Ultrasound,* 3rd Edition. Churchill Livingstone, Elsevier Ltd. 2011.)

- Radiotherapy: Seminomas are radiosensitive and respond well to adjuvant radiotherapy.
- Chemotherapy: typically platinum-based.
- Sperm cryopreservation: prior to initiating therapy, to preserve fertility.

The prognosis is excellent, with 5-year survival >95% and high rates of cure, even in metastatic disease.

SCROTAL DISORDERS

Scrotal massess

There are several benign differentials for scrotal swelling (Table 7.9, Fig. 7.39).

PENILE DISORDERS

The shaft of the penis is composed of corpus cavernosum, the erectile tissue and corpus spongiosum, which keeps the urethra open during ejection. The corpus spongiosum forms the glans penis at the distal end. The glans penis is defined by the coronal sulcus, covered by the foreskin and contains the external urethral meatus (Fig. 7.40).

Balanitis

Balanitis is the inflammation of the glans penis. Balanoposthitis is inflammation of the glans and the foreskin. It is typically caused by bacterial or yeast infections, though it can relate to contact irritants or as a drug reaction. Failure to retract the foreskin and regularly clean the glans promotes development of infection.

Symptoms and signs

Balanitis presents with:

- Pain and erythema of the glans and foreskin
- Penile discharge
- Ulcerated lesions
- Systemic features including fever and malaise (Fig. 7.41)

Management

Balanitis is a clinical diagnosis, and no investigations are required. Management includes:

- Daily foreskin retraction and bathing of the glans
- Topical antifungal/antibacterials for infective causes
- Topical steroids and emollients for inflammatory causes

Table 7.9 Scrotal masses

Diagnosis	Inguinoscrotal hernia	Epididymal cyst	Hydrocele	Varicocele
Aetiology	Protrusion of abdominal contents through inguinal canal	Idiopathic Spermatocele – obstruction to spermatic drainage	Congenital – persist patency of the processus vaginalis Acquired – infection, tumour, trauma	Proximal obstruction of the spermatic vein – abnormal dilation and tortuosity of the pampiniform plexus
Clinical features	Cannot get above the mass Positive cough impulse May be reducible, irreducible or tender	Small firm, painless Palpable within epididymis	Painless swelling of affected scrotum May or may not be reducible Positive transillumination	Painless heaviness of affected testis (more common on LHS) 'Bag of worms' Reducible lying flat Negative transillumination
Mx	Conservative Typically require mesh/ open repair	Conservative Surgical excision if symptomatic	May close spontaneously Hydrocelectomy Aspiration	Scrotal support Varicocelectomy Embolization

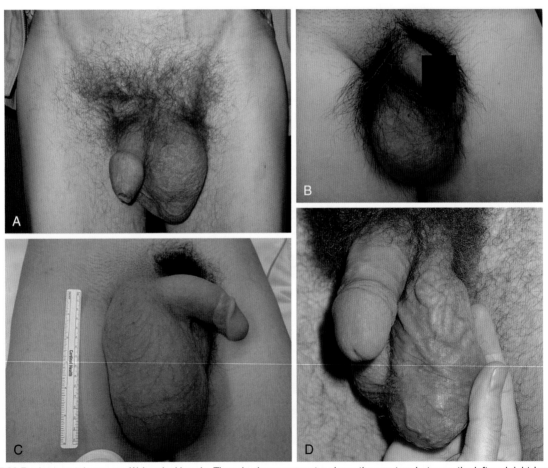

Fig. 7.39 Benign scrotal masses. (A) Inguinal hernia. There is clear asymmetry above the scrotum between the left and right-hand side, and the hernia is seen descending into the scrotum. (B) Epididymal cyst. Small mass in the right hemiscrotum. (C) Hydrocele. Large swelling in the left hemiscrotum. (D) Varicocele. Abnormal dilation and tortuosity of veins in the left hemiscrotum. (From A. de Beaux AC, Paterson HM, Paterson-Brown S. *Core Topics in General and Emergency Surgery,* 6th Edition. Elsevier; 2019. B. Young CJ, Gladman MA. *Examination Surgery: A Guide to Passing the Fellowship Examination in General Surgery*. Elsevier; 2013. C. Kryger JV, Basel D, Jarosz SL, Bordini BJ, Kliegman RM, Toth H. *Nelson Pediatric Symptom-Based Diagnosis: Common Diseases and their Mimics,* 2nd Edition. Elsevier; 2023. D. Shiland BJ. *Mastering Healthcare Terminology,* 7th Edition. Elsevier; 2023.)

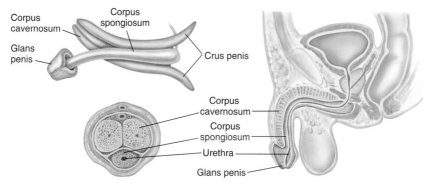

Fig. 7.40 Anatomy of the penis. Engorgement of the corpus cavernosum occurs following parasympathetic stimulation. (From Ball JW, et al. *Seidel's Guide to Physical Examination: An Interprofessional Approach,* 9th Edition. Elsevier; 2019.)

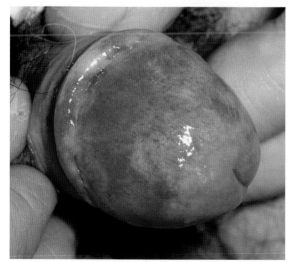

Fig. 7.41 Balanitis. Swollen, tender and erythematous Glans penis. (From Micheletti RG, et al. *Andrews' Diseases of the Skin Clinical Atlas,* 2nd Edition. Elsevier; 2023.)

Complications

Significant or recurrent episodes predispose to complications:

- Phimosis (constriction and inability to retract the foreskin)
- Recurrent UTIs
- Obstructive uropathy
- Penile cancer: a rare squamous cell carcinoma that typically occurs in uncircumcised elderly men, associated with balanitis and HPV infection

Phimosis and paraphimosis

Phimosis describes difficulty or the inability to retract the foreskin over the glans. Paraphimosis describes an inability to return a retracted foreskin to its original position. Paraphimosis can occur as the result of trauma, including iatrogenically in genitourinary procedures, or forceful foreskin retraction (Fig. 7.42, Table 7.10).

RED FLAG

- Paraphimosis is a urological emergency, due to the risk of penile necrosis.
- Urgent manual or surgical reduction is essential.

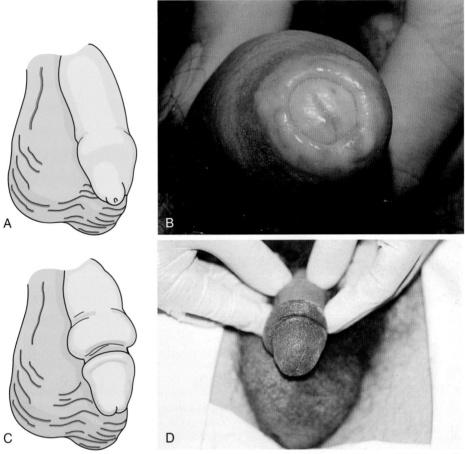

Fig. 7.42 Phimosis and paraphimosis. (A, B) Phimosis. (C, D) Paraphimosis. (From Craft JA, Huether SE, Hogarth K, et al. *Understanding Pathophysiology,* Australia and New Zealand Edition. 4th edition. Elsevier Australia; 2023.)

Table 7.10 Phimosis and paraphimosis

	Phimosis	Paraphimosis
Aetiology	Postbalanoposthitis Congenital Scarring (trauma/circumcision)	Complication of phimosis Trauma – iatrogenic/forceful retraction
Clinical features	Difficulty or inability to retract the foreskin Painful erection Dyspareunia	Inability to return the foreskin to its normal position Constricting tissue at coronal sulcus Oedema and pain of the glans
Mx	Conservative – high likelihood of spontaneous resolution Surgical – vertical incision or circumcision	Conservative – manual reduction and analgesia Surgical – incision of constricting band or circumcision
Complications	Foreskin tear Paraphimosis	Urinary retention Penile ischemia and necrosis

Chapter Summary

- UTIs may present atypically in older adults and are commonly associated with delirium.
- Pyelonephritis presents with fevers, rigors and loin pain, and is a risk factor for urosepsis.
- Cauda equina syndrome can present with sudden onset urinary retention or urinary incontinence.
- Renal colic is the cardinal feature of renal stones. PR diclofenac is the most effective analgesic.
- Unexplained haematuria in an older adult is a red flag feature for urological cancer.
- A PSA can be raised in nearly all prostate conditions, and cannot reliably diagnose or exclude prostate cancer.
- Prostate cancer is associated with sclerotic bony metastasis typically in the lumbosacral and pelvic bones.
- Testicular torsion is a urological emergency, with a 6-hour window to save the testis and preserve fertility.
- A young male presenting with a firm, painless nodule on the testis is likely to represent testicular cancer.
- Paraphimosis is a urological emergency with a risk of penile necrosis. Urgent manual reduction or surgery is required.

UKMLA Conditions
Acute kidney injury
Adverse drug effects
Benign prostatic hyperplasia
Bladder cancer
Dehydration
Epididymitis and orchitis
Frailty
Loss of libido
Metastatic disease
Prostate cancer
Sepsis
Testicular cancer
Urethral discharge and genital ulcers/warts
Urinary incontinence
Urinary symptoms
Urinary tract calculi
Urinary tract infection

UKMLA Presentations
Abnormal urinalysis
Acute kidney injury
Dehydration
Electrolyte abnormalities
Erectile dysfunction
Fever
Haematuria
Loin pain
Loss of libido
Night sweats
Oliguria
Pelvic pain
Scrotal/testicular pain and/or lump/swelling
Sepsis
Urinary incontinence
Urinary symptoms
Weight loss

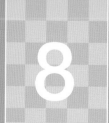

Ear, nose and throat

CLINICAL ANATOMY

The ear

The ear regulates the auditory and vestibular systems. The vestibular system regulates rotatory perception, postural control and coordination of head position and eye movement, to provide balance.

The auditory system transmits external sound waves into nerve impulses interpreted as sounds in the brain, to provide hearing. The external auricle captures sound waves which are directed via the external acoustic canal (EAC) to the tympanic membrane (TM) (Fig. 8.1). The EAC contains hair cells and sweat glands which produce cerumen (ear wax). The TM vibrates to transmit sound waves to the middle ear, an air-filled space that transmits vibrations to the ossicles, three small, interconnected bones called the malleus, incus and stapes, known as the ossicular chain. The pharyngotympanic tube (Eustachian tube) equalizes middle ear pressure and drains fluid from the middle ear. The air-filled mastoid cells lie behind the middle ear, and aid vocal resonance and warm and humidify inhaled air (Fig. 8.2).

> **CLINICAL NOTES**
>
> Normal human hearing ranges between 20-20,000 Hz (pitch) and 0-130 dB (intensity).

The internal ear is composed of a bony labyrinth of the semicircular canals, cochlea and vestibule which contain an internal membranous labyrinth filled with endolymph (Fig. 8.3). The vestibulocochlear nerve enters the internal acoustic meatus and divides into vestibular and cochlear branches, which regulate balance and hearing, respectively. Vibrations of the ossicular chain are transmitted to the endolymph in the membranous labyrinth and then to hair cells within the cochlea, and cochlear nerve, producing the perception of sound. Changes in head position change the flow of endolymph in the membranous labyrinth, transmitting proprioceptive information via the vestibular nerve to the cerebellum, brainstem and spinal cord for the regulation of rotary perception, postural control and balance (Fig. 8.4).

Nose and paranasal sinuses

The nasal cavities form the upper aerodigestive tract and regulate olfaction. They are formed from the frontal, ethmoid and sphenoid bone, and nasal cartilage, and inferiorly by the hard palate. The respiratory region is lined by mucus-secreting ciliated respiratory epithelium and goblet cells. The olfactory region at the apex of the nasal cavity contains olfactory receptors, which transmit to the olfactory cortex to provide the conscious sense of smell (Fig. 8.5).

The paranasal sinuses are four paired air-filled spaces within the skull, including the ethmoidal cells, and sphenoidal, axillary and frontal sinuses. They are lined by mucous-secreting respiratory mucosa and assist in the warming and humidifying of inhaled air and providing vocal resonance, and excretion of inhaled debris, forming part of the mucosal humoral immune system (Fig. 8.6).

The oral cavity and salivary glands

The oral cavity is the opening of the aerodigestive tract. The three paired salivary glands secrete saliva into the oral cavity to assist with digesting and moistening food boluses to aid deglutition, and act as a barrier to pathogens as part of the humoral immune system. The submandibular and sublingual glands sit on the medial aspect of the mandible and drain into the floor of the oral cavity. The parotid gland secretes into the parotid duct just adjacent to the upper molars. The facial nerve courses through the inner ear and facial canal before passing into the parotid gland, where it divides into five terminal branches, the temporal, zygomatic, buccal, marginal mandibular and cervical branches, respectively (Fig. 8.7).

The pharynx

The pharynx is a muscular tube that provides a pathway for air and food to pass from the oral cavity into the lungs and gastrointestinal tract, respectively. The nasopharynx is continuous with the oropharynx. The laryngopharynx is the point at which the pharynx divides into the larynx anteriorly and the oesophagus posteriorly. Upon swallowing, the soft palate elevates, and the epiglottis closes over the laryngeal intel, protecting the airway and directing food into the oesophagus via the oropharynx (Fig. 8.8).

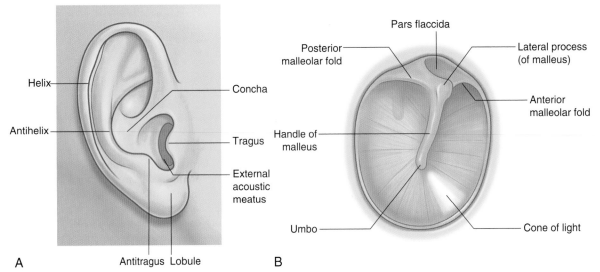

Fig. 8.1 The auricle and tympanic membrane. (A) The auricle of the ear. (B) The tympanic membrane. The cone of light is visible when examined with an otoscope. (From Drake RL, Mitchell AWM, Vogl AW. *Gray's Anatomy for Students,* 5th Edition. Elsevier; 2024.)

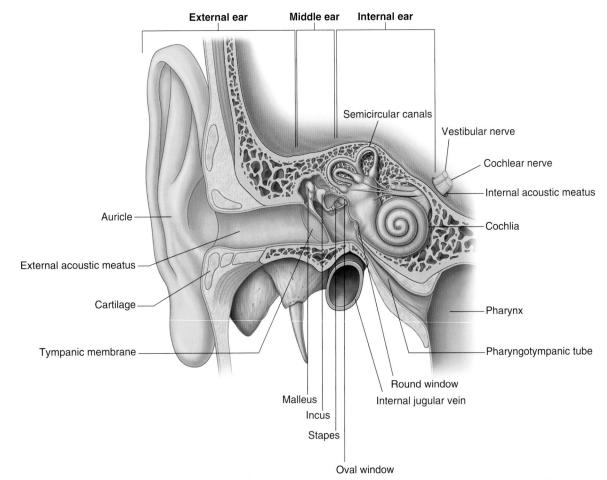

Fig. 8.2 Anatomy of the auditory and vestibular system. (From Mitchell AWM, Vogl AW, Drake RL. *Gray's Anatomy for Students,* 5th Edition. Elsevier; 2024.)

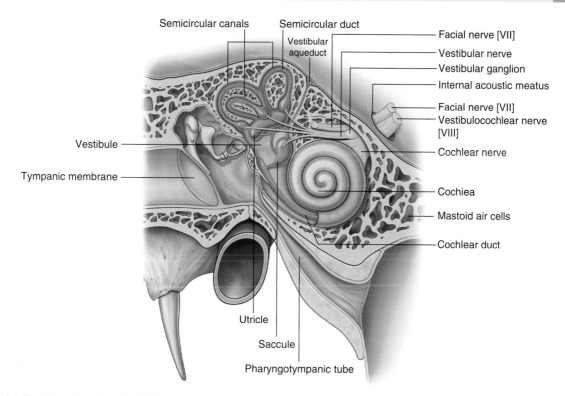

Fig. 8.3 The internal ear. (From Vogl AW, Mitchell AWM, Drake RL. *Gray's Anatomy for Students Flash Cards,* 4th Edition. Elsevier; 2020.)

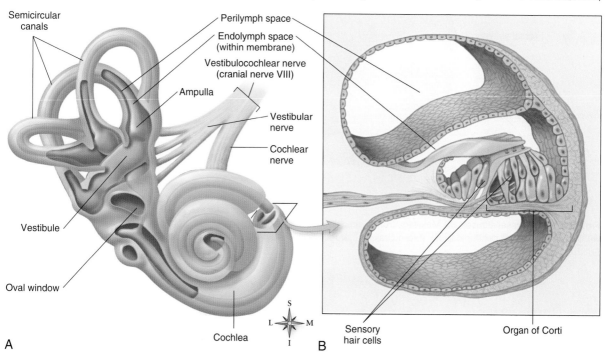

Fig. 8.4 The membranous labyrinth. (A) Structures of the inner ear. (B) Cross-section of the cochlea, depicting the inner hair cells and organ of Corti. (From Patton KT, Thibodeau GA. *Human body in health and disease,* 7th Edition. St. Louis, Elsevier; 2018.)

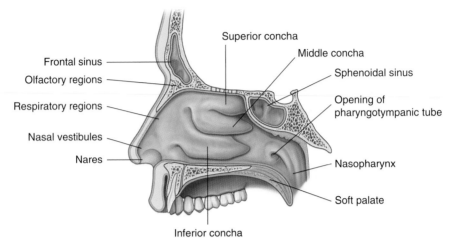

Fig. 8.5 The nasal cavity. (From Drake RL, Vogl AW, Mitchell AWM. *Gray's Anatomy for Students Flash Cards,* 5th Edition. Elsevier; 2024.)

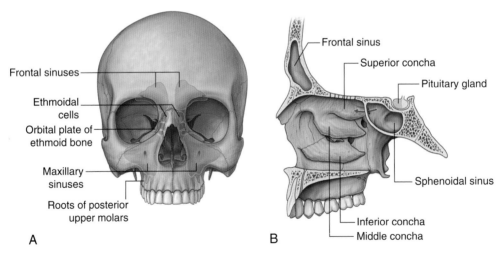

A   B

Fig. 8.6 The paranasal sinuses. (A) Maxillary, frontal sinuses and ethmoid air cells. (B) The sphenoidal sinus is situated posteriorly within the body of the sphenoid bone. (From Drake RL, Vogl AW, Mitchell AWM. *Gray's Anatomy for Students Flash Cards,* 5th Edition. Elsevier; 2024.)

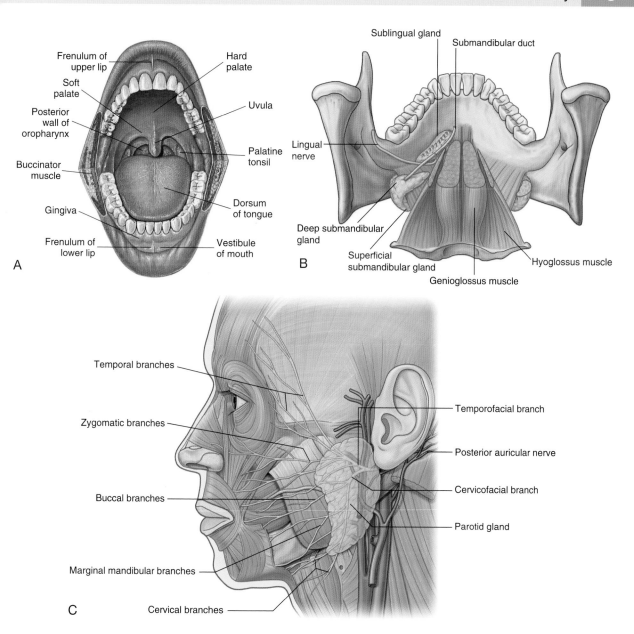

Fig. 8.7 The oral cavity, salivary glands and facial nerve. (A) The oral cavity. (B) The submandibular and sublingual glands, which secrete onto the floor of the mouth. (C) The facial nerve courses through the parotid gland, making it vulnerable to parotid pathology. (From A. Solomon BS, Ball JW, Dains JE, Flynn JA, Stewart RW. *Seidel's Guide to Physical Examination: An Interprofessional Approach,* 10th Edition. Elsevier; 2023. B. Vogl AW, Mitchell AWM, Drake RL, *Gray's Anatomy for Students,* 4th Edition. Elsevier; 2020. C. Drake RL, Vogl AW, Mitchell AWM. *Gray's Anatomy for Students,* 5th Edition. Elsevier; 2024.)

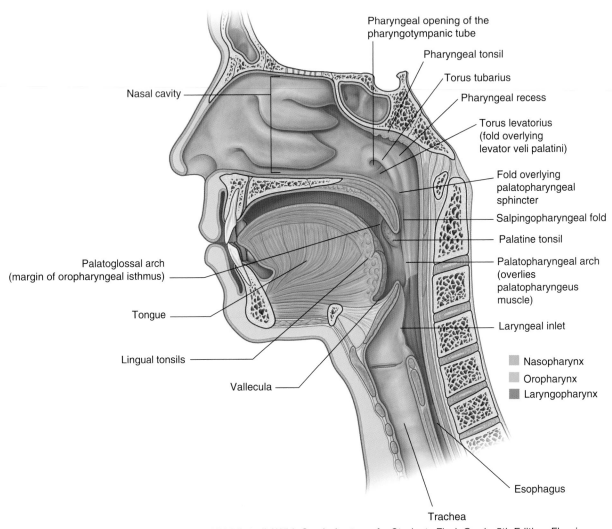

Fig. 8.8 The pharynx. (From Drake RL, Vogl AW, Mitchell AWM. *Gray's Anatomy for Students Flash Cards,* 5th Edition. Elsevier; 2024.)

The larynx

The larynx is a muscular cartilaginous tube that provides phonation and protects the airway when swallowing. Closure of the arytenoid cartilages and vibration of the vocal folds produces sound, which is modified into voice by structures in the upper airway and oral cavity (Fig. 8.9).

The sympathetic chain

The sympathetic chain descends from the skull to the coccyx as two parallel cords on each side of the vertebral column. The neuronal cell bodies are in the lateral horn of the spinal cord. Preganglionic axons exit the ventral roots of the spinal cord and synapse with postganglionic axons at the paravertebral ganglia, which form the sympathetic chain (Fig. 8.10).

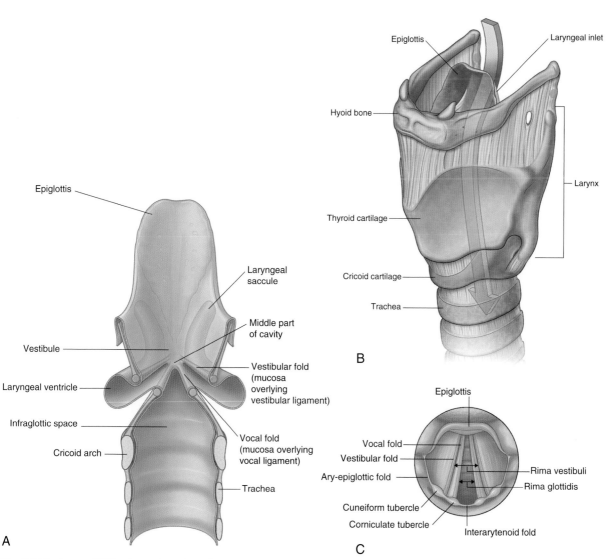

Fig. 8.9 The larynx. (A) The internal surface of the larynx. (B) The laryngeal cartilages. (C) The vocal cords. (From Drake RL, Vogl AW, Mitchell AWM. *Gray's Anatomy for Students,* 5th Edition. Elsevier; 2024.)

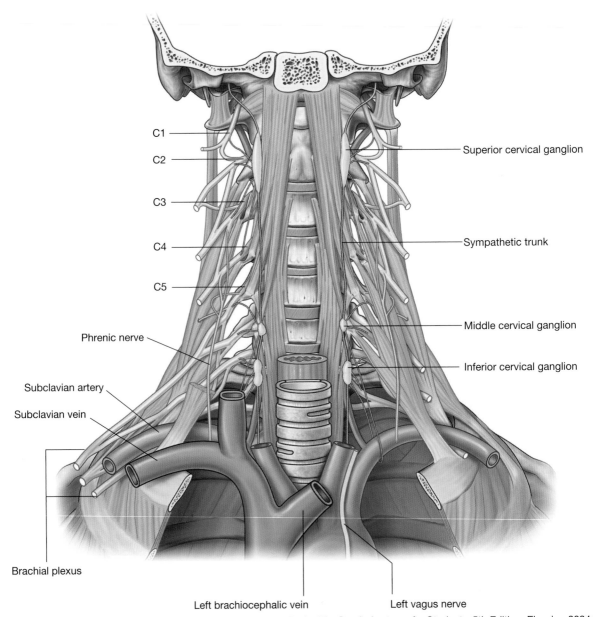

Fig. 8.10 The sympathetic chain. (From Mitchell AWM, Vogl AW, Drake RL. *Gray's Anatomy for Students,* 5th Edition. Elsevier; 2024.)

EAR, NOSE AND THROAT PRESENTATIONS

History taking

Opening the consultation
Introduce yourself and confirm the patient's details.

Presenting complaint (PC)
Ask open questions to identify the presenting complaint.

History of presenting complaint (HPC)
Explore the presenting complaint in-depth using SOCRATES (Table 8.1).

> **HINTS AND TIPS**
>
> - Screen for ear, nose and throat symptoms in all ENT presentations.
> - The close anatomical relationship of head and neck structures means symptoms and pathologies often overlap.

> **RED FLAG**
>
> Red flags in ENT histories include:
> - Ears – persistent unilateral hearing loss/tinnitus, central vertigo, facial nerve palsies, foul otorrhoea, mastoid swelling and pain
> - Nose – blood-stained rhinorrhoea, unilateral nasal polyp, posterior nosebleed
> - Throat – new hoarseness, dysphagia/odynophagia, stridor, growing neck lump

Table 8.1 Common symptoms of ENT pathology

Ears	Hearing loss, otalgia, otorrhoea, tinnitus, vertigo, facial weakness, headache
Nose Paranasal sinuses	Nasal obstruction, rhinorrhoea, sneezing, anosmia, facial pain, swelling or numbness, epistaxis, headache, snoring
Oral cavity Salivary glands	Pain, dysarthria, dysphagia, halitosis swelling
Pharynx Larynx	Dysphagia, odynophagia, dysphonia, choking, stridor, hoarseness, haematemesis, haemoptysis, cough, neck lump

Ideas, concerns and expectations
Understanding the patient's ideas, concerns and expectations early can help you identify concerns you can address, or specific aims for the consultation.

Systemic enquiry
Screen for related symptoms from other body systems and constitutional features.

> **HINTS AND TIPS**
>
> Screen for key symptoms from related body areas, including the cardiovascular, respiratory, gastrointestinal, neurological and dermatological systems, and constitutional features including **FLAWS**:
> - **F** – **F**ever
> - **L** – **L**ethargy
> - **A** – **A**norexia
> - **W** – **W**eight loss
> - **N** – **N**ight sweats

Past medical history
Enquire about previous episodes of similar symptoms, other medical conditions, surgical history, hospital admissions or outpatient procedures.

Drug history
Obtain a list of prescribed medications, and check compliance, recent changes and over-the-counter medication use. Check allergy status and document the nature of reactions.

> **HINTS AND TIPS**
>
> Side effects of intranasal, inhaled or intraaural medications may cause symptoms in the relevant area.

Family history
Screen for family members with similar or related symptoms, which may point toward inherited conditions or infective pathology.

Social history
Gain an overview of the social status:

- Alcohol: quantify amount and type of alcohol consumed.
- Smoking: a significant risk factor for head and neck malignancy.
- Diet and weight: poor diet and obesity can increase the risk of many pathologies or contribute to the worsening of associated medical conditions.
- Occupation: occupational exposures can highlight relevant risk factors.

Closing the consultation
Summarize the history, thank the patient and answer any questions.

DIFFERENTIAL DIAGNOSIS

Otalgia

Otalgia, or ear pain, is typically related to infective pathology, but there is a range of significant pathologies or causes of referred pain which must be excluded (Fig. 8.11).

Investigations for otalgia
Investigations are not typically required, unless there are severe, refractory symptoms or diagnostic uncertainty.

1. Bedside
   - Observations: pyrexia indicates infective pathology. Haemodynamic compromise indicates severe infection or sepsis.
   - Pure tone audiometry: to evaluate hearing loss.
   - EAC MC&S: EAC swabs and cultures can be sent to guide treatment if there is a poor response to antibiotic therapy or suspicion of fungal infection.
   - Middle ear MC&S: tympanocentesis can be used to extract middle ear fluid, indicated in severe infection, poor response to initial antibiotic therapy, or immunocompromise.
2. Bloods
   - FBC/CRP: may show raised inflammatory markers.
   - Blood cultures: only in severe infection.
3. Imaging
   - CT temporal bone: to detect extracranial complications including mastoiditis and osteomyelitis.
   - MRI brain, head and neck: to evaluate for intracranial lesions including acoustic neuroma, malignant otitis externa and head and neck malignancy.

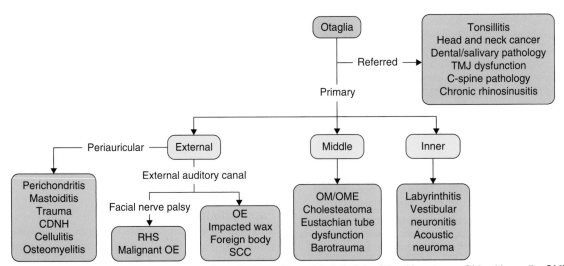

Fig. 8.11 Differential diagnosis of otalgia. *CDNH,* Chondrodermatitis nodularis helicis; *OE,* otitis externa; *OM,* otitis media; *OME,* otitis media with effusion; *RHS,* Ramsay hunt syndrome; *TMJ,* temporomandibular joint dysfunction.

- Panendoscopy: to visualize the entire upper aerodigestive tract, to confirm suspected head and neck malignancy.

Hearing loss

Hearing loss can be divided into conductive hearing loss (CHL), impaired sound wave conduction from the EAC to the cochlea, or sensorineural hearing loss (SNHL), caused by damage to the inner ear labyrinth or cochlear nerve. There can be a mixed picture. Sudden hearing loss may represent life-threatening pathology and requires urgent assessment and treatment. Gradually progressive hearing loss typically relates to benign pathology (Figs 8.12-8.13).

RED FLAG

- Sudden unilateral SNHL with tinnitus and vertigo is an ENT emergency.
- Prompt steroid administration can result in spontaneous recovery within weeks.
- Delay in treatment may result in permanent hearing loss.

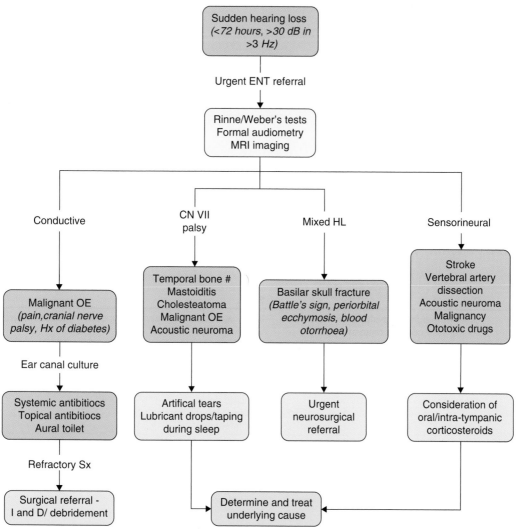

Fig. 8.12 Differential diagnosis of sudden-onset hearing loss. *HL*, Hearing loss; *I&D*, incision and drainage; *OE*, otitis externa; *Sx*, symptoms.

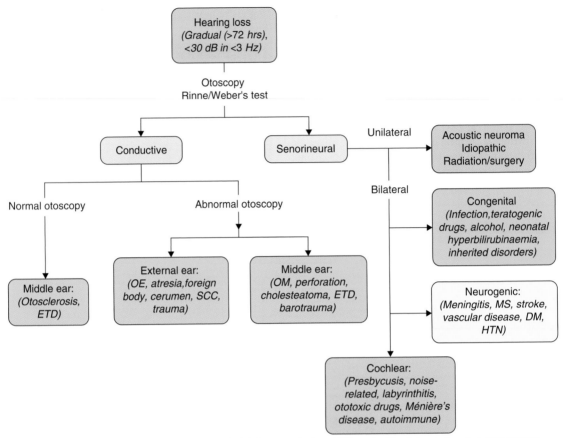

Fig. 8.13 Differential diagnosis of gradual hearing loss. *CMV*, Cytomegalovirus; *ETD*, eustachian tube dysfunction; *HIV*, human immunodeficiency virus; *HTN*, hypertension; *MS*, multiple sclerosis; *OE*, otitis externa; *OM*, otitis media; *SCC*, squamous cell carcinoma.

Table 8.2 Conductive and sensorineural hearing loss

	CHL	SNHL
Pathology	Outer or middle ear dysfunction → disrupted sound wave conduction to inner ear	Inner ear or cochlear nerve dysfunction → reduced neuronal transmission to the brain
Aetiology	Impacted ear wax Otitis externa Otitis media Barotrauma Otosclerosis	Presbycusis (age-related hearing loss) Ménière's disease Noise-induced hearing loss Acoustic neuroma Ototoxic drugs Autoimmune disorders Viral infections
Tuning fork tests	Weber's lateralizes to affected ear Rinne's negative in affected ear	Weber's lateralizes to unaffected ear Rinne's positive in both ears
Symptoms	No sound distortion Normal volume voice Hearing improves in noisy environments EAC pathology on examination	Loss of higher frequencies first Sound distortion Loud voice Tinnitus Hearing worse in noisy environments
Audiometry	Increased air-bone gap	Air and bone auditory thresholds proportionally increased, worse at higher frequencies

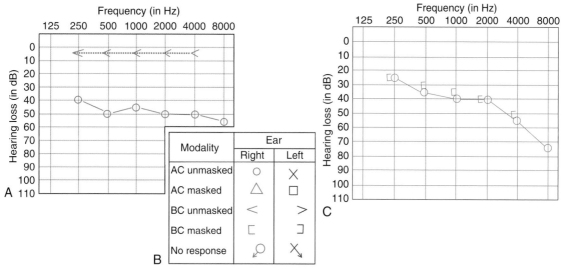

Fig. 8.14 Audiograms (A) CHL, with increased air-bone gap. (B) Symbols used in audiograms. Masked refers to putting noise in the opposing ear while testing one ear. (C) SNHL, with increased auditory thresholds, with the higher frequencies predominantly affected. (From Dhingra S, Dhingra PL. *Diseases of Ear, Nose and Throat & Head and Neck Surgery*, 8th Edition. Elsevier; 2022.)

Investigations for hearing loss

Rinne and Weber's tests should be used to differentiate between CHL and SNHL Table 8.2.

Further investigations include:

1. Beside
   - Pure tone audiometry: to determine the level of hearing loss and likely aetiology Fig. 8.14.
   - Oto-acoustic emissions: faint sounds produced by hair cells in the cochlea. Can confirm SNHL. Often used to detect congenital hearing loss and monitor recovery from ototoxic drug damage.
   - Ear swabs: if there is ongoing discharge not responding to antibiotic therapy, which may suggest fungal infection.
2. Bloods
   - FBC, CRP: infection may show raised inflammatory markers.
   - Blood cultures: in severe systemic infection.
3. Imaging
   - CT temporal bone: to assess for conductive pathologies or mixed hearing loss.
   - CT head: to assess for acute intracranial pathology.
   - MRI brain/internal auditory canals: for suspected intracranial soft tissue pathology including acoustic neuroma or MS, or vascular lesions.

- Pneumatic otoscopy: to check TM compliance and presence of middle ear effusion.

CLINICAL NOTES

- Prompt treatment in children with hearing loss is essential to avoid speech delay.
- Hearing aids are used initially, which amplify sounds.
- Cochlear implants are used for profound hearing loss, with surgical prosthesis to stimulate the auditory nerve.

Tinnitus

Tinnitus is the internal perception of sound including ringing, buzzing, clicking, hissing or pulsing. It may be objective, where it can be heard by others, or subjective, where it is only heard by the patient. Pulsatile tinnitus is heard in time with the heartbeat. Tinnitus can be unilateral, bilateral, acute, chronic, intermittent or constant (Fig. 8.15).

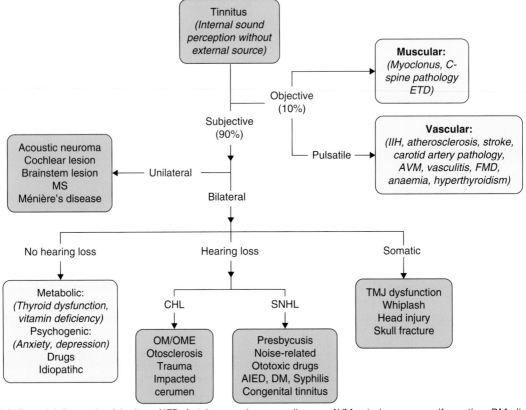

Fig. 8.15 Differential diagnosis of tinnitus. *AIED*, Autoimmune inner ear disease; *AVM*, arteriovenous malformation; *DM*, diabetes mellitus; *ETD*, eustachian tube dysfunction; *FMD*, fibromuscular dysplasia; *MS*, multiple sclerosis; *OM/OME*, otitis media/otitis media with effusion; *TMJ*, temporomandibular joint.

Investigations for tinnitus

1. Bedside
   - Pure tone audiometry: hearing loss is the most common cause of tinnitus.
   - VDRL test: to assess for syphilis if there are relevant risk factors and symptoms.
2. Bloods
   - FBC: anaemia can cause pulsatile tinnitus.
   - TFTs: both hypo and hyperthyroidism can cause tinnitus.
   - CBG: ↑ may indicate diabetes.
   - Lipid profile: elevated cholesterol is a risk factor for stroke.
   - Autoimmune screen: to assess for associated autoimmune disease.
3. Imaging
   - Tympanometry: to assess for middle ear effusion.

- CTA brain/neck: for all patients with pulsatile tinnitus, to assess for vascular pathology.
- CT temporal bones: if there is concurrent conductive hearing loss.
- MRI head: to assess for intracranial pathology.
- Carotid angiography: to detect carotid artery pathology.

CLINICAL NOTES

- Unilateral, asymmetrical or pulsatile tinnitus, or focal neurological deficits are red flags requiring further investigation.
- If the aetiology remains unclear management is supportive, including hearing aids and cochlear implants.

Vertigo

Vertigo is the perception of the environment rotating around. It may result from peripheral inner ear pathology or central vestibular dysfunction. Peripheral causes of vertigo are typically benign, however central causes may be life-threatening and warrant urgent hospital admission for assessment and treatment, so differentiating between the two is essential (Fig. 8.16).

COMMON PITFALLS

- 'Vertigo' is often used incorrectly to describe dizziness or light-headedness.
- Rotatory dizziness associated with nausea and postural instability, is more likely to be true vertigo.

Investigations for vertigo

1. Bedside
   - Pure tone audiometry: essential to assess for hearing loss.
   - ECG: can be considered to rule out cardiac syncope or arrhythmias.
   - Urine drug screen: several recreational drugs can cause vertigo.
   - CBG: rule out hypoglycaemia as a cause of dizziness.
2. Bloods -
   - FBC/CRP: ↑ inflammatory markers suggest infection. Anaemia may cause light-headedness.
   - Vitamin B_{12}: ↓B_{12} anaemia can produce symptoms of vertigo.
3. Imaging
   - MRI brain +/- MRA: to assess for intracranial causes of vertigo (Table 8.3).

HINTS AND TIPS

Vertigo associated with the **5 D's** suggests a central cause:

- **D – D**ysphagia
- **D – D**ysarthria
- **D – D**iplopia
- **D – D**ysmetria
- **D – D**ownbeat nystagmus

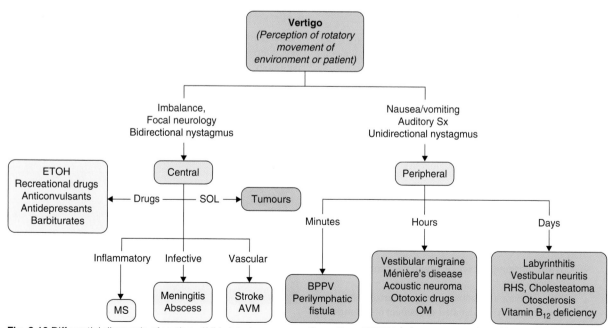

Fig. 8.16 Differential diagnosis of vertigo. *AVM*, Arteriovenous malformation; *BPPV*, benign paroxysmal positional vertigo; *ETOH*, alcohol; *MS*, multiple sclerosis; *OM*, otitis media; *RHS*, Ramsay Hunt syndrome.

Table 8.3 Causes of vertigo

	Benign paroxysmal positional vertigo	Ménière's disease	Vestibular neuritis
Symptoms	Vertigo, nystagmus, postural instability, nausea	Vertigo, tinnitus and SNHL, + nystagmus, aural fullness, nausea	Vertigo, nystagmus, postural instability, nausea
Vertigo features	Episodic, sudden onset, paroxysmal, recurrent	Sudden onset, recurrent	Severe, persistent, continuous
SNHL	Absent	Unilateral, fluctuating, progressing to deafness	Absent SNHL in labyrinthitis
Triggers	Changes in head position	Unknown	Viral URTI
Timescale	Seconds to minutes	Minutes to hours	Hours to days
Diagnosis	Dix-Hallpike manoeuvres	Clinical features, + audiometry	Clinical features
Management	Epley manoeuvre	Vestibular rehabilitation, trigger avoidance Medical and surgical options if refractory	Vestibular rehabilitation Vestibular suppressants

Anosmia and nasal obstruction

Anosmia has a range of causes. Acute anosmia commonly relates to a simple upper respiratory tract infection (URTI) and will resolve with the resolution of infection. Chronic anosmia relates to chronic nasal obstruction and may be reversible with adequate treatment of the condition and relief of the obstruction (Fig. 8.17).

Investigations for anosmia

Persistent anosmia associated with red flag features may suggest more significant underlying pathology, warranting further investigations.

1. Bedside
   - Chemosensory testing: for validated loss of smell identification testing.
   - CBG: symptomatic hyperglycaemia (>11 mmol/L) is diagnostic of diabetes.
   - Schirmer's test: to screen for Sjogren syndrome.
2. Bloods
   - Autoimmune antibodies: to diagnose vasculitis and autoimmune disorders.
   - Vitamin B_{12}/copper/zinc levels: severe vitamin or mineral deficiencies can result in anosmia.
3. Imaging
   - CT/MRI imaging: to exclude sinonasal or intracranial pathology.
   - CXR: hilar lymphadenopathy suggests sarcoidosis.
   - Nasal endoscopy: for detailed assessment of intranasal lesions and take soft tissue biopsies for histology.

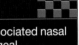

RED FLAG

Persistent anosmia with or without an associated nasal polyp is a red flag feature for nasopharyngeal carcinoma.

Facial pain

Facial pain can relate to internal or external facial pathology, referred pain from local organs, or neuropathic pain and pathology. It is most commonly benign, however there are several significant causes of facial pain which require urgent assessment and treatment (Fig. 8.18).

RED FLAG

Life-threatening causes of facial pain include:
- Head trauma
- Meningitis
- Giant cell arteritis
- Orbital cellulitis
- Glaucoma
- Herpes zoster ophthalmicus.

Any patient presenting with head trauma should be managed as per the ATLS algorithm with C-spine immobilization and a primary survey.

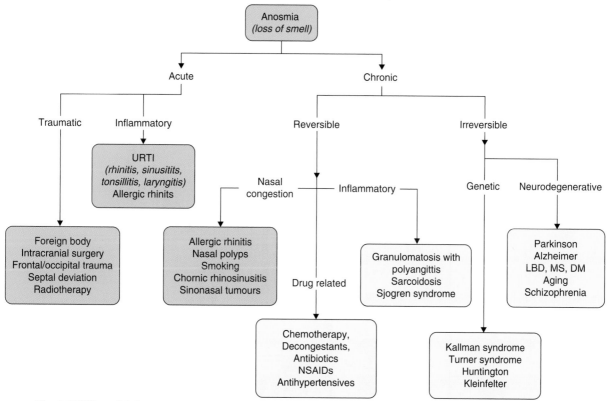

Fig. 8.17 Differential diagnosis of anosmia. *DM*, Diabetes mellitus; *LBD*, Lewy body dementia; *MS*, multiple sclerosis.

Investigations for facial pain

1. Bedside
   - Observations: severe infection may be associated with fever and haemodynamic instability.
   - Tonometry: to diagnose raised intraocular pressure associated with glaucoma.
   - Sinus culture: for refractory sinusitis with poor response to antibiotic therapy.
   - Allergy testing: to confirm allergens in allergic rhinitis.
   - Lumbar puncture: CSF MC&S, cytology and glucose can differentiate between bacterial, viral or aseptic meningitis, to guide treatment.
2. Bloods
   - FBC: ↑ WCC indicates infection. Anaemia may relate to malignancy.
   - U&Es/LFTs: essential in the workup of severe infection or malignancy.
3. Imaging
   - Intraoral US: to assess for salivary gland pathology.
   - Intraoral X-ray: to exclude dental pathologies.
   - CT head and neck: to assess for traumatic, structural or malignant lesions.
   - MRI: for more details assessment of intracranial soft tissue lesions.
   - Nasal endoscopy: for detailed assessment of sinonasal tumours and take tissue biopsies for histology.

DIFFERENTIALS

- Dental pathology is often overlooked and can cause significant pain radiating through the jaw, skull, ears and neck.
- Severe tooth decay, periodontal disease, and abscesses can spread intracranially, causing osteomyelitis.
- Haematogenous bacterial spread risks sepsis and endocarditis.

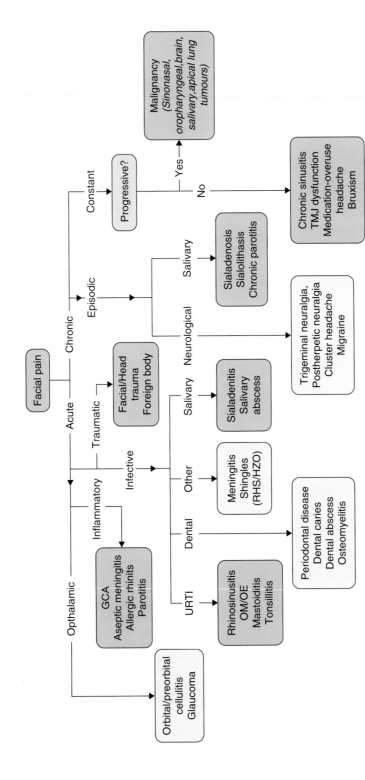

Figure 8.18 Differential diagnosis of facial pan. (Bruxism is a condition in which you constantly grind or clash your teeth, often unconsciously during sleep. It can cause chronic facial pain.). *GCA*, Giant cell arteritis; *HZO*, herpes zoster ophthalmicus; *OE*, otitis externa; *OM*, otitis media; *RHS*, Ramsay- Hunt syndrome; *TMJ*, temporomandibular joint.

Epistaxis

Epistaxis describes a nosebleed. Epistaxis, or nose bleeding is common. Anterior epistaxis account for 95% of bleeds, and arise from the anterior nasal septum, in Little's area where the Kiesselbachs plexus is located, the site of anastomosis for the vessels supplying the nasal mucosa. They typically relate to local trauma or benign pathology. Posterior epistaxis is much less common, and develop from Woodruff's plexus, the site at the back of the nasal passages where the sphenopalatine and posterior ethmoidal arteries converge. Posterior nosebleeds are typical associated with more significant nasal or intracranial pathology, including malignancy (Figs 8.19-8.20).

> **RED FLAG**
> - Anterior epistaxis presents with visible external nasal bleeding.
> - Posterior epistaxis presents insidiously, with bleeding down the back of the throat, haemoptysis and melaena if significant blood is digested.
> - Severe or recurrent posterior nose bleeding is a red flag feature for nasopharyngeal carcinoma.

The approach to epistaxis involves stabilizing the patient and achieving haemostasis (Fig. 8.21).

> **CLINICAL NOTES**
> - Stable patients can be discharged several hours after haemostasis has been achieved.
> - If anterior packing is used, follow-up for pack removal is required.

Investigations for epistaxis

Investigations are not typically required, unless there is severe, recurrent or unexplained bleeding.

1. Bedside
   - ECG: to screen for underlying cardiovascular disease.
2. Bloods
   - FBC: anaemia indicates significant acute blood loss. ↑ WBC suggests infection.
   - G&S: in significant blood loss, send two group and saves and consider cross-matching for transfusion.

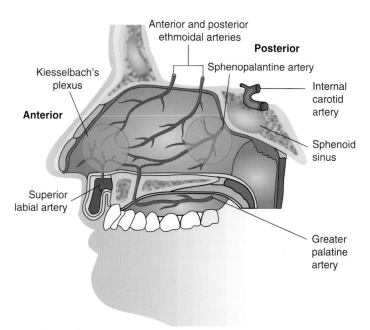

Fig. 8.19 Sites of anterior and posterior nosebleeds. (From Lakshmanaswamy A. *Textbook of Pediatrics,* Elsevier; 2022.)

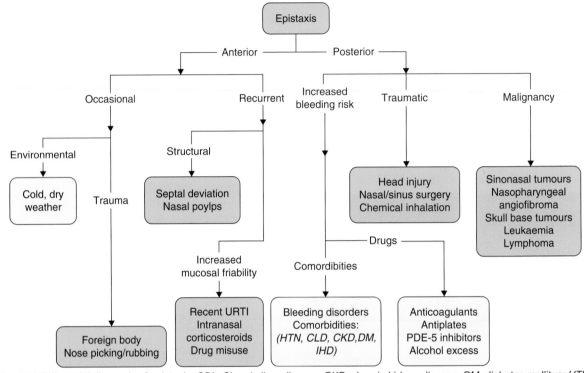

Fig. 8.20 Differential diagnosis of epistaxis. *CDL*, Chronic liver disease; *CKD*, chronic kidney disease; *DM*, diabetes mellitus; *HTN*, hypertension; *IHD*, ischaemic heart disease; *PDE-5,* phosphodiesterase-5; *URTI*, upper respiratory tract infection.

- Clotting studies: coagulopathy may suggest significant bleeding or underlying risk factors.
- U&Es: ↑ urea/creatinine suggests acute kidney injury (AKI) which can relate to significant blood loss, for chronic renal impairment, which may relate to CKD, diabetes mellitus or hypertension.
- LFTs: underlying liver disease can result in coagulopathy.
3. Imaging
   - CT paranasal sinuses: to accurately locate and assess trauma.
   - MRI: if there are concerns of underlying malignancy.

Consider ENT referral for patients with recurrent or posterior epistaxis, or haematology if there is suspicion of underlying bleeding disorders or concurrent anticoagulation therapy.

Sore throat and vocal hoarseness

An acute sore throat most commonly relates to a benign URTI. An acute sore throat presenting with vocal changes or airway obstruction is a red flag for more significant lfie-threatening causes. Chronic throat soreness and vocal changes suggest chronic laryngeal irritation, as the result of benign, ulcerating or malignant pathology (Fig. 8.22).

HINTS AND TIPS

- Vocal hoarseness can relate to recurrent laryngeal or direct laryngeal irritation.
- In isolated hoarseness, consider compressive pathology or injury following head and neck surgery.

RED FLAG

Life-threatening presentations of sore throat and vocal hoarseness include:
- Anaphylaxis
- Epiglottis
- Peritonsillar or retropharyngeal abscesses
- Systemic inflammatory blistering conditions such as Steven-Johnson syndrome.

Urgent intervention is required to prevent airway loss.

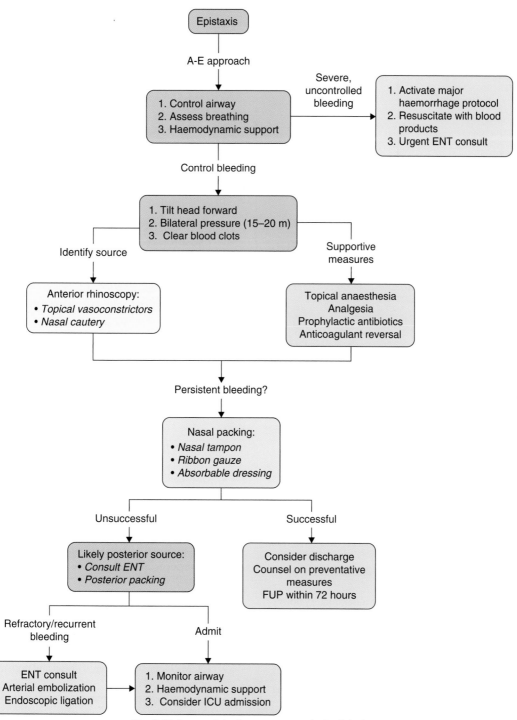

Fig. 8.21 Approach to the management of epistaxis.

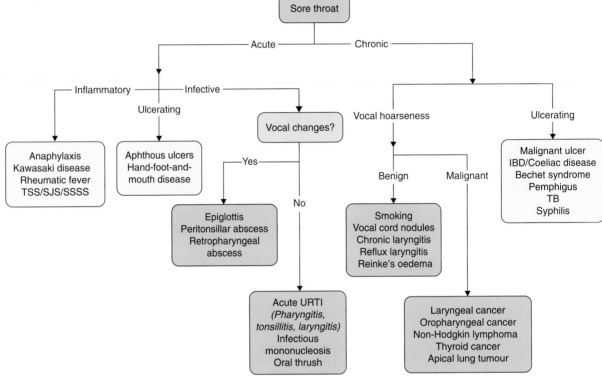

Fig. 8.22 Differential diagnosis of sore throat and hoarseness. *IBD*, Inflammatory bowel disease; *SJS*, Steven-Johnson syndrome; *SSSS*, Staphylococcal-scalded-skin-syndrome; *TB*, tuberculosis ; *TSS*, toxic shock syndrome; *URTI*, upper respiratory tract infection.

Investigations for sore throat and vocal hoarseness

1. Bedside
   - Throat swabs and culture: rapid antigen testing can be performed for Group A streptococcal (GAS) infection, and cultures to diagnose STIs.
   - Serum monospot test: to identify EBV infection in persistent pharyngitis.
   - Faecal calprotectin: to screen for inflammatory bowel disease (IBD) in chronic oral ulceration.
   - VDRL testing: syphilis may present with oral ulceration.
   - HIV testing: a risk factor for recurrent pharyngitis and aphthous ulcers.
2. Bloods
   - FBC: ↓ Hb indicates anaemia, a red flag for underlying malignancy.
   - U&Es/LFTs: important as a baseline for treatment in malignant pathology.
   - CRP/ESR: elevated in inflammatory and autoimmune conditions.
   - Antistreptolysin O titres: to confirm a diagnosis of invasive GAS.
   - Blood cultures: will be positive in for Staphylococcus or Streptococci species in toxic shock syndrome (TSS) and Staphylococcal-scalded-skin-syndrome (SSSS).
3. Imaging
   - CXR: to identify apical lung lesions that may compress on the recurrent laryngeal nerve, or evidence of tuberculosis.
   - Lateral neck X-ray: to look for the steeple sign of acute epiglottitis.
   - CT/MRI imaging: to identify head and neck malignancy, or mediastinal masses.
   - Echocardiogram: to screen for aneurysms in Kawasaki disease.
   - Nasal endoscopy: to visualize nasopharyngeal or sinus lesions and take tissue samples for biopsy if required.

- Laryngoscopy: for direct visualization of laryngeal lesions and to take tissue biopsies for histology.
- Skin biopsy: for diagnosis of blistering skin disorders.

CLINICAL NOTES

- Group A streptococcus (GAS) is a common cause of pharyngitis (Strep throat).
- Invasive GAS infection can develop, with complications including glomerulonephritis, rheumatic fever and toxic shock syndrome.
- Accurate diagnosis and timely treatment are essential to avoid systemic spread of infection.

ENT EXAMINATIONS

Introduction
Prepare for the examination by gathering equipment, introducing yourself and gaining consent.

HINTS AND TIPS

Prepare your equipment appropriately before you approach the patient. A head torch may be invaluable!

General inspection
Begin with an end-of-the-bed assessment, to look for mobility aids, monitoring devices and medications that may give clues as to underlying pathology.

Examining the ears

To examine the ears, you will require a 512 Hz tuning fork, and an otoscope.

Hearing assessment
Begin with a gross hearing assessment:

- Ask if there have been any recent changes in their hearing.
- Position yourself 60 cm behind the patient. Test their better side first.
- Explain to the patient you are going to whisper some numbers to them, and they should repeat it back if they can hear them.

- Rub the tragus of the opposite ear to prevent sounds from being heard in that ear.
- Whisper a number or word. If the patient can repeat it back to you, record the result and test the other ear.
- If the patient cannot repeat it, use a conversational voice, then a loud voice.
- If the patient remains unable to hear, repeat the test at 15 cm, again starting with a whisper, then conversational, then loud voice.
- Record the best result for each ear.

CLINICAL NOTES

- At 60 cm, hearing a whisper indicates hearing of 12 db or better.
- Hearing conversational voice only indicates hearing of 48 db or worse.
- Hearing a loud voice only indicates hearing of 76 db or worse.

Rinne and Weber's test
Assess the hearing using a 512 Hz tuning fork.

HINTS AND TIPS

- A 512 Hz tuning fork is small, and vibrates at a high frequency, useful for assessing hearing. In neurological exams, a 128 Hz tuning fork is used, which is large and vibrates at a lower frequency, useful for assessing vibration sensation.

Weber's test assesses for unilateral SNHL or CHL.

- Pinch the tuning fork and place it in the middle of the forehead.
- Ask the patient where they hear the sound.
- If they can hear it louder in one ear, this is described as 'lateralization'.

Rinne's test assesses the difference in bone and air conduction (The 'air-bone gap'):

- Move to the side which Weber's test lateralizes to.
- Pinch the tuning fork and place it on the mastoid process (testing bone conduction).
- Confirm the patient can hear the sound and ask them to tell you when they can no longer hear it.

Table 8.4 Rinne and Weber's test

	Weber's	Rinne's
Normal	No lateralization	Air conduction > bone conduction (Rinne's positive)
SNHL	Louder in the normal ear	Air conduction > bone conduction (Rinne's positive)
CHL	Louder in the affected ear	Bone conduction > air conduction (Rinne's negative)

- When they can no longer hear it, move the tuning fork in front of the ear (testing air conduction).
- If the patient can hear the sound again, this suggests air conduction is better than bone conduction, which is normal. This is described as 'Rinne's positive' (Table 8.4).

CLINICAL NOTES

- In SNHL, air and bone conduction are reduced equally, as the impairment is within the vestibulocochlear nerve.
- Weber's lateralizes to the unaffected ear and Rinne's test is positive, as the 'air-bone gap', or the difference between air and bone conduction remains the same.
- In CHL, air conduction is reduced, but bone conduction is normal.
- Weber's test lateralizes to the louder in the affected ear, as ambient background noise is reduced, amplifying the perception of sound received via bone conduction to the cochlea. The 'air-bone' gap is increased, therefore Rinne's is negative.

Examining the ear

Inspection
Inspect the external aspect of the ear

- Pinna: look for asymmetry, deformity, erythema, swelling, scars or skin lesions.
- Auricle: look for erythema, skin lesions or haematomas.
- Mastoid: inspect for erythema, swelling and scars.
- EAC: erythema and discharge may be evident externally (Fig. 8.23).

Palpation
Palpate the external ear:

- Tragus: tenderness is associated with underlying infection.
- Lymph nodes: preauricular and postauricular lymphadenopathy may suggest infection.

Otoscopy
If there is pain, examine the nonpainful ear first.

- Turn on the light of the otoscope and apply a sterile speculum.
- Hold the otoscope in your right hand when examining the right ear, and vice versa.
- Hold the otoscope like a pencil, and stabilize your hand against the patient's cheek.
- Pull the pinna upwards and backwards to straighten the EAC.
- Advance the otoscope slowly and gently into the ear, and once in place look through the viewing window (Fig. 8.24).

External auditory canal
Inspect the EAC:

- Ear wax: excessive ear wax is a common cause of conductive hearing loss.
- Discharge: sloughy white discharge is associated with infection. Mucus or blood suggests TM perforation.
- Erythema and swelling: inflammation and oedema suggest infection. Significant swelling may obstruct the view of the TM.
- Foreign bodies: may be evident within the canal and produce hearing loss.

Tympanic membrane
The TM should be systematically assessed for signs of underlying pathology:

- Colour: a normal TM is pearly grey and translucent. Erythema suggests acute infection.
- Shape: Bulging or retraction indicates increased or decreased middle ear pressure, seen in infection or eustachian tube dysfunction, respectively.
- Perforation: perforation of the TM can occur as the result of large effusion and increased pressure in the middle ear, trauma or insertion of tympanostomy tubes.
- Scarring: scarring of the TM (tympanosclerosis) occurs following significant or recurrent infection, or surgery (Figs 8.25-8.26).

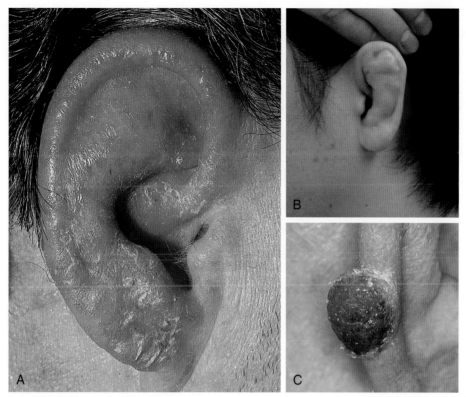

Fig. 8.23 Inspection of the external ear. (A) Erythema and swelling of the auricle, indicating severe external ear infection. (B) Repeated haematomas can result in chronic remodelling of auricular cartilage, known as 'cauliflower ear'. It is common in athletes following repeated blunt trauma. (C) Skin lesion on the helix, suspicious of underlying squamous cell carcinoma. (From A. Dinulos JGH. *Habif's Clinical Dermatology: A Color Guide to Diagnosis and Therapy*, 7th Edition. Elsevier; 2021. B. Manske RC, Magee DJ. *Orthopedic Physical Assessment*, 7th Edition, *South Asia Edition*. Elsevier; 2021. C. Shiland BJ, Zenith. *Medical Assistant: Integumentary, Sensory Systems, Patient Care and Communication—Module A*. Elsevier; 2016.)

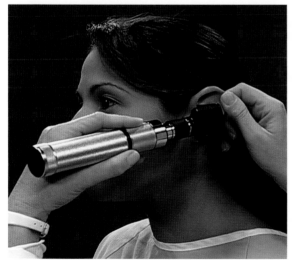

Fig. 8.24 Using an otoscope. Proper positioning of an otoscope, with pencil grip and gentle retraction of the pinna. (From Leonard PC. *Building a Medical Vocabulary: With Spanish Translations*, 11th Edition. Saunders, Elsevier Inc. 2022.)

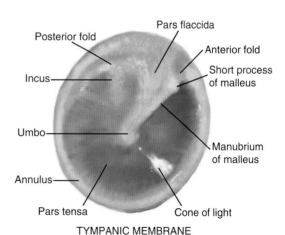

Pars flaccida

Posterior fold

Anterior fold

Short process of malleus

Incus

Manubrium of malleus

Umbo

Annulus

Pars tensa

Cone of light

TYMPANIC MEMBRANE

Fig. 8.25 The normal tympanic membrane. Tympanic membrane of the right ear. (From Lewis SL, Roberts D, Harding MM, Heitkemper MM, Kwong J, Bucher L. *Medical-Surgical Nursing: Assessment and Management of Clinical Problems*, 10th Edition. Elsevier; 2017.)

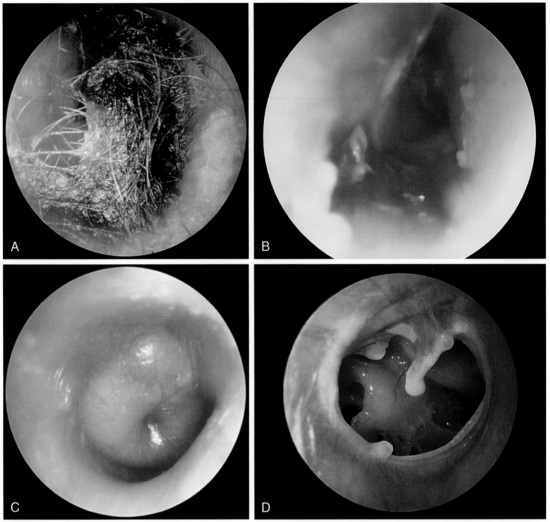

Fig. 8.26 Otoscopy findings in ear pathology. (A) Cerumen (ear wax) obstructing the EAC. (B) In otitis externa, the canal will be erythematous, swollen and full of debris, but the TM, if visible, will not bulge. In otitis media (C) effusion within the middle ear will result in painful swelling behind the tympanic membrane, and visible erythema. (D) TM perforation. (From A. Swartz MH. *Textbook of Physical Diagnosis: History and Examination,* 8th Edition. Elsevier; 2021. B. Nowalk AJ, Chi DH, Tobey A, McIntire SC, Zitelli BJ, Garrison J. *Zitelli and Davis' Atlas of Pediatric Physical Diagnosis,* 8th Edition. Elsevier; 2023. C. Chenot JF, Scherer M. *Allgemeinmedizin, 1. Auflage.* Elsevier; 2022. D. Ignatavicius DD, Rebar CR, Ignatavicius DD, Workman ML, Borchers AA, Heimgartner NM. *Medical-Surgical Nursing: Concepts for Interprofessional Collaborative Care,* Tenth Edition. Elsevier; 2021.)

HINTS AND TIPS

- The cone of light appears in the inferior anterior quadrant, on the left in the left ear, and on the right in the right ear.
- An absent of the cone of light indicates increased middle ear pressure, typically seen in otitis media with middle ear effusion.

Once you have finished inspecting the TM, withdraw the otoscope, change the speculum and repeat the examination on the other side.

Completing the examination

Thank the patient, wash your hands and summarize your findings.

Further tests include:

- Pure tone audiometry: to objectively assess hearing.

- Tympanometry: to assess TM compliance.
- Neurological examination: to identify neurological pathologies associated with symptoms.

HINTS exam

The HINTS exam is used to differentiate between central (life-threatening) and peripheral (typically benign) causes of vertigo. The HINTS exam includes assessment of head impulse, nystagmus and test of skew, and has a high sensitivity and specificity for diagnosing central vertigo. It is used in patients with persistent vertigo, nystagmus and a normal neurological exam.

Head-impulse test

Performing the head-impulse test when patients are actively experiencing vertigo:

- Move the patient's head from side to side with their neck relaxed.
- Then ask them to fix their eyes on your nose.
- Rapidly move the patient's head slightly side to side.

If a corrective saccade occurs (the eyes move with the head, then saccade back to the fixed point) the test is positive. This indicates disruption to the vestibulo-ocular reflex, reassuring for ipsilateral vestibulocochlear pathology.

Nystagmus

Assess for nystagmus:

- Ask the patient to look straight ahead and observe their primary gaze.
- Ask the patient to look left to right without fixating on an object.
- Ask the patient to look at a fixed point away from centre.
- Check for repetitive back-and-forth movements of the eyes at each point.

Unidirectional nystagmus is reassuring for peripheral pathology. Bidirectional or vertical nystagmus is associated with central pathologies. Gaze-evoked nystagmus (occurring when looking at a fixed point away from centre) is strongly suggestive of stroke.

Test of skew

The test of skew test includes

- Cover one of the patient's eyes and ask them to look at your nose.
- Quickly move your hand to cover the other eye.
- Observe the uncovered eye for any vertical or diagonal corrective movement.
- Repeat on the other side.

Table 8.5 HINTS examination findings

	Peripheral	Central
Head impulse	Positive	Negative
Nystagmus	Unidirectional/absent	Bidirectional/vertical
Test of skew	Absent	Vertical skew

Vertical or diagonal movements indicate an abnormal deviation of the eye while it is being covered, and correction when it is uncovered. This suggests a central cause.

Completing the examination

Thank the patient and summarize your findings Table 8.5. Further tests include:

- Examination of the nose and oral cavity: complete assessment is essential for any patient presenting with ENT pathology.
- Assessment of gait: to assess balance, coordination and proprioception.
- Romberg's test: ask the patient to stand with their feet together, hands by their sides and close their eyes. Loss of balance with loss of a visual stimulus indicates a vestibular lesion. The patient will fall to the affected side.
- Dix-Hallpike test: to assess for benign paroxysmal positional vertigo (BPPV) (Table 8.5).

Rhinoscopy

External nose inspection

Inspect the external aspect of the nose:

- Skin changes: skin lesions may suggest dermatological pathology including basal or squamous cell carcinoma.
- Deformities: assess for septal or nasal bone deviation.
- Epistaxis: anterior bleeding may be visible externally.

Nasal cavity inspection

Use a nasal speculum to widen the nasal cavity and inspect the cavities using a head torch.
Using a nasal speculum:

- Insert your index finger into the bend of the speculum and stabilize it with your thumb.
- Use your middle and ring fingers to compress the speculum prongs.
- Insert it gently and slowly into the patient's nose then reduce your grip slightly to widen the prongs and view of the nasal cavity through the gap between your fingers.

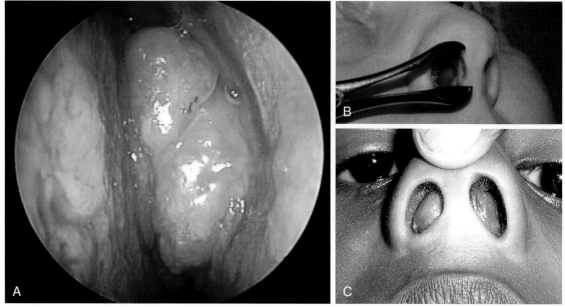

Fig. 8.27 Rhinoscopy. (A) A single, pale grey mass presenting a nasal polyp arising from the middle nasal meatus. (B) Evidence of septal perforation. (C) A large septal haematoma visible in both nasal cavities. (From A. Hauser LJ, Ramakrishnan VR, Scholes MA, Kingdom TT. *ENT Secrets,* 4th Edition. Elsevier; 2016. B. Complications in rhinoplasty. *CPS* 2022. C. Cornelius J, Devaji Rao S. *Clinical Manual of Surgery.* Elsevier; 2014.)

Assessing the nasal cavities:

- Nasal vestibules: assess for inflammation, oedema or mucosal lesions.
- Nasal septum: assess for polyps, deviation, haematomas or perforation.
- Inferior turbinates: inspect for inflammation, polyps or asymmetry (Fig. 8.27).

Palpation

Palpate the nasal bones, cartilage and infraorbital ridges carefully:

- Alignment: septal deviation may be palpable. Malalignment suggests previous fracture.
- Tenderness: may indicate acute nasal or sinus infection.
- Irregularity: suggestive of nasal or orbital fracture.

Nasal airflow

Assess nasal airflow:

- Compress the nostril not being assessed to occlude airflow.
- Ask the patient to breathe through their nose.
- Assess airflow using the feeling of the breath on your hand.
- Repeat on the other side.

Disparity in airflow indicates unilateral nasal obstruction.

Completing the examination

Thank the patient, wash your hands and summarize your findings. Further tests include:

- Examination of the ears and oral cavity.
- Regional lymph node examination: lymphadenopathy is associated with infection.
- Objective olfactory assessment: for formal assessment of hyposmia and anosmia.
- Flexible nasendoscopy: for direct visualization of the posterior nasal cavity.

Examining the oral cavity

HINTS AND TIPS

Equipment required includes:
- Head torch
- Tongue depressor
- PPE (gloves, mask and visor)
  Be sure to remove dentures or implants before proceeding!

General inspection

Inspect the patient's face and oral cavity for signs of pathology.

- Salivary gland swelling: swelling of the cheek or below the jaw may indicate parotid or submandibular pathology.
- Angular stomatitis: inflammation at the corners of the mouth indicating nutrient deficiencies.
- Ulceration: can develop on the lips, gums, tongue or buccal mucosa as the result of trauma, infection or malignancy.
- Teeth: missing or decaying teeth indicate poor oral hygiene. Nicotine staining occurs with smoking, a significant risk factor for head and neck malignancy.
- Gums: inflamed and tender gums indicate gingivitis, which can progress to periodontitis, gum recession and tooth loss, if untreated.
- Parotid duct: swelling indicates infection or calcification.

Tongue and palate

Inspect the superior surface of the tongue and palate:

- Oral thrush: white slough on the tongue associated with fungal infection.
- Glossitis: erythema and enlargement of the tongue related to vitamin deficiencies.
- Hairy leucoplakia: white patches on the tongue associated with EBV infection.
- Palatal vessels: palatal telangiectasia can occur in autoimmune disorders.
- Skin changes: primary palatal neoplasms, malignant skin lesions and papilloma can present with palatal skin changes (Fig. 8.28).

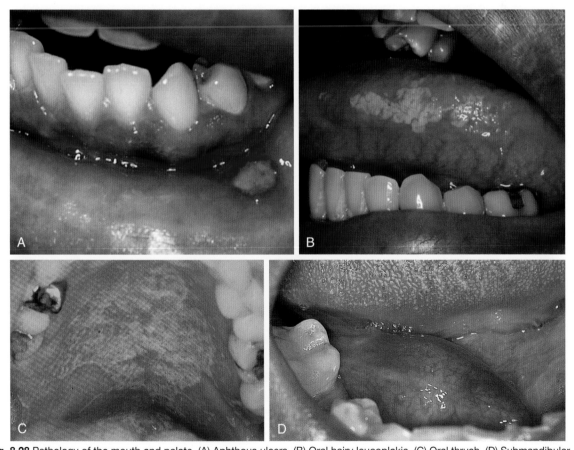

Fig. 8.28 Pathology of the mouth and palate. (A) Aphthous ulcers. (B) Oral hairy leucoplakia. (C) Oral thrush. (D) Submandibular obstruction/swelling. (From A. Zitelli BJ, McIntire SC, D'Alesio A, et al. *Zitelli and Davis' Atlas of Pediatric Physical Diagnosis,* 8th Edition. Elsevier; 2023. B. Ibsen OAC, Peters SM. *Oral Pathology for the Dental Hygienist: With General Pathology Introductions,* 8th Edition. Elsevier; 2023. C. Jones S, Merrick ST, Goldman L, Schafer AI, Glesby MJ. *Goldman-Cecil Medicine, 2-Volume Set,* 26th Edition. Elsevier; 2020. D. Carrozzo M, Flaitz CM, Scully C, Gandolfo S, Bagan JV. *Pocketbook of Oral Disease.* Churchill Livingstone, Elsevier; 2013.)

Tonsils, pharynx and uvula

Inspect the tonsils and uvula for abnormalities:

- Swelling: swelling can occur in infection, stones or malignancy.
- Exudate: erythema and exudate indicate acute infection.
- Calcifications: mineralization of tonsillar debris forms stones, known as tonsilloliths.
- Erythema: pharyngeal erythema occurs as the result of infection or irritation.
- Uvula deviation: a peritonsillar abscess results in deviation of the uvula away from the abscess. Vagus nerve pathology causes deviation away from the lesion because of impaired soft palate elevation (Fig. 8.29).

Salivary glands

Inspect the floor of the mouth for salivary pathology:

- Sialolithiasis: calcification and stone formation obstructing the salivary ducts.
- Sialadenitis: infection of a salivary gland, associated with erythema and discharge.

Palpation

If appropriate and with consent, bimanual palpation of the mouth can be performed.

- Palpate identified lumps to assess the size, texture, consistency and tenderness.

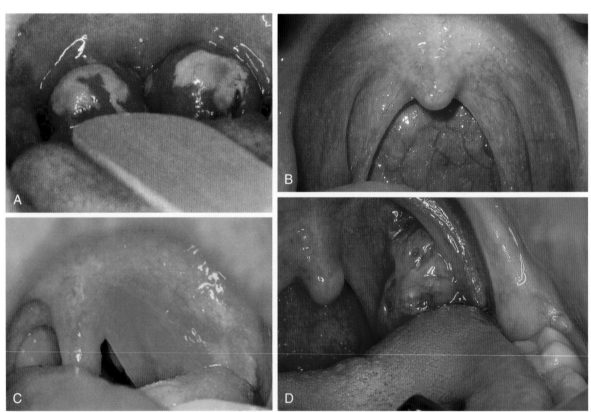

Fig. 8.29 Tonsillar pathology. (A) Tonsillar exudate. (B) Pharyngeal inflammation, indicating pharyngitis. (C) Uvula deviation, indicating a potential underlying peritonsillar abscess. (D) Enlarged palatine tonsil with prominent crypts exhibiting focal yellowish-white calcifications, indicating tonsilloliths. (From A. Epstein-Barr viral infectious mononucleosis. *YMHN* 1995. B. Mayatepek E, Knuf M. *Repetitorium Facharztprüfung Kinder- und Jugendmedizin, 1. Auflage.* Elsevier Urban-Fischer Germany; 2021. C. Ausiello D, Tami TA, Goldman L. *Cecil Medicine,* 23rd Edition. Elsevier; 2008. D. Neville BW, Chi AC, Allen CM, Damm DD. *Color Atlas of Oral and Maxillofacial Diseases.* Elsevier; 2019.)

- Palpate the walls and floor of the mouth to assess for salivary swelling and obstruction.

Completing the examination

Thank the patient, wash your hands and summarize your findings. Further tests include:

- Ear and nose examination.
- Flexible nasal endoscopy: to assess the posterior oral cavity.
- Dental X-ray: to assess for dental abnormalities or caries.
- Ultrasound neck: to further characterize neck lumps or salivary gland swelling.
- CT/MRI imaging: essential if oropharyngeal malignancy is suspected.

DISORDERS OF THE EAR

External ear disorders
Otitis externa

Otitis externa (OE) is the inflammation of the EAC. It typically results from bacterial infection, including Pseudomonas, Staphylococcus and Escherichia coli infection. Fungal infections (otomycosis) are common in immunosuppressed patients. Risk factors include water entry into the ear (swimmer's ear) or chronic skin disorders including seborrheic dermatitis. Chronic OE is inflammation lasting >6 weeks.

Symptoms and signs

Typical symptoms and signs include:

- Severe otalgia
- Conductive hearing loss
- Otorrhoea
- Intense itching
- Crusting and auricular erythema (Fig. 8.30)

Investigations

Investigations are only required in recurrent or refractory disease, diagnostic uncertainty or risk factors for severe infection.

- Ear MC&S: if there are risk factors for antibiotic resistance, insufficient response to initial treatment, or suspected intracranial complications.
- Tympanometry: If there is diagnostic uncertainty between OE and otitis media (OM), tympanometry can be performed, to assess tympanic membrane mobility and to confirm the presence of a middle ear effusion.

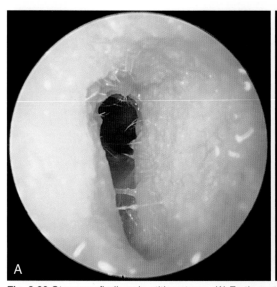
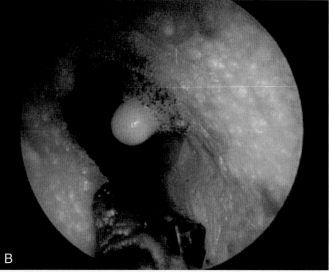

Fig. 8.30 Otoscopy findings in otitis externa. (A) Erythematous and swollen EAC with sloughy discharge, indicating OE. (B) Black spores are typical of fungal infection, commonly aspergillus. (From A. Swartz MH. *Textbook of Physical Diagnosis: History and Examination,* 8th Edition. Elsevier; 2021. B. Dhillon RS, East CA. *Ear, Nose and Throat and Head and Neck Surgery: An Illustrated Colour Text,* 4th Edition. Elsevier; 2012.)

Management

Management includes supportive therapy and topical antibiotics:

- Analgesia: over-the-counter analgesia, with short courses of opioids for significant pain.
- Aural toilet: warm water lavage to clear debris from the EAC.
- Topical antibiotics: ciprofloxacin or gentamicin drops, for 7-14 days.
- Topical steroids: offered in combination with antibiotics to reduce swelling and pain.
- Topical antifungals: typically clotrimazole, used in otomycosis.

If symptoms fail to improve after a 14-day antibiotic course, consider ENT referral. Systemic antibiotics are used in systemic illness, intracranial spread of infection or immunocompromised patients.

COMMON PITFALLS

- Ear drops should be used while lying down.
- The ear should be filled with drops and tragus gently manipulated to encourage penetration into the ear.
- It is important to remain lying down for several minutes to ensure drops don't flow out of the ear.
- Review ear drop technique if symptoms fail to resolve following initial treatment!

Complications

Complications of otitis externa include:

- Cellulitis: extension of infection to the skin outside the EAC.
- Abscess: local collections of pus, that may require drainage.
- Ear canal stenosis: chronic OE can result in scarring and narrowing of the EAC, which presents with CHL and recurrent ear infection. Surgery can be performed to widen the canal and improve hearing.
- TM perforation: spread of infection to the eardrum can result TM perforation, which typically resolves spontaneously within several months, or can be surgically repaired.
- Malignant otitis externa (MOE): necrotizing intracranial spread of infection that can result in osteomyelitis of the skull base, meningitis and cerebral abscess (Figs 8.31-8.32).

RED FLAG

- Severe otalgia, hearing loss, otorrhea, periauricular erythema and facial nerve palsies suggests MOE.
- There is a high risk of overwhelming systemic infection and death without prompt recognition and management.
- Risk factors include immunocompromise, typically diabetes.

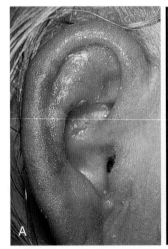
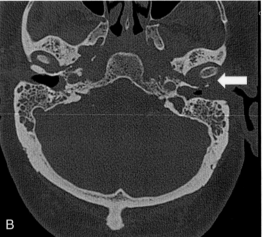

Fig. 8.31 Malignant otitis externa. (A) External appearance of MOE. (B) CT of the temporal bone in a diabetic patient demonstrating bony erosion of the left anterior ear canal (arrow) and soft tissue filling the external auditory canal (EAC). (From A. Habif TP. *Skin Disease: Diagnosis and Treatment,* 3rd Edition. Elsevier; 2011. B. Ruckenstein MJ, Lund VJ, Thomas JR, et al. *Cummings Otolaryngology: Head and Neck Surgery,* 7th Edition. Elsevier; 2021.)

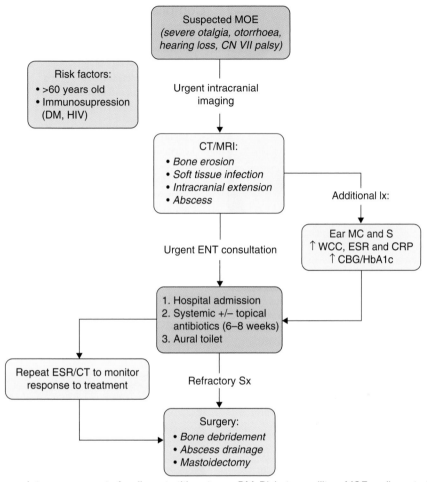

Fig. 8.32 Approach to management of malignant otitis externa. *DM*, Diabetes mellitus; *MOE*, malignant otitis externa.

Middle ear disorders
Otitis media

Otitis media (OM) is an acute infection of the middle ear. It typically develops following a viral URTI and subsequent bacterial superinfection, typically Streptococcus pneumoniae or Haemophilus influenza infection. It is most common in children between 6-24 months.

Symptoms and signs

Typical features include (Fig. 8.33):

- Otalgia
- Hearing loss in the affected ear
- Fever

CLINICAL NOTES

Infants may present with ear tugging, reduced oral intake, vomiting, incessant crying and irritability, fever and febrile seizures.

Investigations

Investigations are only indicated in severe infection, unclear diagnosis or suspected complications:

- Middle ear fluid MC&S: to guide antibiotic therapy if there is poor initial response.

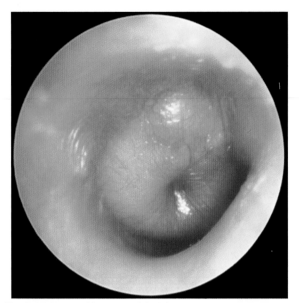

Fig. 8.33 Acute otitis media. A bulging, erythematous tympanic membrane (TM). Perforation may occur, associated with purulent discharge in the EAC and otorrhoea. (From Chenot JF, Scherer M. *Allgemeinmedizin, 1. Auflage*. Elsevier; 2022.)

- Blood cultures: if there is evidence of severe systemic infection.
- CT/MRI brain and temporal bone: if intracranial complications (i.e., mastoiditis, meningitis or cerebral abscess) are suspected.
- Tympanometry: to confirm middle ear effusion.

Management

OM is typically self-limiting within 1 week and can be managed conservatively. Antibiotics are indicated in the following circumstances:

- Bilateral symptoms
- TM perforation
- Systemic illness
- Cochlear implants
- Very young children or adults

COMMUNICATION

- Advise patients that antibiotics offer no benefit in viral infections, and have associated side effects.
- If the patient is very anxious and resistant to conservative measures, a backup antibiotic prescription can be considered.

Complications

Complications include:

- Mastoiditis: spread of infection into the mastoid air cells, resulting in severe otalgia, boggy mastoid swelling and forward protrusion of the pinna.
- Labyrinthitis: inflammation of the inner ear labyrinth, associated with vertigo, nystagmus, and sensorineural hearing loss.
- Facial nerve palsy: a rare complication, treated with corticosteroids.
- TM perforation: typically resolves spontaneously with antibiotic treatment. The ear should be kept clean and dry. Tympanoplasty can be performed if the TM fails to repair after several months.
- Chronic infection: chronic infection can develop following repeated episodes, including chronic suppurative otitis media (CSOM) and otitis media with effusion (OME).
- Cholesteatoma: destructive proliferation of keratinizing squamous epithelium in the middle ear, presenting with painless, foul otorrhea and progressive hearing loss. Surgical removal with tympanomastoidectomy is required to limit bony erosion (Figs 8.34-8.36).

RED FLAG

Mastoiditis is a medical emergency, due to the risk of intracranial spread and severe systemic infection. In patients with persistent or worsening OM, and evidence of mastoid swelling or pinna displacement, have a low threshold for hospital referral.

HINTS AND TIPS

- CSOM is a chronic middle ear infection associated with nonhealing TM perforation.
- Symtoms include persistent otorrhoea and CHL.
- Management includes topical antibiotics and tympanoplasty.
- OME is a chronic noninfective middle ear effusion. Symptoms include CHL and delayed speech development in children.
- Management includes watchful waiting for 3 months, followed by tympanostomy tube insertion to drain middle ear fluid if symptoms fail to resolve.

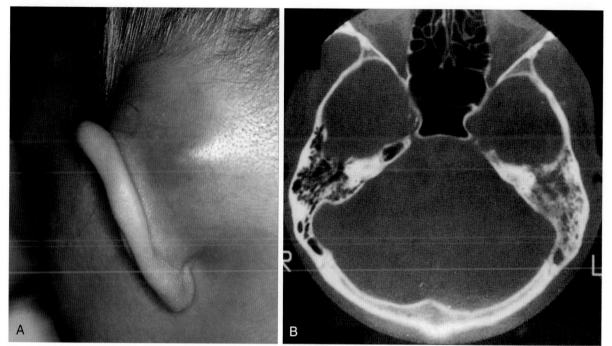

Fig. 8.34 Clinical findings in mastoiditis. (A) Erythema and swelling of the mastoid, with forward protrusion of the pinna. (B) CT scan showing destruction of the mastoid air cells on the left-hand side and collection of pus in the cavity. (From A. Omar AM. *USMLE Step 2 CK Plus.* Elsevier; 2023. B. Long SS, Conway JH, Kimberlin DW, Prober CG, Wald ER. *Principles and Practice of Pediatric Infectious Diseases,* 6th Edition. Elsevier; 2023.)

Otosclerosis

Otosclerosis is the abnormal growth of bone in the inner ear labyrinth. Impaired ossicular vibration results in reduced sound wave transmission to the inner ear and a progressive conductive hearing loss (CHL). Symptoms are commonly bilateral. The cause is unknown.

Symptoms and signs

Symptoms include

- Progressive CHL which will result in deafness
- Tinnitus
- Vertigo
- Quiet speech, due to increased perception of noise heard by bone conduction

Investigations

Audiometry will reveal CHL, with decreased air conduction (Fig. 8.37).

Management

Otosclerosis is typically managed with surgery. Hearing aids may be useful to compensate for hearing loss but cannot influence progression.

- Stapedectomy: removal of the osteosclerotic stapes bone and prosthesis replacement.
- Cochlear implant: for patients with profound bilateral deafness.

Inner ear disorders
Acoustic neuroma

An acoustic neuroma is a benign, slow-growing tumour arising from Schwann cells in the vestibulocochlear nerve. Tumours can form at any point along the nerve, and may extend into the cerebellopontine angle, the triangular space bounded by the cerebellum, brainstem and temporal bone. Unilateral tumours are typically sporadic. Bilateral tumours are closely associated with neurofibromatosis type 2.

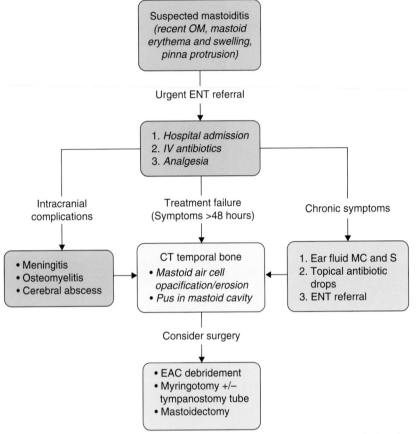

Fig. 8.35 Approach to the management of mastoiditis. *EAC*, External auditory canal; *OM*, otitis media.

Symptoms and signs

Symptoms relate to the mass effect of the tumour and the structures affected:

- CN VIII: SNHL tinnitus, vertigo, postural instability. Most commonly affected.
- CN V: unilateral facial paraesthesia and pain.
- CN VII: unilateral facial weakness, that can progress to paralysis.
- Cerebellum: ataxia.
- Ventricular system: obstructive hydrocephalus.

Investigations

Assessment should start with a complete cranial nerve exam. Further tests include:

- Audiometry: to detect unilateral or bilateral SNHL, which will be present in the majority of patients.
- MRI contrast: to confirm the diagnosis and locate the tumour (Fig. 8.38).

Management

Management options include:

- Watchful waiting: for patients with small tumours, minimal hearing loss or advanced age, with surveillance every 6-12 months.
- Surgical resection: for those with large tumours with compressive symptoms or significant hearing loss. Adjuvant radiotherapy can be offered.

Acoustic neuromas have a good prognosis, low recurrence rates and high rates of cure.

Benign paroxysmal positional vertigo

Benign paroxysmal positional vertigo (BPPV) is a common inner ear disorder presenting with paroxysmal episodes of vertigo triggered by changes in head position. Dislodging of otoconia, small crystals within the otolith organs into the semicircular canals disrupt endolymph flow and result in vertigo. The aetiology is unclear. BPPV has been associated with head trauma,

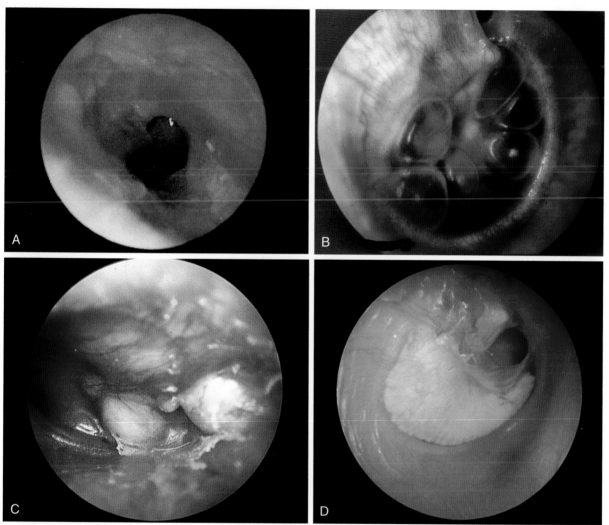

Fig. 8.36 Chronic otitis media infections and complications. (A) CSOM, with evidence of TM perforation, otorrhoea and inflammation of the external auditory canal. (B) Otitis media with effusion. Bubbles and air fluid levels are evidence behind the retracted TM. (C) Abnormal skin growth and bony erosions in the middle ear, indicating cholesteatoma. (D) Chalky white plaques on the TM, with small perforation, indicating tympanosclerosis. (From A. Dhillon RS, East CA. *Ear, Nose and Throat and Head and Neck Surgery: An Illustrated Colour Text,* 4th Edition. Churchill Livingstone, Elsevier; 2012. B. Dhingra S, Dhingra PL. *Diseases of Ear, Nose and Throat & Head and Neck Surgery,* 8th Edition. Elsevier; 2022. C. Nowalk AJ, McIntire SC, Chi DH, Zitelli BJ, Garrison J, Tobey A. *Zitelli and Davis' Atlas of Pediatric Physical Diagnosis,* 8th Edition. Elsevier; 2023. D. Glynn M, Wareing MJ, Warner E, Drake WM. *Hutchison's Clinical Methods: An Integrated Approach to Clinical Practice,* 25th Edition. Elsevier; 2023.)

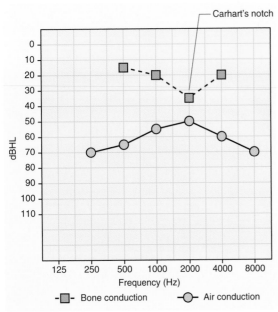

Fig. 8.37 Audiogram in otosclerosis. Audiogram showing decreased air conduction relative to bone conduction. The Carhart's notch is a decrease in bone conduction at 2000 Hz, commonly seen in patients with otosclerosis. (From Keegan D, et al. *Crash Course: Ophthalmology Dermatology ENT,* 3rd Edition. Elsevier; 2009.)

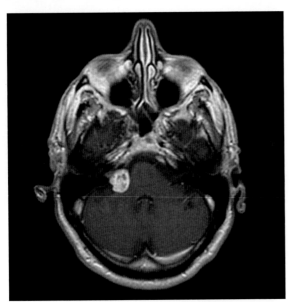

Fig. 8.38 MRI in acoustic neuroma. Contrast MRI demonstrating a large right acoustic neuroma originating from the internal auditory canal. The tumour extends into the cerebellopontine angle, where it is compressing the brain stem. (From Goldman L, DeAngelis LM, Schafer AI. *Goldman-Cecil Medicine, 2-Volume Set,* 26th Edition. Elsevier; 2020.)

intracranial surgery and other inner ear disorders, and risk factors including female sex, increasing age and osteoporosis.

Symptoms and signs

Symptoms include sudden onset, recurrent episodes of vertigo precipitated by changes in head position relative to gravity, with spontaneous resolve within minutes. Further symptoms include:

- Nystagmus (toward the affected ear)
- Postural instability
- Nausea and vomiting

Investigations

Diagnostic criteria include:

- A history of episodic vertigo triggered by changes in head position.
- Vertigo and rotatory nystagmus triggered by provoking manoeuvres.
- Resolution of symptoms within 60 seconds of onset.

Dix Hallpike manoeuvre

The Dix-Hallpike manoeuvre is the first-line provoking manoeuvre. Performing the manoeuvre involves:

1. Sit the patient upright on the examination bed.
2. Rotate the head to 45 degrees on the affected side.
3. Lay the patient down quickly, keeping the head rotated and slightly extending the neck.
4. Hold the position, examine the eyes for nystagmus and enquire if the patient has vertigo.

If the test is negative, repeat with the head turned to the unaffected side at step 2. If the test is positive, wait for nystagmus to resolve, and perform the Epley repositioning manoeuvre, which follows from step 4 of the Dix-Hallpike manoeuvre.

Epley manoeuvre

1. Turn the patient's head by 90 degrees to the unaffected side, and hold for 30 seconds.
2. Turn the patient's head and body by 90 degrees again so that they are lying on their unaffected side with their face turned toward the ground, and hold for 30 seconds.
3. Bring the patient back to a seated, upright position with the head at neutral.
4. Ask the patient to rest in that position for several minutes.

If the Dix-Hallpike test is positive, the Epley manoeuvre should rapidly resolve symptoms (Fig. 8.39).

If the Dix-Hallpike manoeuvre is negative, further tests include:

- Head-roll test: for diagnosing lateral semicircular canal BPPV.

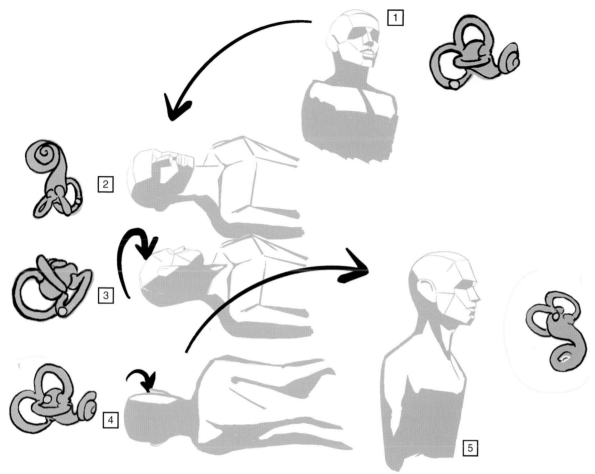

Fig. 8.39 Dix-Hallpike and Epley manoeuvres. The Dix-Hallpike manoeuvre (steps 1–2) triggers displacement of the otoconia into the semicircular canals. The Epley manoeuvre (steps 3–5). (From Armbruster BA, et al. *Medicine in a Day: Revision Notes for Medical Exams, Finals, UKMLA and Foundation Years*. Elsevier; 2023.)

- Audiometry: to rule out differentials. Typically, normal in BPPV.
- Vestibular function tests: to diagnose vestibular pathology.
- MRI head: to exclude central causes of vertigo.

Management

Conservative measures are preferred first-line, and include:

- Watchful waiting: mild, infrequent BPPV can be managed with observation alone.
- Epley repositioning manoeuvres: either performed by a medical professional or the patient themselves at home, if recurrences are frequent.
- Vestibular rehabilitation therapy: a set of physical exercises to treat dizziness and imbalance that the patient can perform at home as an adjunctive measure.

CLINICAL NOTES

- Medical vestibular suppressants are avoided where possible due to their side effect profile.
- They may be used for short durations if repositioning manoeuvres are not possible, for example in C-spine injury.
- Surgery, including vestibular neurectomy or semicircular canal occlusion, is indicated only for intractable BPPV with frequent, disabling recurrences.

Many cases spontaneously resolve within months. There is an annual recurrence rate of approximately 15%.

Complications

Complications include:

- Postural instability/falls: subsequently leading to fractures, dislocations or head injury.
- Psychological effects: BPPV can result in depression, anxiety and social avoidance, due to the unpredictable nature of symptoms.

Ménière's disease

Ménière's disease results from impaired endolymph flow in the inner ear. The aetiology is unclear. It is common in women aged between 40-50 years and has been associated with viral infection and autoimmune disease.

Symptoms and signs

Ménière's disease presents with attacks of the 'Ménière's triad', of sudden onset severe vertigo, tinnitus and unilateral fluctuating SNHL lasting for minutes to hours. Further symptoms include:

- Horizontal rotatory nystagmus
- Aural fullness
- Nausea and vomiting

> **HINTS AND TIPS**
>
> - Symptoms of Ménière's disease are severe, and often completely debilitating.
> - SNHL will progressively worsen with each attack.

Investigations

Ménière's disease is diagnosed by the characteristic clinical features, supported by audiometry. Diagnostic criteria include:

- >2 attacks of spontaneous vertigo lasting minutes to hours.
- Audiometry demonstrating SNHL in the affected ear before, during or after an episode.
- Fluctuating symptoms in the affected ear.
- Exclusion of other causes of vertigo.

Further investigations are not typically indicated, unless required to rule out other differentials.

Management

Management focuses on symptom control and avoidance of attacks. There is no cure.

- Conservative management: lifestyle modifications, including stress reduction and trigger avoidance, and vestibular rehabilitation.
- Medical management: vestibular suppressants including betahistine. Intratympanic gentamicin or steroid injections can be considered for refractory symptoms (Fig. 8.40).
- Surgical management: labyrinthectomy (sacrifices hearing) or vestibular neurectomy (preserves hearing).

Hearing aids and cochlear implants can be used if permanent hearing impairment develops.

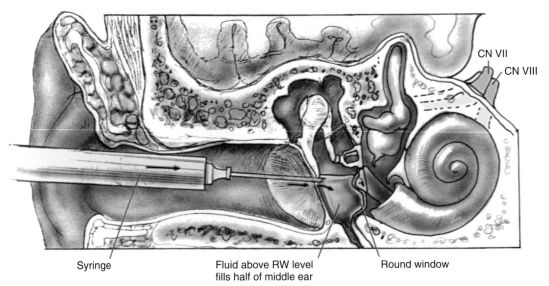

CN VII
CN VIII

Syringe   Fluid above RW level   Round window
                 fills half of middle ear

Fig. 8.40 Intratympanic injections. Intratympanic gentamicin injection. Typically well tolerated and associated with great reduction in intensity and frequency of symptoms. (From Brackmann D, et al. *Otologic Surgery*, 5th Edition. Elsevier; 2023.)

Vestibular neuritis

Vestibular neuritis is the inflammation of the vestibular nerve. It commonly develops following a viral URTI. It is the second most common cause of vertigo. Symptoms typically develop over several hours, last for days to weeks, and may persist for months.

Symptoms and signs

Vestibular neuritis presents with an acute vestibular syndrome:

- Severe vertigo, that is persistent and continuous
- Nystagmus
- Nausea and vomiting
- Postural instability and falls

If hearing loss is present, it is referred to as labyrinthitis.

DIFFERENTIALS

- Perform a thorough neurological examination to exclude life-threatening causes of acute vestibular syndrome, including cerebellar stroke or lateral medullary syndrome.
- If there are neurological symptoms, urgent cranial imaging is required.

Management

Vestibular neuritis is a clinical diagnosis. Vestibular rehabilitation therapy should be initiated as soon as possible, and includes:

- Repositioning manoeuvres
- Habituation exercises, with repetition exposure to symptom triggers
- Gaze stabilization exercises
- Postural control exercises
- Falls prevention techniques

Medical options include:

- Vestibular suppressants: can be considered acutely for symptomatic control.
- Oral steroids: may improve one-month recovery. Not used routinely.
- Intratympanic gentamicin injections: for refractory, unresolving cases.

The prognosis is good. Most patients recover spontaneously after several days, with a low risk of recurrence. Some patients may develop BPPV, which may persist for several months.

DISORDERS OF THE NOSE AND PARANASAL SINUSES

Rhinitis and sinusitis

Rhinitis is the inflammation of the nasal mucosa. It is classified as allergic or nonallergic. Allergic rhinitis develops following allergen exposure. Nonallergic rhinitis typically relates to infection, most commonly viral URTIs, and commonly occurs with concurrent paranasal sinus inflammation (sinusitis), described as rhinosinusitis. There are several other, noninfective but less common subtypes of nonallergic rhinitis Tables 8.6-8.7 and Figs 8.41-8.42.

DIFFERENTIALS

- Bacterial superinfection can develop presenting with worsening symptoms, fever and purulent rhinorrhoea.
- Chronic rhinosinusitis presents with low grade symptoms for >12 weeks, in those with a history of recurrent, untreated episodes of acute sinusitis.

RED FLAG

- Severe, poorly treated bacterial or fungal rhinosinusitis may progress to intracranial or orbital complications, including meningitis, orbital cellulitis or intracerebral abscesses.
- Sepsis and multiorgan failure may subsequently develop.
- Red flags include focal neurology, altered mental state, visual changes or features of systemic infection.
- Urgent hospital admission, intracranial imaging and ENT consult are required if red flag features develop.

Nasal polyps

Nasal polyps are benign growths that develop following chronic inflammation of the nasal mucosa or paranasal sinuses. They commonly occur bilaterally. Risk factors include chronic rhinosinusitis, cystic fibrosis, atopic history and NSAID use.

Symptoms and signs

Symptoms include:

- Nasal congestion
- Hyposmia and anosmia
- Postnasal drip
- Recurrent acute rhinosinusitis/chronic rhinosinusitis

Table 8.6 Allergic rhinitis and rhinosinusitis

	Allergic rhinitis	Infective (rhinosinusitis)
Aetiology	T1 hypersensitivity reaction to allergen (dust, animal fur, mould, pollen)	Viral (most common), bacterial or fungal infection (rare)
Risk factors	Atopic history (asthma, dermatitis) Otitis media Allergic conjunctivitis Maternal smoking	Preexisting URTI Nasal obstruction Atopic history (including allergic rhinitis) Immunosuppression
Symptoms	Sneezing/nasal itching Nasal congestion Rhinorrhoea Postnasal drip	Purulent rhinorrhoea Nasal obstruction/anosmia Postnasal drip Facial pain/pressure, erythema
Signs	Pale, boggy nasal mucosa Hypertrophic turbinates, nasal polyps Pharyngeal cobblestoning	Purulent, oedematous nasal mucosa Hypertrophic turbinates Nasal polyps
Classification	Episodic/seasonal/perennial Intermittent/persistent Mild/moderate/severe	Acute – viral, bacterial, fungal (<4 weeks) Chronic – >12 weeks, low-grade symptoms Recurrent acute – >4 episodes in 1 year
Investigations	Allergen skin testing Nasal endoscopy if diagnosis unclear	Chronic/recurrent – CT scan/nasal endoscopy can be considered
Management	Allergen avoidance Nasal irrigation Oral/intranasal antihistamines Nasal decongestants Persistent Sx – intranasal corticosteroids	Viral – typically self-limiting, conservative Bacterial – antibiotics with 7-day follow-up Fungal – urgent ENT consult, surgical debridement Chronic – intranasal corticosteroids (12 weeks)

Table 8.7 Noninfective subtypes of nonallergic rhinitis

	Clinical features	Aetiology
NARES	Increased eosinophils in the nasal mucosa Chronic rhinitis with nasal polyps and hyposmia	Unknown
Drug induced	Recurrent rhinitis associated with medication sensitivity	NSAIDs, PDE-5 inhibitors Antidepressants
Hormonal	Increased oestrogen release leading to increased blood flow to nasal mucosa	Pregnancy Oral contraceptives Hypothyroidism
Gustatory	Muscarinic receptors stimulation → cholinergic response → rhinorrhoea	Spicy food Alcohol
Atrophic	Rhinitis with atrophy and sclerosis of the nasal mucosa Foul-smelling nasal cavity, hypertrophic turbinates, green crusting, epistaxis	Primary – idiopathic Secondary – granulomatous nasal disease
Vasomotor	Parasympathetic stimulation and vasodilation of mucosal blood vessels	Irritants, temperature changes, drugs, emotions

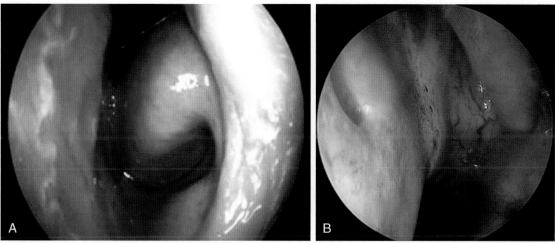

Fig. 8.41 Anterior rhinoscopy in rhinitis. (A) Pale mucosa and clear secretions in children with allergic rhinitis. (B) Mucopurulence in the nasal cavity in a patient with acute bacterial rhinosinusitis. (From A. Wilmott RW, et al. *Kendig's Disorders of the Respiratory Tract in Children,* 9th Edition. Elsevier; 2019. B. Management of the upper airway distress during pregnancy. *IAC* 2023.)

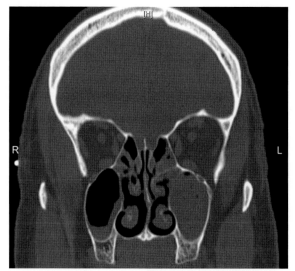

Fig. 8.42 CT scan in chronic rhinosinusitis. The maxillary sinuses (lateral to the nasal cavity) and ethmoid sinuses (medial to the orbital cavities) exhibit mucosal thickening and accumulation of obstructed secretions consistent with inflammatory changes within the paranasal sinuses. (From Rich RR, Corry DB, Corry DB, et al. *Clinical Immunology: Principles and Practice,* 6th Edition. Elsevier; 2023.)

Investigations

Anterior rhinoscopy will show bilateral nasal hypertrophy and polyposis. Further investigations are indicated if there is diagnostic uncertainty:

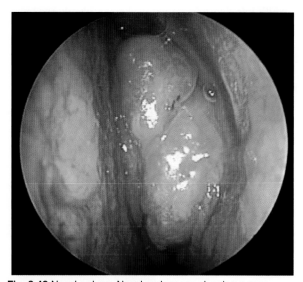

Fig. 8.43 Nasal polyps. Nasal endoscopy showing a grey mucosal hypertrophy, indicating a nasal polyp arising from the middle nasal meatus. (From Scholes MA, Ramakrishnan VR. *ENT Secrets,* 4th Edition. Elsevier; 2016.)

- Sweat test: ↑ chloride levels are diagnostic for cystic fibrosis.
- Nasal cytology: ↑ eosinophils are associated with polyp severity.
- Nasal CT: to determine location and extent of polyps, and exclude other differentials.
- Nasal endoscopy: to visualize polyps directly (Fig. 8.43).

Management

Medical management includes:

- Intranasal corticosteroids: an initial low-dose 3-month course for mild to moderate symptoms, or high-dose course for severe symptoms.
- Oral corticosteroids: given alongside high-dose intranasal corticosteroids for severe symptoms.
- Doxycycline: short courses can provide symptomatic benefit.

For patients with recurrent or refractory symptoms, surgical polypectomy is indicated, to avoid repeated courses of systemic steroids. Complications are rare, and typically only occur following associated superimposed infection, or complications of steroid therapy or sinus surgery.

Nasopharyngeal carcinoma

Nasopharyngeal carcinoma is a rare form of pharyngeal cancer arising in the nasopharynx. Malignancy of the oropharynx and laryngopharynx is even rarer. Risk factors include chronic HPV and EBV infection, tobacco and alcohol use, obesity and radiation exposure. Squamous cell carcinomas are most common.

Symptoms and signs

Nasopharyngeal carcinoma is initially asymptomatic. When symptoms develop, they include:

- Unilateral nasal discharge and obstruction
- Unilateral nasal polyps
- Posterior epistaxis
- Eustachian tube dysfunction – recurrent OM, OME, CHL and tinnitus
- Painless lymphadenopathy
- Sore throat
- Frontal headache

RED FLAG

- Unilateral nasal polyps and posterior epistaxis are red flag features for nasopharyngeal carcinoma.
- Urgent 2 week wait referral to ENT should be made.

Investigations

Assessment includes anterior rhinoscopy, indirect laryngoscopy and otoscopy. Diagnostic testing incudes:

- Panendoscopy with biopsy: tissue samples should be taken for histology.
- CT/MRI imaging: to assess tumour extent and local invasion (Fig. 8.44).

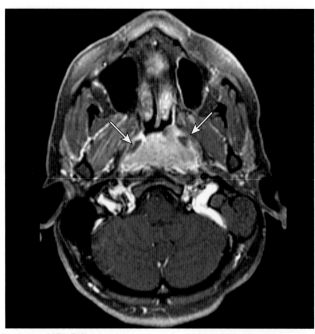

Fig. 8.44 Nasopharyngeal carcinoma on MRI. Diffuse enhancement is evident throughout a large nasopharyngeal mass. (From Müller S, Thompson LDR, Nelson BL. *Diagnostic Pathology: Head and Neck,* 3rd Edition. Elsevier; 2022.)

Management

Management of all malignancy should take an MDT approach, depends on the extent of disease, patient wishes and performance status, and goals of treatment. Options include:

- Localized: high dose radiotherapy to the tumour and surrounding lymph nodes +/– adjuvant chemotherapy.
- Advanced: chemoradiotherapy +/– radical neck dissection.

The prognosis is typically poor, due to late diagnoses at advanced stages. For localized lesions, there is a 5-year survival rate of approximately 80%.

DISORDERS OF THE THROAT

Tonsillitis and pharyngitis

Tonsillitis is the acute inflammation of the palatine tonsils. It commonly develops alongside acute pharyngeal inflammation, described as tonsillopharyngitis. Tonsillopharyngitis is common among young children, typically related to viral infection or invasive group A streptococci (GAS) bacteria (strep throat).

CLINICAL NOTES

- iGAS infections are associated with suppurative complications including peritonsillar and retropharyngeal abscess, and invasive complications including rheumatic fever, or post–streptococcal glomerulonephritis.
- Prompt identification and treatment are essential to reduce the risk of systemic spread of infection and complications.

Symptoms and signs

The typical features of tonsillopharyngitis relate to the underlying aetiology.

- Viral: nasal congestion, rhinorrhoea, sneezing and cough. No fever.
- Bacterial: fever, sore throat, dysphagia. No cough (Fig. 8.45).

Investigations

Viral tonsillopharyngitis can be diagnosed clinically. The Fever-PAIN or Centor scoring systems can be used to assess the likelihood of bacterial infection (Table 8.8):

If bacterial infection is likely, further investigations can be performed:

- Rapid antigen detection testing: to diagnose GAS infection.
- Throat swabs and culture: to diagnose the cause if rapid antigen testing is negative.

Table 8.8 FeverPAIN and Modified Centor criteria

	FeverPAIN	Centor
Criteria	**F**ever **P**urulence (tonsillar exudate) **A**ttended rapidly (<3 days) Severe **I**nflamed tonsils **N**o cough or coryza	Age <14 Tonsillar exudate Tender cervical lymphadenopathy Fever of 38°C Absence of cough
Interpretation	0–1 – <20% risk of bacterial infection 2–3 – 40% risk of bacterial infection 4–5 – >60% risk of bacterial infection	<2 – <20% risk of bacterial infection 3–4 – 30%–50% risk of chance of bacterial infection

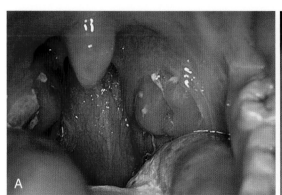
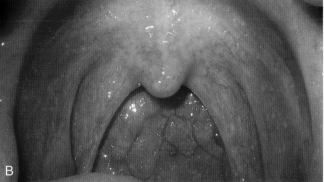

Fig. 8.45 Tonsillitis and pharyngitis. (A) Bacterial tonsillitis with tonsillar exudate, pharyngeal erythema, pus coating inflamed tonsils. (B) Viral pharyngitis with pharyngeal erythema and oedema. (From A. Ahmed AN, Waduud MA, Slater TA. *Pocketbook of Differential Diagnosis,* 5th Edition. Elsevier; 2022. B. Mayatepek E. *Repetitorium für die Facharztprüfung Kinder- und Jugendmedizin*, Urban & Fischer, Elsevier Urban-Fischer Germany; 2021.)

Further investigations including bloods and imaging should be performed if there is evidence of suppurative complications.

Management

Management depends on the aetiology:

- Viral: supportive measures include analgesia, saltwater gargles and throat lozenges.
- Bacterial: antibiotics (phenoxymethylpenicillin) for 10 days.

> **HINTS AND TIPS**
>
> Amoxicillin should be avoided, as in tonsillopharyngitis relating to an underlying EBV infection (infectious mononucleosis), amoxicillin triggers development of a widespread maculopapular rash.

For recurrent tonsillitis, those with chronic symptoms, or evidence of complications of tonsillectomy may be indicated, under the following criteria:

- >7 episodes of tonsillitis in the past year.
- >5 episodes of tonsillitis in the past 2 years.
- >3 episodes of tonsillitis in the past 3 years.

Each episode must be documented by a health professional and treated with antibiotics.

Complications

Complications include:

- Chronic tonsillitis: >2 weeks of symptomatic tonsillitis, with increased risk of superimposed acute infection. Typically associated with structural abnormalities of the upper aerodigestive tract. An indication for tonsillectomy.
- Peritonsillar abscess: associated with GAS infection, presenting with odynophagia, drooling, trismus (lockjaw), vocal changes ('hot potato voice') and uvula deviation. Hospital admission for IV antibiotics and abscess drainage are required.
- Parapharyngeal abscess: a rare abscess of the parapharyngeal space that presents with trismus, respiratory distress and neck stiffness. Urgent surgical drainage is required to avoid airway obstruction, sepsis and death.
- Obstructive sleep apnoea: chronic tonsillitis can result in tonsillar hypertrophy and airway obstruction, with associated cardiovascular complications including hypertension, sudden cardiac death, respiratory insufficiency and obesity.

- Tonsillectomy complications: surgical complications include injury to local structures, nasopharyngeal stenosis, postoperative pain and haemorrhage (Figs 8.46-8.47).

> **RED FLAG**
>
> - Post tonsillectomy haemorrhage can occur as an immediate (<24 hours) or late (>24 hours) complication following tonsillectomy.
> - Small bleeds can be managed expectantly.
> - Profuse haemorrhage warrants resuscitation with airway support and tonsillar packing.

Infectious mononucleosis

Infectious mononucleosis (IM), or 'mono', is an acute tonsillopharyngitis caused by the Epstein-Barr virus (EBV). It is incredibly contagious and spread through infected bodily secretions, typically saliva. It is sometimes referred to as glandular fever.

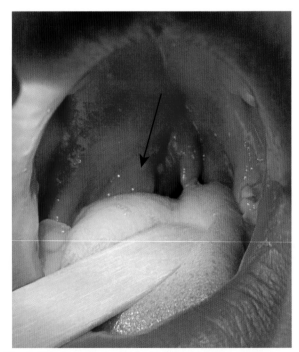

Fig. 8.46 Peritonsillar abscess. Unilateral tonsillar swelling and uvula deviation in peritonsillar abscess. (From Omar AM. *USMLE Step 2 CK Plus*. Elsevier; 2023.)

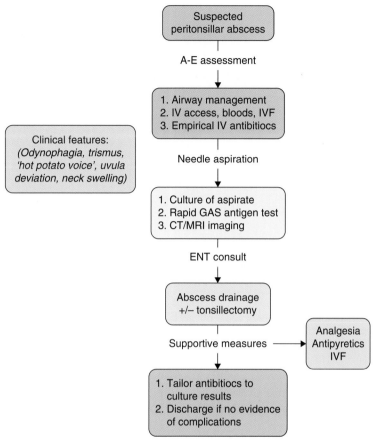

Clinical features:
(Odynophagia, trismus,
'hot potato voice', uvula
deviation, neck swelling)

Suspected
peritonsillar abscess

A-E assessment

1. Airway management
2. IV access, bloods, IVF
3. Empirical IV antibitiocs

Needle aspiration

1. Culture of aspirate
2. Rapid GAS antigen test
3. CT/MRI imaging

ENT consult

Abscess drainage
+/– tonsillectomy

Supportive measures ⟶ Analgesia
Antipyretics
IVF

1. Tailor antibitiocs to
culture results
2. Discharge if no evidence
of complications

Fig. 8.47 Approach to the management of peritonsillar abscess. *GAS*, Group A streptococcus; *IVF*, intravenous fluids.

Symptoms and signs

Typical features include:

- Pharyngitis: with pharyngeal erythema, oedema and grey tonsillar exudate.
- Fever: worse in the first week, and at night.
- Lymphadenopathy: typically posterior cervical chain.
- Malaise: significant fatigue is common, lasting up to 6 weeks (Fig. 8.48).

CLINICAL NOTES

- Transient viral hepatitis can develop presenting with hepatomegaly, jaundice and abdominal pain.
- Splenomegaly can occur, relating to splenic infiltration with lymphocytes and atypical lymphoid cells.

Investigations

Suspected IM infection should be confirmed on laboratory testing:

- Monospot test: tests antibodies to EBV infection. Highly specific.
- Serology: indicated to confirm the diagnosis monospot testing is negative.
- Blood smear: lymphocytosis with >10% atypical lymphocytes.
- LFTs: elevated transaminases indicate hepatitis.

Management

Conservative management is appropriate, include analgesia, rest and adequate hydration. Patients should be advised to avoid contact sports for 6 weeks after the resolution of symptoms due to the risk of splenic rupture.

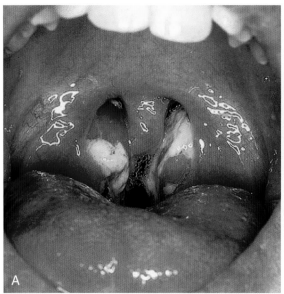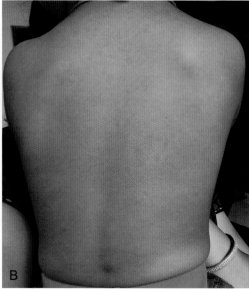

Fig. 8.48 Infectious mononucleosis. (A) Inflamed tonsils with bilateral grey exudate. (B) Widespread maculopapular rash relating to amoxicillin use in a child with IM. (From A. Jäger-Roman E, Rodens K, Fegeler U. *Praxishandbuch der pädiatrischen Grundversorgung, 2. Auflage*. Elsevier; 2020. B. Pharyngitis: Certain clinico-pictorial differentiators. *PID* 2013.)

CLINICAL NOTES

Complications include haemolytic anaemia, Guillain-Barré syndrome, encephalitis, pericarditis, interstitial nephritis and lymphoma.

Obstructive sleep apnoea

Obstructive sleep apnoea (OSA) is a breathing disorder associated with collapse of the pharyngeal muscles during sleep, resulting in apnoeic episodes (complete cessation of breathing for >10 seconds), alveolar hypoventilation and hypoxia. It is much more common in men. Risk factors include obesity, increased neck size, structural abnormalities of the upper airways, and lifestyle factors including alcohol, smoking and sedative use.

DIFFERENTIALS

- OSA in children may relate to laryngomalacia, a congenital laxity of laryngeal cartilage.
- Laryngomalacia is common in trisomy 21, and typically resolves spontaneously by 2 years of age.
- Nonresolving or severe cases are treated with supraglottoplasty.

Symptoms and signs

Characteristic features include:

- Excessive daytime somnolence
- Frequent 'microsleeps' or naps in inappropriate settings (e.g., while driving)
- Restless sleep, with frequent awakenings with gasping or choking
- Loud snoring with apnoeic episodes (observed by a partner)
- Unrefreshing sleep despite adequate sleep opportunity
- Morning headaches
- Impaired concentration and memory
- Low mood, decreased libido

Investigations

A diagnosis of OSA is made with a detailed sleep history, screening questionnaires and sleep studies.

- Sleep history: sleep partner interviews with details about snoring and apnoeic episodes.
- Screening questionnaires: STOP-BANG/Epworth sleepiness scale.
- Sleep studies: polysomnography evidence of >5 apnoeic episodes per hour.

- Criteria on the **STOP-BANG** questionnaire include:
  - **S** – **S**noring loudly
  - **T** – **T**iredness
  - **O** – **O**bserved apnoeic episodes during sleep
  - **P** – high blood **P**ressure
  - **B** – **B**MI >35
  - **A** – **A**ge >50
  - **N** – **N**eck circumference >40 cm
  - **G** – male **G**ender
- A score of <2 is low risk, and >5 high risk for moderate to severe OSA

CLINICAL NOTES

OSA can be graded by severity:
- Mild – 5-15 apnoeic episodes per hour
- Moderate – 15-30 apnoeic episodes per hour
- Severe – >30 apnoeic episodes per hour

Further evaluation for complications and related conditions can be performed:

- BP: secondary hypertension can develop as a response to chronic hypoxia.
- ECG: may indicate right heart strain due to pulmonary hypertension.
- FBC: polycythaemia can develop in response to chronic hypoxia.
- Lipid profile/HbA1c: hypercholesterolemia and diabetes are common comorbidities.

Management

The first-line treatment option is continuous positive airway pressure (CPAP) during sleep. CPAP splints the airway open to prevent collapse and the frequency of apnoeic episodes. BIPAP can also be used.

COMMUNICATION

- CPAP is often poorly tolerated.
- Counsel patients on the importance of compliance and long-term complications associated with untreated nocturnal hypoxia.
- If patients are unable to tolerate CPAP, alternative measures such as oral appliances and positional measures may be considered.

Supportive measures include:

- Lifestyle measures: weight loss, smoking cessation and alcohol reduction.
- Sleep hygiene: including avoidance of sedatives before bed to improve sleep quality.
- Stopping driving: patients must stop driving until symptoms are under control.

Complications

The complications of OSA relate to the duration and severity of symptoms

- Cardiovascular: hypertension, atrial fibrillation, stroke and sudden cardiac death.
- Respiratory: pulmonary hypertension, respiratory insufficiency.
- Haematological: polycythaemia, venous thromboembolism.
- Neurological: depression, vascular dementia.
- Social: car crashes/workplace accidents, increased appetite and obesity, relationship issues.

Laryngitis

Laryngitis is the inflammation of the larynx. Acute laryngitis results to viral infection or vocal overuse. Chronic laryngitis results to chronic laryngeal irritation, typically as the result of GORD, smoking or recurrent URTIs. Acute laryngitis may progress to chronic laryngitis without adequate treatment.

Symptoms and signs

Laryngitis presents with typical features:

- Vocal hoarseness
- Dry, barking cough
- Inspiratory stridor and accessory respiratory muscle use
- Fever in acute infection

Investigations

Laryngitis is a clinical diagnosis. Indirect laryngoscopy can be performed using a small handheld mirror for limited visualization of the larynx to detect laryngeal inflammation.

Direct laryngoscopy is performed for formal diagnosis:

- Flexible endoscopy: performed with the patient awake.
- Rigid laryngoscopy: performed under general anaesthesia (Fig. 8.49).

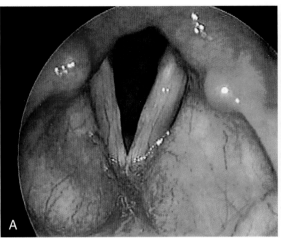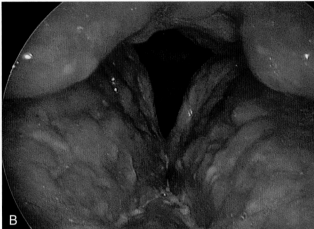

Fig. 8.49 Acute and chronic laryngitis. (A) Erythema, mucous and oedema in acute viral laryngitis. (B) Cobblestoning and mucosal thickening in chronic laryngitis associated with GORD. (From A. Koitschev C, Limberger A, Koitschev A. *Kurzlehrbuch Hals-Nasen-Ohren-Heilkunde*. Elsevier; 2014. B. Laryngeal disorders in people living with HIV. *YAJOT* 2022.)

DIFFERENTIALS

- A vocal cord nodule is a benign fibrotic lesion resulting from chronic vocal cord microtrauma.
- Symptoms include low-pitched vocal hoarseness, with bilateral nodules visible on laryngoscopy.
- Management is with vocal rest and in refractory cases, microsurgical removal.

Management

Management is typically conservative for both acute and chronic laryngitis, including vocal rest, smoking cessation and over-the-counter analgesia. Acid-reducing therapies can be used if GORD is the underlying aetiology.

Laryngeal carcinoma

Laryngeal carcinoma can arise in the glottis, the vocal cords, supraglottis or subglottis. Tumours are almost always squamous cell carcinomas. It is closely associated with smoking and alcohol consumption. Glottic carcinomas have the best prognosis, as symptoms manifest early and they are detected sooner. Supraglottic or supraglottic tumours have significantly poorere prognosis.

Symptoms and signs

Typical features include:

- Vocal hoarseness
- Dysphagia

- Stridor

RED FLAG

- Unexplained hoarseness for over 3 weeks in smokers is a red flag for laryngeal carcinoma.
- Urgent 2 week wait referral is required.

Investigations
Diagnosis involves:

- Direct laryngoscopy and biopsy: for direct visualization of the lesion and to obtain tissue samples for histology.
- CT/MRI imaging: to assess tumour extent and invasion into surrounding structures.

Management
Management of all malignancy should involve an MDT approach and consideration of the patient wishes, performance status and tumour stage.

- Localized: radiotherapy or minimally invasive transoral endoscopic laser resection (voice preserving).
- Advanced: laryngectomy +/– radical neck dissection (voice sacrificing).

Vocal rehabilitation, with speech training, voice prosthesis and electronic speaking aids can be offered following laryngectomy.

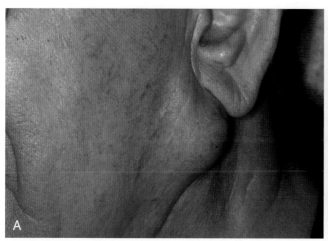
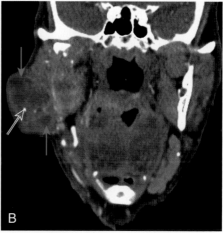

Fig. 8.50 Parotid pleomorphic adenoma. (A) Firm nodular mass of the left parotid gland lifting the earlobe at the angle of the mandible. (B) Right parotid gland mass with cystic degeneration, calcification and necrosis within the central portion of the mass. (From A. Indhu Kannan, Rajeswari Kathiah, Gayathri Devi Thanigaimani. *Textbook of Pathology.* Elsevier; 2022. B. Müller S, Nelson BL, Thompson LDR. *Diagnostic Pathology: Head and Neck,* Third Edition. Elsevier; 2022.)

SALIVARY DISORDERS

There are a range of benign conditions that can affect the salivary glands.

- Sialadenosis: noninflammatory painless swelling of the salivary glands. May be recurrent and is often bilateral, related to diabetes, alcohol, malnutrition or medications.
- Sialadenitis: acute inflammation of the salivary glands, resulting from inflammatory and infectious disorders. Infection is associated with purulent discharge from the gland.
- Sialolithiasis: formation of stones in the salivary ducts which cause pain before and during mastication. Typically managed conservatively.
- Ranula: a rare cyst arising in the sublingual gland, causing painless swelling below the tongue. Treated with surgical removal.

CLINICAL NOTES

- Mumps is a common cause of parotid sialadenitis
- Bilateral painful parotitis starts within a few days of acute infection, and typically resolves within two weeks.

Salivary tumours

Most salivary tumours are benign.

- Pleomorphic adenoma: the most common lesion. Presents with gradual painless unilateral parotid swelling. A small minority may undergo malignant transformation.
- Warthin tumour: the second most common lesion, presenting with painless unilateral parotid swelling. Closely associated with smoking (Fig. 8.50).

HINTS AND TIPS

The rule of 80s applies to salivary tumours:
- 80% are in the parotid
- 80% of parotid tumours are benign
- 80% of parotid tumours are pleomorphic adenomas

CLINICAL NOTES

- Malignant lesions are rare.
- The most common is parotid carcinoma.
- Symptoms include painless mucosal ulceration and swelling, and local infiltrative symptoms including facial nerve palsy.
- Treatment is with curative intent, with gland resection, radical neck dissection and adjuvant radiotherapy.

DISORDERS OF THE FACIAL NERVE

Facial nerve palsy

Facial nerve palsy is the partial or total paralysis of the facial nerve. This occurs as the result of a central upper motor neuron lesion, such as stroke, or a peripheral lower motor neuron lesion, known as Bell's palsy, which is typically idiopathic, but may relate to viral infection. Secondary causes of peripheral facial nerve palsy include trauma, viral infection, diabetes, pregnancy or tumours.

Symptoms and signs

Symptoms relate to paralysis of the muscles of facial expression on the affected side:

- Central facial palsy: lower facial droop only, with forehead sparing due to bilateral motor cortex innervation of the forehead.
- Peripheral facial nerve palsy: complete unilateral facial drop, due to pathology of the lower motor neuron of the facial nerve (Fig. 8.51).

Additional symptoms relate to the wide range of functions of the facial nerve:

- Ear pain: the peripheral fibres of the facial nerve supply the external auditory meatus.
- Taste impairment: sensory fibres of the facial nerve supply the anterior tongue.
- Hyperacusis: denervation of the stapedius muscle results in elevated sound perception.
- Dry mouth: impaired parasympathetic supply results in reduced saliva production.
- Ocular features: including an inability to fully close the eyes, decreased lacrimation, ectropion and keratitis due to corneal dehydration.
- Facial synkinesis: involuntary facial spasms (Fig. 8.52).

DIFFERENTIAL

- Herpes zoster oticus (Ramsay Hunt syndrome) occurs via reactivation of herpes zoster in the geniculate ganglion controlling the facial and vestibulocochlear nerves.
- Symptoms include facial nerve palsy, vertigo, sensorineural hearing loss and a vesicular rash in the auditory canal and pinna.

Investigations

A thorough clinical evaluation is essential to evaluate for central pathology, including neurological examination, cranial nerves, otoscopy and hearing assessment. Further investigations include:

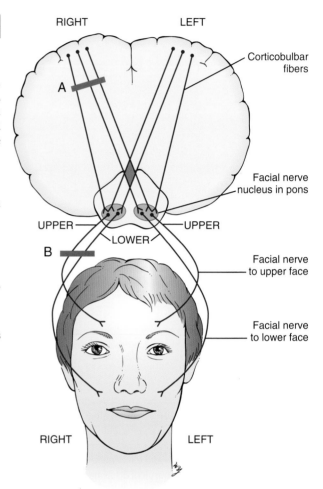

Fig. 8.51 Facial nerve palsy. Upper motor and lower motor neuron lesions of the facial nerve. (From Swartz MH. *Textbook of Physical Diagnosis: History and Examination,* 8th Edition. Elsevier; 2021.)

- Viral PCR: to assess for viral infections associated with Bell's palsy.
- CT head: to assess for acute intracranial pathology, including stroke, space-occupying lesions or trauma.
- Audiology: to evaluate for hearing loss in viral or intracranial pathology.
- Nerve conduction studies: to definitively diagnose nerve palsy.

Management

Conservative management for all patients with facial nerve palsy includes:

- Eye care: artificial tears, ointment and taping close the affected eye.

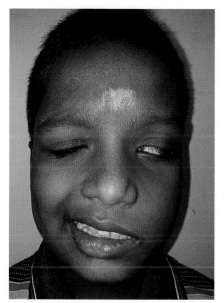

Fig. 8.52 Clinical features of Bell's palsy. The patient is unable to fully close the left eye, or raise the mouth on the left-hand side. (From Thirunavukkarasu AB. *Pediatrics for Medical Graduates*. Elsevier; 2017.)

- Mouth care: lip and oral cavity hydration and moisturization.
- Facial physiotherapy: for persistent symptoms, to improve muscle strength.

For Bell's palsy, specific treatments are indicated:

- Oral corticosteroids: must be started within 72 hours to provide definitive benefit.
- Antivirals: considered as adjuvants to steroid therapy.

Patients with Bell's palsy will typically recover completely within 3 weeks. ENT follow-up for all patients with persistent or unremitting symptoms is advised.

CLINICAL NOTES

Management of secondary facial nerve palsy involves treatment of the underlying cause, with urgent neurological opinion required in central causes.

Chapter Summary

- Pulsatile tinnitus suggests vascular pathology including carotid artery stenosis.
- When assessing a patient with vertigo, perform a HINTS exam and full neurological exam to rule out central causes including cerebellar stroke.
- Unilateral nasal polyps and posterior epistaxis are red flags for nasopharyngeal carcinoma.
- Otitis externa infections in immunocompromised adults risk the development of malignant otitis externa, life-threatening osteomyelitis of the skull base.
- Mastoiditis is a life-threatening complication of otitis media, presenting with mastoid swelling, erythema and the forward profusion of the pinna, requiring treatment with IV antibiotics.
- BPPV presents with sudden onset vertigo with changes in head position and can be diagnosed with the Dix-Hallpike manoeuvre and treated with the Epley manoeuvre.
- Meniere's disease presents with sudden attacks of vertigo, SNHL and tinnitus and can be treated with prophylactic betahistine.
- The FeverPAIN criteria or Centor criteria should be used to guide antibiotic treatment in tonsillitis. Amoxicillin should be avoided, as it can provoke a widespread rash in patients with infectious mononucleosis.
- Obstructive sleep apnoea presents with daytime somnolence and frequent nocturnal apnoeic episodes. The STOP-BANG questionnaire and polysomnography are used for diagnosis, and treatment involves CPAP.
- Hoarseness persistent over 3 weeks with a smoking history is a red flag for laryngeal carcinoma.

Continued

● Chapter Summary—cont'd

UKMLA Conditions

Acoustic neuroma
Adverse drug effects
Allergic disorder
Bell's palsy
Benign paroxysmal positional vertigo
Epistaxis
Infectious mononucleosis
Lymphadenopathy
Ménière's disease
Metastatic disease
Obesity
Obstructive sleep apnoea
Otitis externa
Otitis media
Rhinosinusitis
Sepsis
Tonsillitis
Trigeminal neuralgia
Upper respiratory tract infection
Varicella-zoster

UKMLA Presentations

Allergies
Anosmia/loss of smell and nasal obstruction
Diplopia
Dizziness
Driving advice
Epiglottitis. Ear and nasal discharge
Epistaxis
Facial pain
Facial swelling
Facial weakness/ptosis
Fever
Hearing loss
Hoarseness and voice change
Loss of smell
Lymphadenopathy
Nasal obstruction
Night sweats
Painful ear (otalgia)
Sepsis
Sleep problems
Snoring
Sore throat
Stridor
Swallowing problems (dysphagia)
Tinnitus
Unsteadiness
Vertigo
Weight gain/weight loss

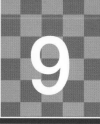
History taking

Opening the consultation

Wash your hands, introduce yourself, confirm patient details and gain consent to proceed.

Presenting complaint (PC)

Begin with an open question to identify the presenting complaint.

> **COMMUNICATION**
>
> - Visible lesions with aesthetic implications can cause a great deal of distress.
> - Allow time for patients to express their concerns in detail, to help you understand the outcome desired.

History of presenting complaint (HPC)

Explore the presenting complaint in more detail.

> **HINTS AND TIPS**
>
> SOCRATES is typically used to explore pain, however, it can be applied to any presenting symptom. Any nonrelevant elements can be excluded.
> - S – Site – location of the lesion
> - O – Onset – when the lesion was first noticed
> - C – Character-specific features, including feel, number and shape of lesions
> - R – Radiation – whether the symptom spreads
> - A – Associated symptoms – including itch, bleeding or pain
> - T – Timing – how the lesion has changed over time, any previous episodes or identifiable triggers
> - E – Exacerbating/relieving factors – anything that makes it better or worse
> - S – Severity – grading out of 10, of the severity of the symptoms

> **HINTS AND TIPS**
>
> In soft tissue injury, clarify:
> - Mechanism of injury.
> - Time scale of associated symptoms (immediate or delayed).
> - Details of first aid performed.

Key symptoms relating to skin surgery include:

- Rash: widespread, localized and associated with itch, erythema, dry skin or discharge.
- Lesions: benign or malignant lesions, associated with pain, bleeding or discharge.
- Wounds: may be open or closed, associated with acute or chronic trauma or infection.
- Blisters: pus-filled vesicles or tense bullae, related to infective or autoimmune pathology.
- Abnormal pigmentation: darkening or lightening of skin, relating to autoimmune pathology or chronic trauma.
- Systemic features: fever, lethargy, appetite and weight change, or night sweats.

> **RED FLAG**
>
> Red flag features in skin histories include:
> - Sudden onset, widespread erythema
> - Pain out of proportion to clinical findings, with blistering, discolouration and systemic illness
> - Clear, haemorrhagic or tense blisters
> - Skin symptoms following drug administration
> - New or changing lesion, that is large, asymmetrical, with irregular pigment

Systemic screen

A thorough systemic screen is essential, due to the number of conditions that may present with cutaneous manifestations.

- Cardiac: endocarditis, rheumatoid arthritis (RA), systemic lupus erythematosus (SLE).
- Respiratory: sarcoidosis, RA, SLE.
- Gastroenterology: inflammatory bowel disease, coeliac disease, hepatobiliary pathology.

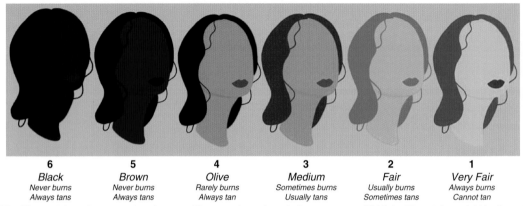

6	5	4	3	2	1
Black	*Brown*	*Olive*	*Medium*	*Fair*	*Very Fair*
Never burns	Never burns	Rarely burns	Sometimes burns	Usually burns	Always burns
Always tans	Always tans	Always tan	Usually tans	Sometimes tans	Cannot tan

Fig. 9.1 The Fitzpatrick scale categorizes human skin tones based on their response to UV light. Type 1 (very fair) is the palest, most likely to burn but less likely to tan. Type 6 (black) is the darkest, is the least likely to burn, and always tan. (From Gwan A. *Equity in visual representation of vulvar conditions in major gynecology textbooks. JNMA.* 2022.)

- Infectious diseases: soft tissue infections, Lyme disease, herpes zoster.
- Endocrinology: diabetes, Addison's disease, thyroid dysfunction.
- Musculoskeletal: RA, SLE, dermatomyositis.
- Neurological: meningococcal sepsis.

Past medical history

Current medical conditions may be a risk factor for the underlying diagnosis.

> **CLINICAL NOTES**
>
> Past medical history may suggest risk factors for the presenting complaint:
> - Atopy - dermatitis
> - Immunosuppression - skin cancer
> - Diabetes - soft tissue infections

Drug history

Clarify medication history, including over-the-counter medications, any recent changes and associated side effects.

> **HINTS AND TIPS**
>
> Check whether they have tried anything for their symptoms, and any positive or negative effects of the treatment.

Family history

Check for any family history of skin disorders or skin symptoms, and the age of development.

Social history

A full social history may highlight associated risk factors for dermatological pathology:

- Functional baseline: assess independence with activities of daily living, accommodation and support network, and any carer input.
- Occupation: there may be occupational exposure to irritants, pathogens or carcinogens.
- Alcohol: record weekly units and type of alcohol consumed.
- Smoking: a key risk factor for malignancy. Record the number of pack years.
- Recreational drugs: intravenous drug use increases the risk of skin infections, and blood-borne diseases.
- Diet: allergies or intolerances in the patient's diet may manifest with skin signs.
- Sun exposure: screen for a history of sun exposure, including foreign holidays, blistering sunburn and sunbed use, and relation of symptoms to the sun.
- Contact history: check for recent contacts with similar symptoms.
- Travel: foreign travel may increase the risk of infective pathology or sun exposure (Fig. 9.1).

> **CLINICAL NOTES**
>
> Ask about previous sun exposure and reaction of skin to sunlight to assess skin type on the Fitzpatrick scale, and the associated malignancy risk.

Ideas, concerns and expectations

Exploring the patient's ideas, concerns and expectations to gauge what they want to get out of the consultation and any particular concerns you can address.

Closing the consultation

Summarize the history back to the patient and thank them for their time.

DIFFERENTIAL DIAGNOSIS OF A SKIN LESION

There is a broad differential diagnosis of a skin lesion. Many lesions can be diagnosed based on their appearance and key characteristics alone (Fig. 9.2).

There are several traumatic skin lesions that require surgical repair (Fig. 9.3).

Fine-line scarring is normal following trauma, and will naturally fade over time. Imbalanced wound healing can result in pathological scarring, with clinical and cosmetic implications (Fig. 9.4).

CLINICAL NOTES

- Medical scar management involves intralesional steroid injections or compression therapy.
- Surgical options include cryotherapy, laser or light therapy or excision.

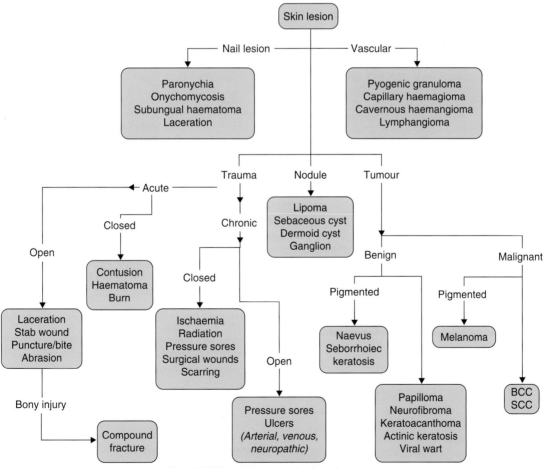

Fig. 9.2 Differential diagnosis of a skin lesion.

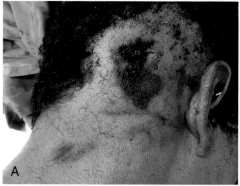
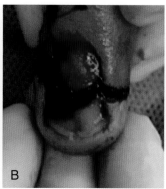
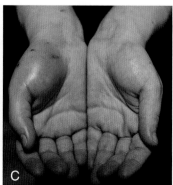

Scalp laceration with associated abrasion and contusion. Managed with washout, debridement and primary closure.

Nailbed laceration and subungual haematoma. Nailbed repair is required.

Infected bite wounds. Exploration and washout are performed to clean the wound and identify underlying injuries before closure.

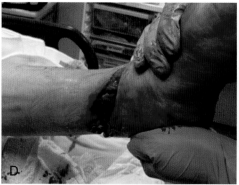
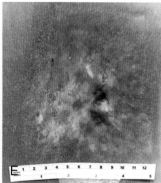
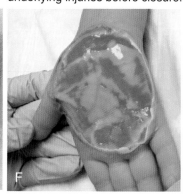

Compound ankle fracture. Staged management with debridement and fixation is required before definitive closure.

Radiation injury, managed with debridement and reconstruction with vascularised tissue.

A contact burn, with red areas of superficial partial thickness and white areas of deep partial thickness injury.

Fig. 9.3 Traumatic skin lesions. (From A. Loftus I, Verster J, Houck MM. *Encyclopedia of Forensic Sciences,* 3rd Edition. Elsevier; 2023. B. Courtesy of Carrie Roth Bettlach, MSN, FNP-C. C. Goldstein EJC, Sykes JE. *Greene's Infectious Diseases of the Dog and Cat,* 5th Edition. Elsevier; 2023. D. Biers SM, Arulampalam THA, Quick CRG. *Essential Surgery: Problems, Diagnosis and Management,* 6th Edition. Elsevier; 2020. E. Wible BC. *Diagnostic Imaging: Interventional Radiology,* 3rd Edition. Elsevier; 2023. F. Urden LD, et al. *Critical Care Nursing: Diagnosis and Management,* 9th Edition. Elsevier; 2022.)

EXAMINATION OF A SKIN LESION

HINTS AND TIPS

The acronym **WIPER** can be used to prepare for the exam:
- **W** – **W**ash your hands
- **I** – **I**ntroduce yourself
- **P** – **P**atient details
- **E** – **E**xplain the procedure and **E**xpose appropriately
- **R** – **R**eposition patient

CLINICAL NOTES

Be sure to consent the patient for a chaperone to be present for any examination involving an intimate area.

General inspection

Inspect the patient from the end of the bed, to assess the number and location of lesions:

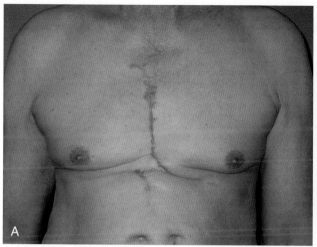

Hypertrophic scars, resulting from high fibroblast proliferation and collagen deposition following skin trauma. Do not extend beyond the site of original injury and will gradually improve.

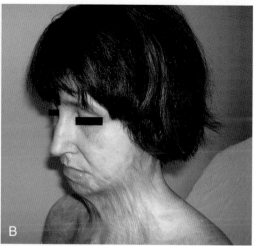

Scar contractures, which often relate to burns. Scar maturation, thickening and tightening during healing results in skin.

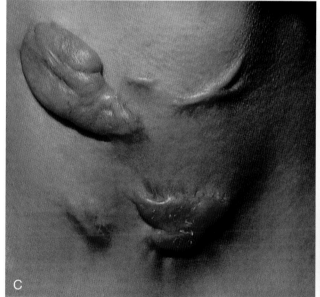

Keloid scars. An abnormal reaction to skin injury, characterized by proliferation of fibroblasts and collagen that extends beyond the margins of the original wound. More common in dark-skinned individuals.

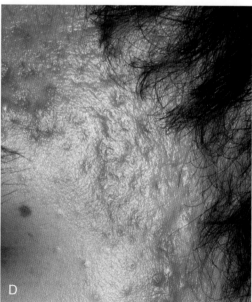

Pitted scars, indented scars that form when the skin cannot regenerate lost tissue. Typically relate to chickenpox or acne.

Fig. 9.4 Scars. (From A. Gurtner GC, Neligan PC. *Plastic Surgery: Volume 1: Principles,* 4th Edition. Elsevier; 2018. B. Pu LLQ. *Atlas of Reconstructive Surgery: A Case-Based Approach.* Elsevier; 2024. C. McIntire SC, Garrison J, et al. (Eds). *Zitelli and Davis' Atlas of Pediatric Physical Diagnosis,* 8th Edition. Elsevier; 2023. D. Dinulos JGH. *Habif's Clinical Dermatology: A Color Guide to Diagnosis and Therapy,* 7th Edition. Elsevier; 2021.)

- Photo distribution: lesions may be in areas of high sun exposure, including the face, ears, nose or limbs.
- Flexural: bilateral symmetrical flexural lesions are suggestive of eczema.
- Extensor: lesions affecting extensor surfaces are suggestive of psoriasis.
- Follicular: lesions may affect areas with a high density of pilosebaceous units.
- Dermatomal: lesions confined to one dermatome that do not cross the midline.
- Acral: lesions specifically affecting the hand and feet.

HINTS AND TIPS

Bedside equipment including medications, mobility aids and monitoring devices will offer insights into functional status and comorbidities.

Close inspection

Inspect the lesion closely:

- Size: measure the width, and height of the lesion if raised.
- Shape: assess the shape of the lesion (linear, discoid, target or annular), any pattern if multiple, and whether lesions are discrete or confluent.
- Symmetry: individual lesion symmetry or a symmetrical pattern if multiple.
- Colour: lesions can be erythematous, hypo- or hyperpigmented, or purpuric.
- Contour: assess for symmetry, elevation, flattening or depression.

RED FLAG

In pigmented lesions, assess for the ABCDE criteria of underlying malignancy
- **A**symmetry – asymmetrical features including size, shape and colour
- **B**order – an irregular border or contour
- **C**olour – irregular pigment with more than two colours
- **D**iameter – large lesions of >6 mm in diameter
- **E**volution – new growth or change in the appearance of a lesion

Palpation

Gently palpate the lesion:

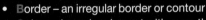

- Consistency: assess if the lesion is soft, firm or hard, or textured with lichenification, scale, crust or ulcerations.
- Temperature: warmth suggests infection or inflammation.
- Tethering: attachment of a lesion to underlying structures, associated with malignancy.
- Tenderness: suggestive of infection.

HINTS AND TIPS

Assess for regional lymphadenopathy if you suspect underlying malignancy.

Systemic examination

There may be associated features on other skin areas:

- Nail: pitting, onycholysis or deformities such as koilonychia.
- Elbows: psoriatic plaques, rheumatoid nodules or gouty tophi.
- Hair: alopecia can manifest with plaques of hair loss or total baldness.
- Scalp: psoriatic plaques present with thick scalp scaling, typically affecting the hairline. Seborrhoeic dermatitis (dandruff) presents with a diffuse, fine scale.
- Mucous membranes: hyperpigmentation, bullae, ulcers and striae can affect the oral mucosa.

Completing the examination

Thank the patient and summarize your findings.

HINTS AND TIPS

The key components to remember when describing a skin lesion can be remembered by the 3S's, 3C's and 3T's.
- **S**ize, **s**hape, **s**ymmetry
- **C**olour, **c**ontour, **c**onsistency
- **T**emperature, **t**ethering, **t**enderness

Further tests include:

- Dermoscopy: to more closely evaluate a lesion.
- Systemic examination: to screen for systemic diseases that may present with skin signs.
- Skin swabs: send for microscopy, culture and sensitivity (MC&S) if there is suspicion of infective aetiology.
- Skin biopsy: for histology analysis, essential if there is a risk of malignancy.

PLASTICS AND SKIN SURGERY DISORDERS

Wound management

A wound is an area of local soft tissue damage relating to acute or chronic mechanical trauma. Acute wounds result from acute disruption of skin and soft tissue structures. Chronic wounds begin as acute wounds and result from impaired healing, chronic inflammation and recurrent infection. Both acute and chronic wounds can be open, with exposure of underlying tissues to the external environment, or closed, where the skin is intact. The clinical significance of a wound relates to the extent of injury and involvement of underlying structures, wound contamination and associated complications (Table 9.1).

Approach to wound management

Acute wounds should be managed with an A–E approach, with appropriate stabilization of the patient and treatment of all identified injuries (Fig. 9.5).

CLINICAL NOTES

Assess the neurovascular status, including sensation, motor function and local capillary refill time.

Investigations

Appropriate investigation can take place once haemodynamic stability has been achieved.

1. Bedside
   - Urinalysis: to assess for haematuria or myoglobinuria relating to rhabdomyolysis.

Table 9.1 Classification of wounds

	Acute	Chronic
Open	Stab wounds Lacerations Punctures Compound fracture	Vascular ulcers (arterial/venous) Neuropathic ulcers Advanced pressure sores
Closed	Contusions (Bruise) Haematoma Blunt trauma Crush injuries	Pressure sores Surgical wounds Ischaemic Radiation injury

- CBG: hyperglycaemia impairs wound healing.
- Compartmental pressures: ↑ pressure suggests compartment syndrome, which warrants urgent fasciotomy to prevent acute limb ischaemia.
- Wound MC&S: to identify associated infection and guide antibiotic therapy.

2. Bloods
   - FBC: anaemia can result from severe haemorrhage.
   - Clotting screen: coagulopathy must be reversed to achieve haemostasis and prior to operative management.
   - G&S: two samples should be sent prior to surgery and to facilitate transfusion.
   - U&Es: acute kidney injury (AKI) can occur with large fluid loss or rhabdomyolysis.
   - CK: ↑CK may occur with skeletal muscle breakdown following crush injuries.
   - Cultures: patients with high-risk wounds or evidence of systemic infection.

3. Imaging
   - X-rays: to identify associated fractures or pneumothorax.
   - Doppler US: in suspected deep vein thrombosis (DVT) or vascular injury.
   - CT traumogram: whole-body CT, performed in significant trauma, to identify bony, vascular and visceral injuries, and intracranial complications.
   - TTE (transthoracic echocardiogram): to identify thoracic injury, pericardial effusion or cardiac tamponade.

Management
Open wounds

The management of open wounds includes:

- Wound cleaning: removal of gross contaminants, large volume irrigation and debridement of devascularized tissue.
- Wound closure: immediate or delayed primary closure or healing by secondary intent.
- Wound reconstruction: via skin grafts or tissue flaps in extensive tissue loss.
- Antibiotic therapy: complicated, contaminated or high-risk wounds (those associated with foreign objects, bite wounds or open fractures) require antibiotic prophylaxis.
- Tetanus prophylaxis: for high-risk wounds including bites or lacerations (Table 9.2, Fig. 9.6).

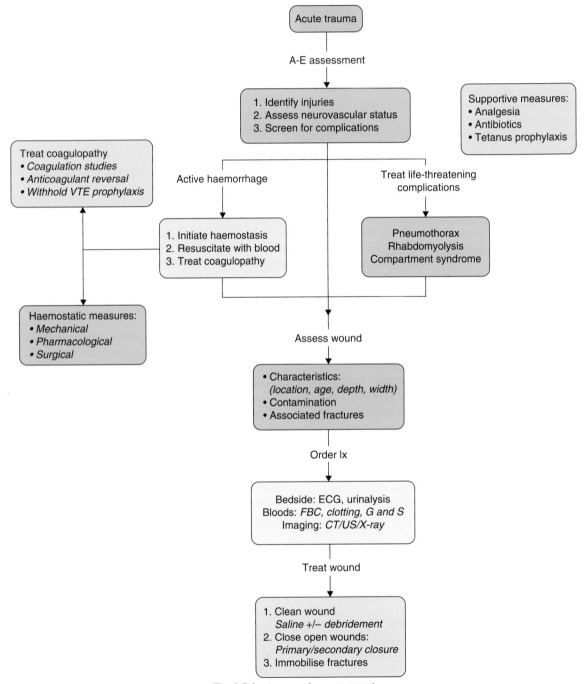

Fig. 9.5 Acute wound management.

Table 9.2 Methods of wound closure

	Primary closure	**Secondary closure**	**Delayed primary closure**
Method	Approximation of edges	Edges not approximated	Delayed approximation
Indications	Clean wounds Young wounds Tension-free approximation possible	Infected/high infection-risk wounds Old wounds Bite wounds Large, irregular wounds	Clean, healthy, wounds, that presented late Contaminated but noninfected wounds
Procedure	Clean wound Excise edges Irrigate wound Approximate edges Apply sterile dressing	Anaesthetize Irrigate wound Debride devascularized tissue Drain wound (+/− NPWT) Apply moist dressing	Clean wound Debride devascularized tissue Approximate edges
Healing	Primary intention Minimal inflammation Minimal scarring	Secondary intention Significant inflammation Significant scarring and granulation tissue	Tertiary intention Significant scarring

Delayed primary closure is performed once healing by secondary intent has already begun, interrupting normal wound healing, hence scarring is the most significant of all closure techniques. NPWT, negative pressure wound therapy, is used to draw out infected fluid from a wound, promoting healing.

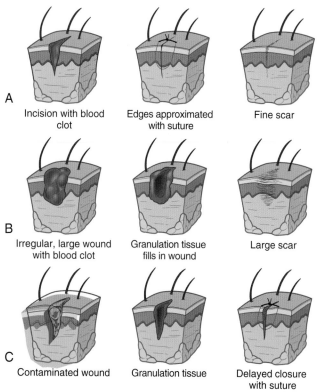

Fig. 9.6 Methods of wound closure. Types of wound healing. (A) Primary intention, with direct closure and minimal scarring. (B) Secondary intention, with significant inflammation, granulation tissue and scarring. (C) Tertiary intention. The wound begins to heal by secondary intent, before primary closure is performed. (From Ratliff CR, Harding MM. *Lewis's Medical-Surgical Nursing: Assessment and Management of Clinical Problems,* 12th Edition. Elsevier; 2023.)

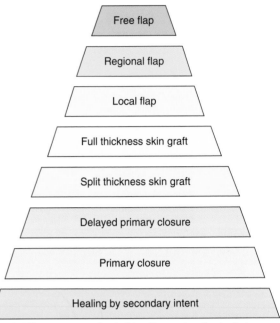

Fig. 9.7 The reconstructive ladder. Reconstructive techniques, increasing in complexity as you ascend up the ladder.

Reconstructive surgery

Reconstructive options relate to the location, complexity and associated wound complications (Fig. 9.7).

Skin grafts

A skin graft involves the removal of healthy skin from a suitable donor site, and transplantation to the wound site, to close a wound, reducing ongoing fluid losses and the risk of wound infection. Grafts can be split-thickness or full-thickness and can be meshed to stretch them up to 6× their original size to improve defect coverage and reduce donor site injury. Suitable donor sites are those with large areas of uninterrupted skin, typically the thigh, abdomen and lateral chest wall (Table 9.3, Figs 9.8 and 9.9).

Skin grafts fail if they do not develop adequate blood supply from the recipient vascular bed. Signs of graft failure include:

- Graft site pallor: indicating graft ischaemia.
- Localized infection: graft failure and incomplete wound coverage increase infection risk.

- Systemic illness: malaise following surgery may indicate imminent graft failure.
- Full thickness necrosis: with death of the donor tissue, requiring operative reintervention.

Table 9.3 Skin graft techniques

	Split thickness	Full thickness
Graft	Epidermis and upper dermis	Epidermis, dermis and dermal appendages
Indications	Large, chronic wounds Flap donor sites	Small, well-vascularised wounds Uncontaminated
Advantages	Better healing potential Superficial injury to donor site	Improved cosmetic outcome
Disadvantages	More significant scarring/skin pigmentation change Risk of contractions	Increased risk of necrosis More significant injury to donor site

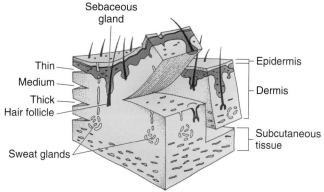

Fig. 9.8 Split and full-thickness skin grafts. A split-thickness skin graft uses the epidermis and part of the dermis. A full-thickness skin graft includes the epidermis and all of the dermis, including pilosebaceous units and apocrine glands. (From Rothrock JC. *Alexander's Care of the Patient in Surgery,* 17th Edition. Elsevier; 2023.)

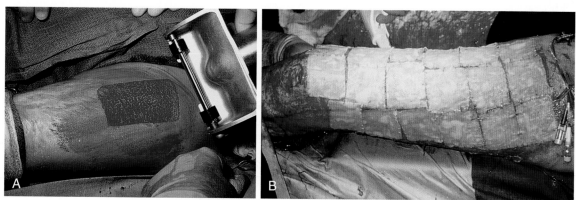

Fig. 9.9 Superficial skin graft technique. (A) Thin sheets of skin are removed with a dermatome then (B) placed over the wound. (From A. Rodgers CC, Wilson D, Hockenberry MJ. *Wong's Nursing Care of Infants and Children,* 11th Edition. Elsevier; 2018. B. Shiland BJ. *Medical Assistant: Integumentary, Sensory Systems, Patient Care and Communication—Module A.* Elsevier; 2016.)

CLINICAL NOTES

- Donor grafts receive their blood supply from the recipient skin bed.
- Thorough debridement of devascularized and necrotic tissue prior to transplantation is essential to allow adequate graft blood supply and encourage graft acceptance.

Skin flaps

Skin flaps involve transferring donor tissue with its corresponding blood supply to a wound if there is deep or extensive tissue loss. Donor tissue can be cutaneous, fasciocutaneous, myocutaneous or muscle, based on the reconstruction outcome and function required.

Flaps can be classified by blood supply:

- Local flap: tissue adjacent to the defect transposed onto the wound, utilizing the local microvasculature.
- Regional (pedicled) flap: regional tissue not directly bordering the defect is raised on a vascular pedicle, with maintenance of blood supply.
- Free flap: complete removal of tissue from a donor site with dissection of the vascular supply, and transposition onto the defect with microsurgical vascular anastomosis (Fig. 9.10).

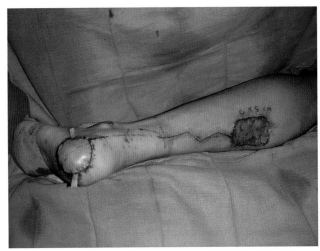

Fig. 9.10 Regional musculocutaneous flap. Regional gastrocnemius flap, with incision for the pedicle dissection, inset onto a calcaneal wound and closure of the donor site using split-thickness skin graft. (From Pu LLQ. *Atlas of Reconstructive Surgery: A Case-Based Approach*. Elsevier; 2024.)

CLINICAL NOTES

Split-thickness skin grafts are used in conjunction with free flaps to cover the donor site or defects not completely covered by the flap.

HINTS AND TIPS

Examples of commonly used flaps include:
- Deep inferior epigastric perforator (DIEP) flap
- Latissimus dorsi flap
- Gracilis flap
- Anterolateral thigh (ALT) flap
- Transverse rectus abdominis myocutaneous (TRAM)

Flap failure is the most significant complication, resulting from arterial or venous insufficiency postoperatively. Reexploration is required.

Complications

Patients with acute and chronic wounds should be followed up regularly, to assess healing, and detect evidence of complications:

- Infections: local infection will impair healing and may result in systemic illness.

- Neurovascular injury: injury to related structures can result in temporary or permanent loss of sensory or motor function, ischaemia and impaired potential.
- Scarring: fibrosis and granulation tissue formation can result in scarring, with cosmetic implications, and associated symptoms including for chronic pain.
- Contractions: fibrosis of connective tissue, resulting in deformity and loss of function.

Surgical complications include:

- Surgical site infection: infection at the site of incision, which can complicate postoperative recovery and delay healing.
- Fistula: abnormal connection between body areas, resulting from impaired healing.
- Wound dehiscence: spontaneous wound breakdown following repair, requiring surgical reintervention and secondary reconstruction.
- Haematoma: collection of blood resulting from a failure of haemostasis. Large collections require surgical drainage.

Benign skin lesions

Benign skin lesions can often be identified from clinical examination alone, assessing physical characteristics of the lesion and associated patient risk factors, but may require biopsy or surgical excision for histological analysis if malignancy cannot be excluded (Figs 9.11 and 9.12).

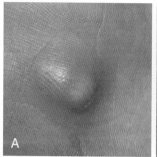

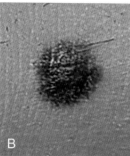

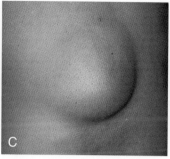

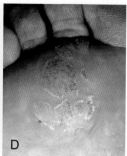

Epidermal (sebaceous) cyst with central punctum. Formed from sebaceous gland obstruction and epidermal debris collection.

Melanocytic naevi, a benign pigmented lesion. Compound naevi have a risk of malignant transformation.

Lipoma, a subcutaneous lobulated fat mass, which may develop into a liposarcoma.

Warts, viral lesions common in the hands and feet causing papillary hyperplasia and keratinisation.

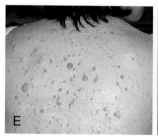

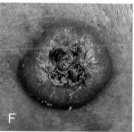

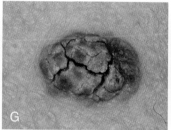

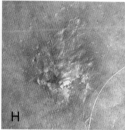

Neurofibroma, benign nerve sheath tumours presenting as a small firm subcutaneous mass.

Keratoacanthoma, a rapidly growing, locally destructive ulcerating lesion that will regress spontaneously.

Seborrhoeic keratosis, a raised, pigmented lesion, with a waxy appearance, common in older adults.

Actinic (solar) keratosis, a hyperkeratotic premalignant lesion common on sun-exposed sites.

Fig. 9.11 Common benign skin lesions. (From A. Weston WL, Morelli JG. *Pediatric Dermatology DDX Deck,* 2nd Edition. Elsevier; 2017. B. Luo J, Liao H, Zhou SK. *Deep Network Design for Medical Image Computing: Principles and Applications.* Elsevier; 2023. C. Rao S, Rao K. *Essentials of Surgery for Dental Students.* 2016. D and G. Elston DM, James WD, McMahon PJ, Micheletti RG, Micheletti R. *Andrews' Diseases of the Skin Clinical Atlas,* 2nd Edition. Elsevier; 2023. E. Dover AR, Innes JA, Fairhurst K. *Macleod's Clinical Examination,* 15th Edition. Elsevier; 2024. F. Wigmore S, Parks RW, Addison P, Garden OJ. *Principles and Practice of Surgery,* 8th Edition. Elsevier; 2023. H. High WA, Kyle WL, Fitzpatrick JE. *Urgent Care Dermatology: Symptom-Based Diagnosis.* Elsevier; 2018.)

Management

Management relates to the lesion size, location and associated complications:

- lesions: cryotherapy, laser therapy or excision for cosmetic regions or associated symptoms, including pain or itch.
- Vascular lesions: excision or cauterization is advised, due to the risk of bleeding.

Necrotizing fasciitis

Necrotizing fasciitis is a life-threatening soft tissue infection resulting in necrosis of the superficial and deep fascia and subcutaneous fat. Immunosuppressed patients, including those with diabetes, malignancy or intravenous drug users, or those with open wounds, are at the greatest risk. It commonly relates to group A streptococcal infection and carries a significant mortality risk without urgent assessment and treatment.

Symptoms and signs

Necrotizing fasciitis presents as severe cellulitis, with a poor response to antibiotic therapy:

- Erythema: significant, diffuse and fast spreading.
- Tissue induration: induration of the subcutaneous tissue larger than visible skin affected.
- Skin emphysema: gas-forming organisms cause skin crepitus and bullae formation.
- Purple/black skin discolouration: relating to necrosis and ecchymosis.

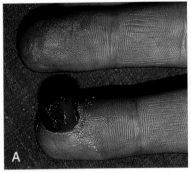

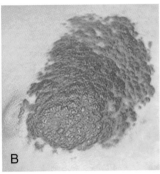

Pyogenic granuloma, a highly vascularised mass of granulation tissue that develops after trauma, and bleeds easily and excessively.

Capillary haemangioma (port wine stain), resulting from congenital capillary malformation.

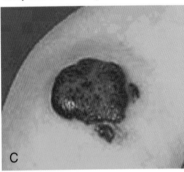

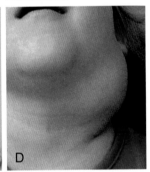

Cavernous haemangioma, a localised collection of dilated veins with a high risk of ulceration and bleeding.

Lymphangioma, fluid filled lymphatic channels relating to lymphatic malformation.

Fig. 9.12 Common vascular skin lesions. (From A. Kinross J, Chaudry MA, Rasheed S. *Clinical Surgery,* 4th Edition. Elsevier; 2023. B. Woodman I, McKinney O. *Crash Course: Pathology,* 5th Edition. Elsevier; 2019. C. Randall D, Waterhouse M. *Kumar & Clark's Clinical Medicine,* 7th Edition. Elsevier; 2009. D. Paige DG, Kumar P, Wakelin SH, Clark M. *Kumar & Clark's Clinical Medicine,* 9th Edition. Elsevier; 2017.)

- Severe pain: classically out of proportion to clinical findings (Fig. 9.13).

Management

Necrotizing fasciitis is a surgical emergency. Urgent debridement and antibiotic therapy are essential (Fig. 9.14).

Complications

Complications of necrotizing fasciitis include:

- Limb amputation: for severe necrosis of the limbs.

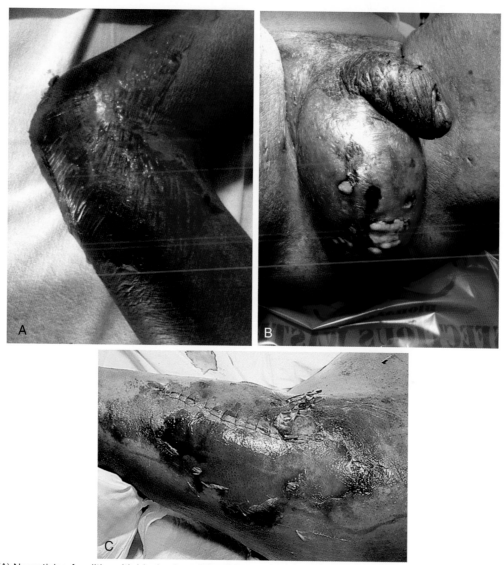

Fig. 9.13 (A) Necrotizing fasciitis, with blackening of the skin, exudation and bullae formation. (B) Fournier's gangrene, necrotizing fasciitis of the perineum, which can rapidly spread to involve the abdominal wall and gluteal muscles. (C) Necrosis overlying a hip joint following hip surgery, with significant erythema, necrosis and skin sloughing. (From A. Garden OJ, Addison P, Parks RW. *Principles and Practice of Surgery,* 7th Edition. Elsevier; 2018. B. Townsend CM, Mattox KL, Evers BM, Coburn M, Townsend C, Beauchamp RD. *Sabiston Textbook of Surgery: The Biological Basis of Modern Surgical Practice,* 19th Edition. Elsevier; 2012. C. Spicer WJ. *Clinical Microbiology and Infectious Diseases: An Illustrated Colour Text,* 2nd Edition. Churchill Livingstone, Elsevier Ltd. 2008.)

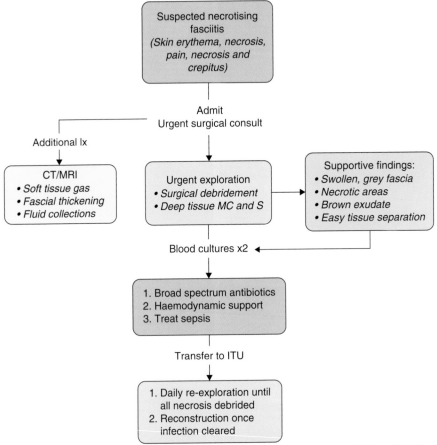

Fig. 9.14 Approach to the management of necrotizing fasciitis. Urgent surgical debridement is indicated in all suspected cases, and will confirm or exclude the underlying diagnosis.

- Abdominal evisceration: due to severe necrosis of the perineal and abdominal skin.
- Renal failure: acute kidney injury (AKI) and subsequent renal failure.
- Sepsis: resulting in multiorgan dysfunction and death.

Pressure ulcers

Pressure ulcers develop due to chronic local pressure resulting in skin ischemia and necrosis, typically over bony areas. They are common in older, immunocompromised and malnourished patients who have been immobilized for long periods.

Symptoms and signs

Features include:

- Focal erythema: with or without associated oedema.

- Pain: chronic or transient pain that can be severe.
- Decreased skin perfusion: nonblanching skin with increased capillary refill time.

Features of advanced ulcers include:

- Eschar: dark dead tissue that sloughs off the ulcer bed.
- Visible deep tissues: muscle and bone may be evident if the ulcer is severe.
- Local infection: purulence, odour and systemic illness indicate wound infection (Fig. 9.15).

Pressure ulcers can be staged depending on the depth of the ulcer:

- Stage 1: nonblanching erythema with intact skin.
- Stage 2: partial thickness skin loss (epidermis).
- Stage 3: full thickness skin loss (epidermis and dermis, fascia intact).

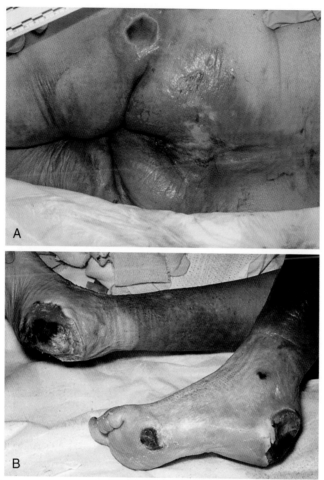

Fig. 9.15 (A) Large pressure ulcer over the sacrum, with evidence of pus and slough indicating infection. The greater trochanter has a full-thickness injury as indicated by the waxy-white appearance, demonstrating complete skin loss. (B) Bilateral calcaneal pressure ulcers with evidence of skin necrosis, slough and erythema. (From A. Eckhardt A, Jarvis C. *Physical Examination & Health Assessment,* 9th Edition. Elsevier; 2024. B. Edwards S, Drake WM, Glynn M. *Hutchison's Clinical Methods: An Integrated Approach to Clinical Practice,* 25th Edition. Elsevier; 2023.)

- Stage 4; full thickness skin loss (fascial erosion, muscle, tendon and bone exposure).

Management
Management involves wound care, prevention strategies and treatment of complications.

- Superficial, clean wounds: regular cleaning and wound dressings.
- Deep, infected or necrotic wounds: debridement, antibiotics and wound dressings.

CLINICAL NOTES

- Silver dressings are often used due to their broad-spectrum antimicrobial activity.
- Negative pressure wound therapy (NPWT) can be applied to infected ulcers to drain infected fluid and promote healing.

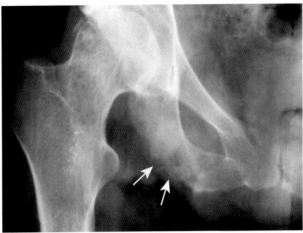

Fig. 9.16 Severe pressure ulcers may result in osteomyelitis. X-ray findings include focal osteopenia, cortical destruction and periosteal reaction. (From Deakin PJ, et al. *Essential Surgery: Problems, Diagnosis and Management,* 6th Edition. Elsevier; 2020.)

Once healing has begun, delayed primary closure can be considered. For frail patients with guarded prognoses, conservative management may be appropriate.

Supportive measures include:

- Pressure relief: frequent position changes, pressure mattresses and padding over the affected area.
- Skin care: maintaining clean, moisturized skin, to reduce the risk of erosion.
- Pain management: pain may be significant and require opioid analgesia.
- Optimization of risk factors: good medical management of comorbidities is essential.
- Nutritional support: to support wound healing and reduce risk of further ulcers including protein supplementation, multivitamin replacement and increased calorie intake.

Complications

Complications relate to skin breakage and increased risk of infection:

- Soft tissue infection: including cellulitis or local abscess.
- Osteomyelitis: infection spreading to involve the bone.
- Sepsis: systemic infection can result from deep, poorly managed ulcers.
- Marjolin's ulcer: squamous cell carcinoma arising from chronic, nonhealing wounds (Fig. 9.16).

Malignant skin lesions

Malignant skin lesions can occur anywhere, however, they are more common in sun-exposed sights. Other risk factors include radiation, carcinogen exposure and chronic wounds.

Basal cell carcinoma

Basal cell carcinoma (BCC) is the most common malignant skin lesion. They typically arise in sun-exposed sites, particularly the face. They grow slowly, have a low risk of metastasis, and have excellent prognosis.

Symptoms and signs

BCC has distinctive clinical features:

- Pink nodule with surface sheen
- Ulcerated areas with a rolled edge
- Superficial telangiectasia
- Surface scale or crust

They are typically painless (Fig. 9.17).

Management

All suspected BCCs should be excised with adequate tissue margins, and histological confirmation of the diagnosis. Additional measures include:

- Radiotherapy: if complete surgical removal is not possible, or for hard-to-reach lesions.
- Cryoablation: application of liquid nitrogen to freeze and destroy malignant cells.
- Topical chemotherapy: using imiquimod or 5-flurouacil, for small, superficial lesions.

Squamous cell carcinoma

Cutaneous squamous cell carcinoma (SCC) is the second most common cutaneous malignancy. Risk factors include excess sunlight, chemical carcinogens, radiation, chronic wounds and

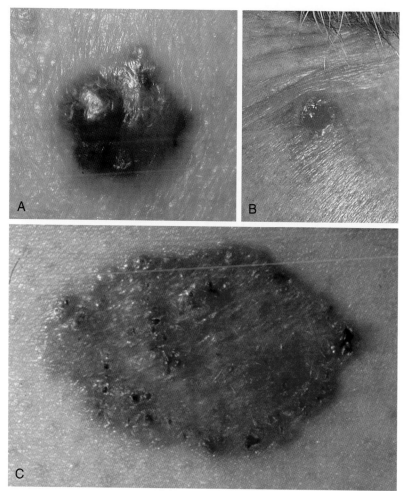

Fig. 9.17 Types of basal cell carcinoma (BCC). (A) nodular BCC, with multiple telangiectasia and surface sheet. (B) ulcerated BCC, with a central crater and rolled edge. (C) Superficial BCC, with surface crust and telangiectasia. (From A and C. James WD, Micheletti RG, McMahon PJ, Elston DM. *Andrews' Diseases of the Skin Clinical Atlas,* 2nd Edition. Elsevier; 2023. B. Craft JA, Huether SE, Tiziani A, Brashers VL, Gordon CJ, McCance KL. *Understanding Pathophysiology,* 4th Edition. Elsevier; 2023.)

immunosuppression. They are slow growing and locally invasive, with a risk of regional lymphatic metastasis.

> **HINTS AND TIPS**
>
> Actinic keratosis is a premalignant lesion that can develop into Bowen's disease (SCC in situ) before progressing to invasive SCC.

Symptoms and signs

SCC typically presents with painless, nonhealing ulcers. Further features include:

- Inflammation and erythema
- Indurated lesion with everted edges
- Granulation tissue
- Friable, easy bleeding lesion (Fig. 9.18)

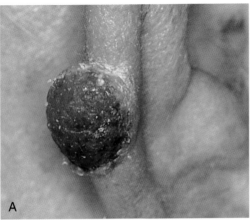
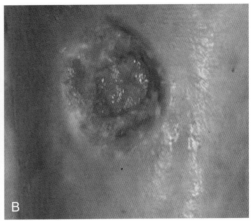

Fig. 9.18 Squamous cell carcinoma. (A) Inflamed, indurated, everted lesion with granulation tissue on the ear, resembling SCC. (B) Chronic ulcer with associated SCC (Marjolin ulcer). (From A. Shiland BJ. *Medical Assistant: Integumentary, Sensory Systems, Patient Care and Communication—Module A.* Elsevier; 2016. B. Shin L, Sidawy AN, Woelfel SL, Armstrong DG, Perler BA. *Rutherford's Vascular Surgery and Endovascular Therapy,* 10th Edition. Elsevier; 2023.)

Management

All lesions suspicious for SCC should be excised with adequate tissue margins, and histological confirmation of the diagnosis. Additional measures include:

- Cryotherapy: suitable in cases of Bowen disease (SCC in situ).
- Radiotherapy: primary or adjunctive measure in large or inoperable tumours.
- Topical chemotherapy: adjuvant measure, or for those with systemic metastasis.

CT, MRI or lymph node biopsy can be performed to detect regional metastasis.

Melanoma

Melanoma is a tumour arising from epidermal melanocytes. It is very common, particularly in light-skinned individuals with a history of excessive sun exposure. Other risk factors include age, family history, immunosuppression and the presence of dysplastic naevi. Melanoma are life-threatening, due to their rapid spread and high risk of metastasis.

Clinical features

All pigmented lesions should be evaluated for the risk of melanoma using the ABCDE criteria:

- **A** – **A**symmetry
- **B** – **B**order (irregular, with unclear margins)
- **C** – **C**olour change, new or varying pigmentation
- **D** – **D**iameter >6 mm
- **E** – **E**volution – changing size or shape of a lesion (Fig. 9.19).

Management

Management of suspected melanoma involves full-thickness excisional biopsy with 3 mm margins. Following histological confirmation of the diagnosis, surgical resection with wide local excision is performed.

CLINICAL NOTES

Full thickness biopsy allows estimation of the Breslow thickness (tumour depth), to guide the safety margin required during excision.

Staging investigations can diagnose regional or distant metastasis, which can occur almost anywhere in the body, including the regional lymph nodes, liver, lung, brain and bone.

The prognosis is variable, related to the speed of diagnosis and the presence of metastasis. Breslow thickness is the most important prognostic factor, with increasing tumour depth associated with significantly worse outcomes (Fig. 9.20).

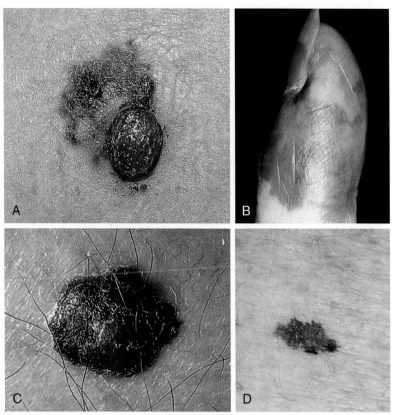

Fig. 9.19 Malignant melanoma. (A) Superficial spreading melanoma, an asymmetric nodular and flat lesion with irregular border and colour. (B) Acral lentiginous melanoma, with periungual spread of pigmentation to the proximal and lateral nail folds. (C) Nodular melanoma, with asymmetrical border and dark pigmentation. (D) Lentigo maligna (melanoma in situ), an irregular, pigmented patch, with horizontal growth. (From A and C. Kinross J, Rasheed S, Chaudry MA. *Clinical Surgery,* 4th Edition. Elsevier; 2023. B. Dinulos JGH. *Habif's Clinical Dermatology: A Color Guide to Diagnosis and Therapy,* 7th Edition. Elsevier; 2021. D. Huether SE, Gordon CJ, Brashers VL, McCance KL, Tiziani A, Craft JA. *Understanding Pathophysiology,* Australia and New Zealand Edition, 4th Edition. Elsevier. Australia; 2023.)

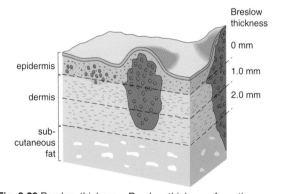

Fig. 9.20 Breslow thickness. Breslow thickness from the granulation layer to the lowest detectable tumour cell. Determines appropriate safety margins, risk of metastasis and prognosis of disease. (From Shaikh H, et al. *Crash Course Pathology,* 5th Edition. Elsevier; 2020.)

Burns

Burns are tissue injuries caused by heat, radiation or chemicals. Significant clinical sequelae can result from large burns due to inflammatory mediator release and systemic inflammation. The significance of a burn relates to the depth and body surface area involved (Table 9.4, Fig. 9.21).

CLINICAL NOTES

Burns which involve >50% BSA are typically lethal.

Investigations

Investigations are indicated to monitor for complications

1. Bedside
   - Pulse oximetry: to assess for systemic and limb hypoxaemia.
   - Wound swabs: if local infection is suspected.

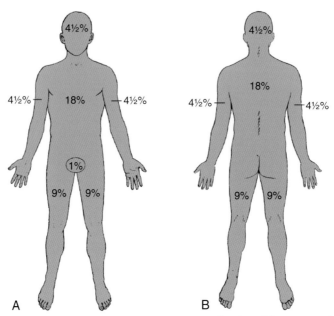

Fig. 9.21 Rule of nines. Division of the body into 11 areas of 9% allowing estimation of the amount of skin surface burned in an adult. (From Rogers JL. *McCance & Huether's Pathophysiology: The Biologic Basis for Disease in Adults and Children,* 9th Edition. Elsevier; 2024.)

Table 9.4 Burn depth

Depth	Affected skin layer	Clinical features	Prognosis
1st-degree (superficial)	Superficial epidermis	Localized pain and erythema No blistering Blanching, rapid CRT	Healing in 3–6 days No scarring
2nd-degree (superficial partial thickness)	Epidermis, upper dermis	Localized pain, erythema, swelling and heat Bullae formation Blanching, slow CRT	Healing in 1–3 weeks Pigmentation changes No scarring
2nd-degree (deep partial thickness)	Deeper dermis	Minimal pain, mottled red/white skin Fragile bullae Nonblanching	Healing >3 weeks Scarring
3rd-degree	Subcutaneous tissue	No pain, tissue necrosis, black/grey eschar Nonblanching	No spontaneous healing

2. Bloods
   - ABG: to assess for respiratory failure and metabolic acidosis.
   - FBC: systemic inflammation can result in haemolytic anaemia.
   - U&Es: fluid losses result in hyperkalaemia and hyponatraemia, and AKI.
   - LFTs: hypoalbuminaemia can result from fluid losses and tissue damage.

- Blood cultures: if there is evidence of systemic infection.

Management
Minor burns can be managed with local cooling with running water, topical moisturizers and dressings. Severe burns should be managed with airway support, fluid resuscitation and debridement and reconstruction of burnt skin (Fig. 9.22).

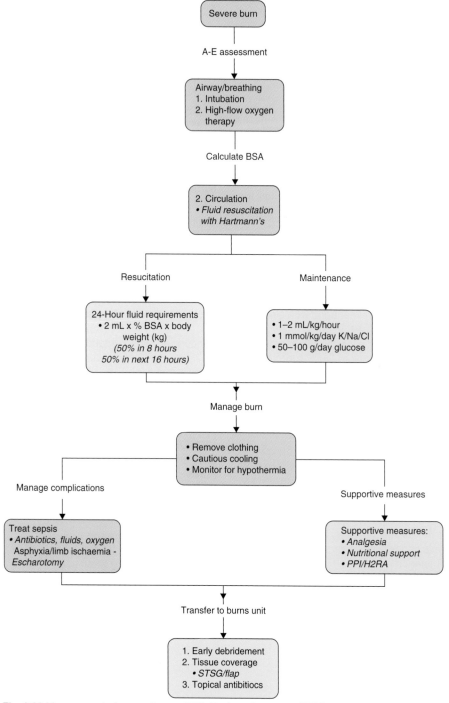

Fig. 9.22 Management of severe burns. *BSA,* Body surface area; *STSG,* split-thickness skin graft.

CLINICAL NOTES

The Parkland formula is no longer used, due to frequent over-resuscitation and associated complications including pulmonary oedema and compartment syndrome.

Complications

Complications of severe burns include:

- Hypovolaemic shock: severe fluid losses can result in shock and oliguria.
- Acute respiratory distress syndrome (ARDS): resulting from systemic inflammation.

- Sepsis: bacterial infection can result in systemic inflammation, disseminated intravascular coagulation and acute organ failure.
- Inhalation injury: ARDS related to smoke and gas inhalation.
- Postburn hypermetabolism: state of hypermetabolism following burn injury resulting in severe protein catabolism, muscle wasting and multiorgan dysfunction.
- Eschars: constrictive effects may result in asphyxia, compartment syndrome or acute limb ischaemia, requiring escharotomy or fasciotomy.

The prognosis depends on the extent of the burns, the age of the patient and comorbidities. There is a 50% mortality rate for burns covering more than 50% BSA.

● Chapter Summary

- Open wounds must be managed with cleaning, debridement and wound closure, with antibiotic therapy for high-risk wounds.
- Necrotizing fasciitis is a life-threatening deep tissue infection requiring urgent debridement and systemic antibiotics.
- The most significant risk factor for cutaneous malignancy is sun exposure.
- The ABCDE criteria is used to evaluate pigmented lesions for malignancy.
- Severe burns should be managed with respiratory support, fluid resuscitation and debridement of necrotic tissue.

UKMLA Conditions
Atopic dermatitis and eczema
Basal cell carcinoma
Cellulitis
Compartment syndrome
Contact dermatitis
Cutaneous fungal infection
Hyperthermia and hypothermia
Malignant melanoma
Necrotizing fasciitis
Pressure sores
Psoriasis
Squamous cell carcinoma
Urticaria

UKMLA Presentations
Bites and stings
Burns
Chronic rash
Lacerations
Massive haemorrhage
Nail abnormalities
Scarring
Shock
Skin or subcutaneous lump
Skin ulcers
Soft tissue injury
Trauma

Cardiothoracic surgery 10

CLINICAL ANATOMY

Cardiac anatomy

The heart is a muscular organ which connects the systemic and pulmonary circulation. The four chambers of the heart contract to pump blood from the deoxygenated systemic circulation to the lungs, where it is oxygenated before being pumped into the systemic circulation.

The right atrium receives deoxygenated blood from the systemic circulation via the superior and inferior vena cava. Blood flows into the right ventricle and is pumped into the pulmonary circulation via the pulmonary veins, where gas exchange takes place, and the blood becomes oxygenated. Oxygenated blood drains via the pulmonary artery into the left atrium and then the left ventricle, before being pumped into the systemic circulation via the aorta.

The atrioventricular (AV) valves divide the atria and ventricles, and the semilunar (SL) valves divide the ventricle and circulatory system, and open and close to allow blood flow in response to changing intracardiac pressures. The AV valves include the tricuspid valve, which separates the right atrium and ventricle, and the mitral valve, a bicuspid valve that separates the left atrium and ventricle. The subvalvular apparatus includes the papillary muscles and chordae tendineae that prevent AV valve

prolapse during ventricular contraction. The SL valves include the pulmonary valve, which separates the right ventricle and pulmonary vessels, and the aortic valve, which separates the left ventricle and aorta. They are both tricuspid valves (Fig. 10.1).

The walls of the heart consist of three layers, the endocardium, myocardium and pericardium. The endocardium is a thin layer of connective tissue which contains Purkinje cells, modified cardiomyocytes that form part of the cardiac conduction system. The myocardium is a thick muscular layer of cardiomyocytes, which produce the force of heart muscle contraction and release hormones including atrial natriuretic peptide (ANP), which regulates blood pressure. The pericardium is formed of a visceral inner layer and parietal outer layer, in between which is a fluid-filled pericardial space (Fig. 10.2).

Cardiac cycle

The cardiac cycle is divided into systole and diastole. During systole, the ventricular muscles contract, pumping blood into the pulmonary and systemic circulation. Increased intraventricular pressures force the closure of the AV valves, producing the first heart sound (S1) and the SL valves open. At the end of systole, decreased intraventricular pressures result in the closing of the SL valves, producing the second heart sound (S2). Diastole begins with ventricular

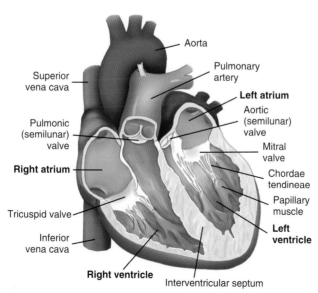

Fig. 10.1 Anatomy of the heart. Anatomy of the heart chambers and the great vessels. (From Harding MM, Kwong J, Hagler D, Reinisch C. *Lewis's Medical-Surgical Nursing: Assessment and Management of Clinical Problems,* 12th Edition. Elsevier; 2023.)

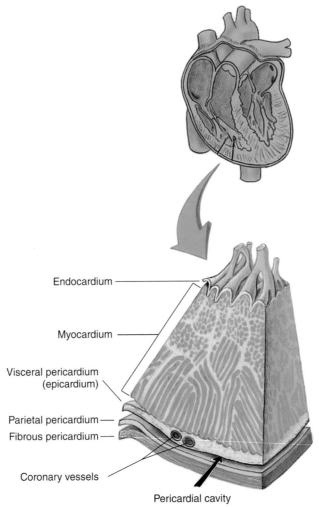

Endocardium

Myocardium

Visceral pericardium
(epicardium)

Parietal pericardium

Fibrous pericardium

Coronary vessels

Pericardial cavity

Fig. 10.2 Layers of the heart wall. Cross-sectional representation of the layers of the heart wall and the surrounding pericardial cavity and vascular structures. (From *ICD-10-CM/PCS Coding: Theory and Practice*. Elsevier; 2023.)

muscle relaxation, and reduced intraventricular pressures result in the opening of the AV valves and the passive flow of blood from the atria to the ventricles. Once the ventricles have filled, the cardiac cycle repeats with systolic contraction (Fig. 10.3).

The cardiac conduction system regulates heart rate (HR). The sinoatrial (SA) node in the right atrium contains specialized pacemaker cells that generate action potentials, which are conducted to the atrioventricular (AV) node in the AV septum as the atria contract. The AV node delays conduction to the ventricles, to allow ventricular diastolic filling. The AV bundle splits into left and right 'bundle branches' to supply each ventricle, with terminal Purkinje fibres in the ventricular endocardium which synchronize ventricular contractions (Fig. 10.4).

Cardiac physiology

Regulation of the cardiac cycle

The autonomic nervous system regulates HR and contractility, which influences stroke volume (SV) and cardiac output (CO). Sympathetic stimulation releases adrenaline and noradrenaline, which bind to β1 adrenergic receptors on cardiac myocytes, resulting in increased calcium and sodium channel conduction, increasing HR, contractility and CO. Parasympathetic stimulation releases acetylcholine, which binds to muscarinic receptors, reducing SA node conduction and resulting in vagal innervation of the AV node, reducing action potential propagation, reducing HR and CO.

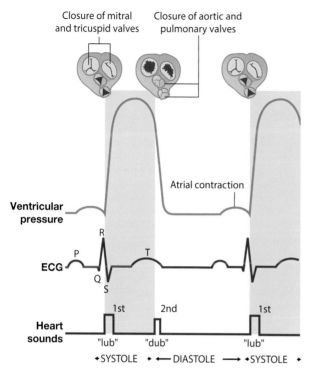

Closure of mitral and tricuspid valves

Closure of aortic and pulmonary valves

Atrial contraction

Ventricular pressure

ECG

Heart sounds

"lub" "dub" "lub"

◄SYSTOLE ► ◄── DIASTOLE ──► ◄SYSTOLE ►

Fig. 10.3 Heart sounds. Closure of the heart valves and the production of heart sounds in relation to the cardiac cycle. (From Vogl AW, Mitchell AWM, Drake RL. *Gray's Basic Anatomy*. Churchill Livingstone, Elsevier Inc. 2013.)

Preload and afterload

Preload and afterload are systemic factors which affect cardiac output. Preload is the final myocardial stretch that occurs at the end of systole, which relates to end-diastolic ventricular volume (EDV). Increased circulating blood volume increases EDV, increasing preload, SV and CO. Afterload is the force that the ventricles contract against to eject blood, which relates to total peripheral resistance (TPR) in the circulatory system. Increased TPR leads to increased afterload, and decreased SV and CO.

Blood pressure (BP) is the pressure generated by heart muscle contraction within blood vessels. Systolic BP is the maximum pressure reached during a cardiac cycle, and diastolic the minimum pressure. Mean arterial pressure (MAP) is a simplified value of systolic and diastolic pressures. Blood pressure is influenced by CO and TPR (Table 10.1).

Coronary circulation

The left coronary artery (LCA) supplies most of the myocardium and gives off the left anterior descending (LAD),

Table 10.1 Cardiac physiology

Term	Definition	Calculation
Heart rate (HR)	The rate of heart contractions per minute (bpm)	Normal – 60–100 bpm
Stroke volume (SV)	The volume of blood pumped into the systemic circulation by each heartbeat	SV = EDV – ESV
Ejection fraction (EF)	The proportion of EDV ejected from the ventricle with each contraction	EF = SV/EDV Normal – 50%–70%
Cardiac output (CO)	The volume of blood pumped into the circulatory system per minute	CO = HR × SV
Blood pressure (BP)	The pressure in the vascular system with each heartbeat	MAP = CO × TPR

EDV, *End-diastolic volume;* ESV, *end-systolic volume;* MAP, *mean arterial pressure.*

which supplies the left atrium and ventricle, and left circumflex (LCX) arteries, which supply the posterior left heart and papillary muscles. The right coronary artery (RCA) gives off the posterior descending artery (PDA), which supplies the posterior heart, and other branches that supply the right side of the heart, AV and SA nodes. The coronary veins include the great, posterior, small and middle cardiac veins, that drain into a single large coronary sinus, which then drains into the right atrium (Fig. 10.5).

CARDIOTHORACIC SURGERY PRESENTATIONS

History taking

Opening the consultation
Wash your hands, introduce yourself and confirm the patient details.

Presenting complaint (PC)
Begin with open questions to identify the patient's primary complaint.

COMMUNICATION

The 'golden minute' is often advised to allow the patient to express their symptoms in sufficient detail.

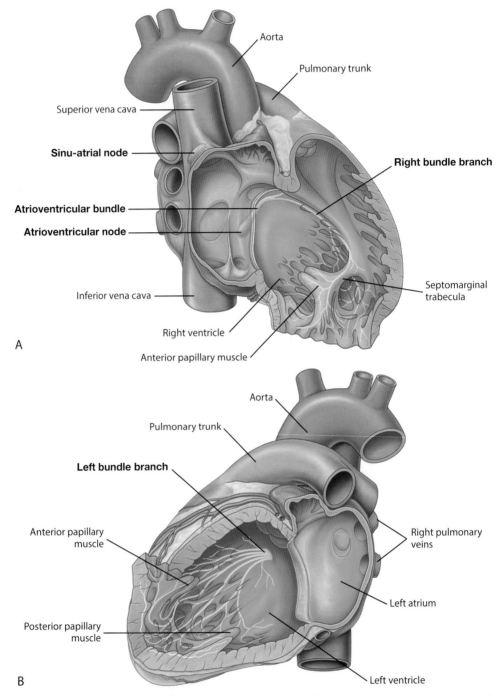

Fig. 10.4 Cardiac conduction system. (A) The right-sided conduction system. (B) The left-sided conduction system. A unidirectional wave of excitation results in synchronized contraction, from the papillary muscles to the apex of the ventricles. (From Vogl AW, Mitchell AWM, Drake RL. *Gray's Basic Anatomy*. Churchill Livingstone, Elsevier Inc. 2013.)

History of presenting complaint (HPC)

Explore the presenting complaint in more detail.

Common presentations in cardiovascular histories include:

- Chest pain: crushing central chest pain radiating to the left arm, neck and jaw is suggestive of acute coronary syndrome (ACS). Sharp pleuritic pain may indicate pulmonary embolism (PE) and tearing substernal pain aortic dissection (AD).

- Dyspnoea: shortness of breath, worse on exertion or worse lying flat (orthopnoea).
- Palpitations: a fast, pounding or fluttering heartbeat. May be regular or irregular.
- Syncope: an episode of transient loss of consciousness, with spontaneous and complete recovery.

Systemic screen

A brief systemic screen can offer invaluable insights into the potential differential diagnosis. Include a few key symptoms from each relevant system:

- Respiratory: shortness of breath, cough, wheeze, sputum and haemoptysis can all be associated with acute and chronic cardiac conditions.

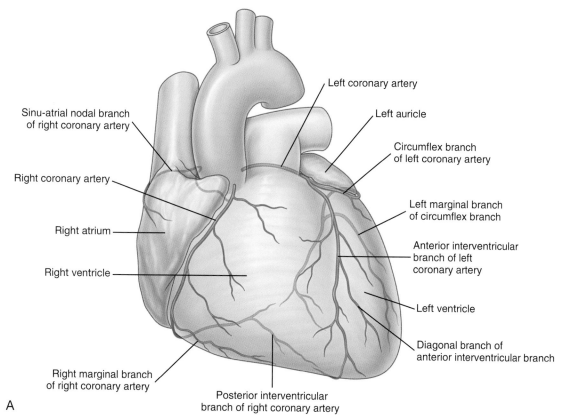

A

continued

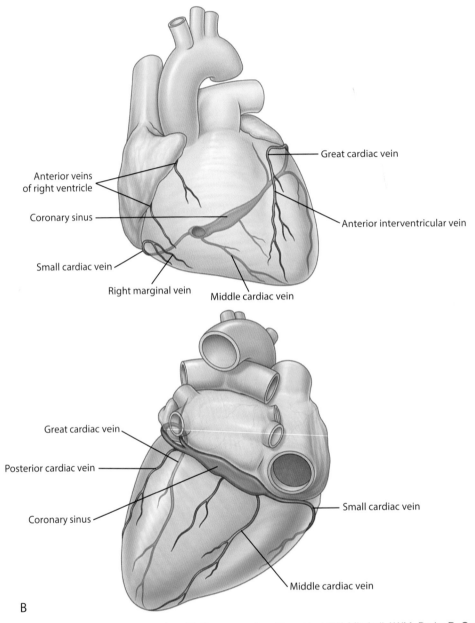

Great cardiac vein

Anterior veins
of right ventricle

Coronary sinus

Small cardiac vein

Right marginal vein

Middle cardiac vein

Anterior interventricular vein

Great cardiac vein

Posterior cardiac vein

Coronary sinus

Small cardiac vein

Middle cardiac vein

B

Fig. 10.5 Coronary vasculature. (A) Coronary arteries. (B) Coronary veins. (From Vogl AW, Mitchell AWM, Drake R. *Gray's Basic Anatomy*. Churchill Livingstone, Elsevier Inc. 2013.)

- Gastroenterology: dyspepsia, nausea and vomiting, can relate to acute cardiac events.
- Neurology: visual changes or postural instability can indicate cerebral hypoperfusion, which may be secondary to cardiac pathology.
- Urological: polyuria and recurrent UTIs suggest diabetes, and oliguria chronic kidney disease, both important comorbidities which increase cardiovascular risk.
- Dermatology: skin and nail changes may be associated with endocarditis.

- Musculoskeletal: peripheral oedema can occur in congestive heart failure. Cramping muscle pain on exertion suggests claudication related to peripheral vascular disease.

> **HINTS AND TIPS**
>
> Screen for constitutional features (FLAWS) suggestive of underlying systemic illness or malignancy:
> - **F** – Fever
> - **L** – Lethargy
> - **A** – Appetite loss
> - **W** – Weight change
> - **S** – Night sweats

Past medical history

Enquire about past and current medical and surgical history, including hospital admissions, complications and procedures.

> **HINTS AND TIPS**
>
> - Salient medical history may be forgotten, particularly for conditions that have been resolved.
> - Check the GP records for current and previous conditions, operations and investigations.

Drug history

Obtain a complete drug history, assessing compliance, side effects, use of over-the-counter or complementary medications, and allergies.

Family history

Screen for a family history of cardiac disease or important comorbidities, including myocardial infarction, valvular disorders, hypertension, hyperlipidaemia and diabetes.

> **DIFFERENTIALS**
>
> - Check the age of presentation for relevant family history.
> - Inherited cardiac conditions commonly present young.
> - A history of sudden death in young relatives may suggest inherited channelopathies or myopathies.

Social history

Screen for relevant cardiovascular risk factors:

- Smoking: a significant cardiovascular risk factor. Record the number of pack years.

- Alcohol: record the type consumed, and units per week. Excessive alcohol use is associated with dilated cardiomyopathy.
- Drugs: intravenous drug use increases the risk of endocarditis. Stimulants can cause hypertension, palpitations and chest pain. Opiates can cause bradycardia and syncope.
- Diet and weight: obesity and high salt or fat diets are modifiable risk factors for cardiovascular disease.
- Exercise: appreciating the extent of exercise a patient does and can do is important to understand symptom impact and cardiovascular risk.
- Occupation: patients in high-risk occupations (operating machinery or driving heavy vehicles) may need to stop working until their symptoms are controlled.
- Performance status: assess the patient's independence with activities of daily living and support needs, including mobility, carers and social support.

> **HINTS AND TIPS**
>
> - Always offer smoking cessation advice if relevant.
> - It is a useful opportunity for health promotion and will gain you marks in exams.

Ideas, concerns and expectations

Assess the patient's ideas, concerns and expectations to gain insight into any relevant concerns and what they hope to get out of the consultation.

Closing the consultation

Summarize the history, answer any questions and thank the patient for their time.

DIFFERENTIAL DIAGNOSIS

Chest pain

The characteristics of chest pain as well as ECG findings can help narrow down the differential diagnosis and rule out immediate life-threatening causes (Fig. 10.6).

Investigations for chest pain

1. Bedside
   - Observations: tachycardia and hypotension indicate haemodynamic compromise. Fever may be present in acute infection or malignancy.
   - ECG: the most important initial investigation to identify ACS.

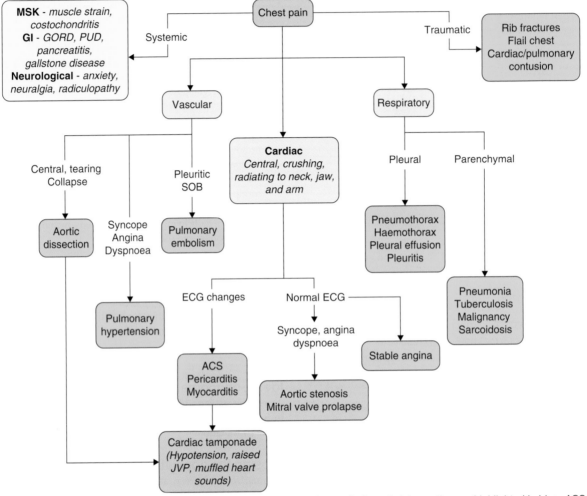

Fig. 10.6 Differential diagnosis of chest pain. Conditions that may require cardiothoracic intervention are highlighted in blue. *ACS*, Acute coronary syndrome; *GORD*, gastroesophageal reflux disease; *JVP*, jugular venous pressure; *PUD*, peptic ulcer disease; *SOB*, shortness of breath.

2. Bloods
   - Serial troponins: at presentation and hourly intervals afterwards. Rising troponins suggest ACS.
   - FBC/CRP: ↓ Hb suggests anaemia or acute blood loss. ↑ WCC and CRP indicate acute infection.
   - U&Es: baseline test to detect acute or chronic renal impairment.
   - ABG: ↑ lactate and acidosis suggest sepsis. Acute hypoxia may indicate PE.
   - BNP: ↑ BNP is indicative of heart failure, associated with angina.
   - LFTs/amylase: to rule out cholecystitis or pancreatitis.
3. Imaging
   - Chest X-ray (CXR): to diagnose pulmonary infection, effusion or mass. A widened mediastinum may indicate AD, and a large bottle-shaped heart is classic for pericardial effusion. Absent lung marking suggests pneumothorax or atelectasis.
   - Coronary angiography +/- percutaneous coronary intervention (PCI): to diagnose and treat STEMI or NSTEMI with high-risk features.
   - CT angiography (CTA): to diagnose thoracic aneurysms or AD.
   - CT pulmonary angiogram (CTPA): filling defects within the pulmonary vasculature indicate PE.
   - Transthoracic echocardiography (TTE): to assess cardiac function and aid diagnosis of pericardial or valvular conditions.

Dyspnoea

Acute dyspnoea can relate to acute cardiovascular or respiratory conditions, systemic infection or neurological disorders, and is a common feature of many conditions causing pain or anxiety. Chronic dyspnoea typically relates to chronic cardiac or respiratory disease (Figs 10.7-10.8).

RED FLAG

- Acute dyspnoea (seconds to minutes) represents immediately life-threatening conditions including AD and PE.
- Subacute dyspnoea (hours to days) typically relates to significant (and potentially life-threatening) pathology including acute asthma or COPD exacerbation.
- Both are medical emergencies.

Investigations for dyspnoea

1. Bedside
   - Observations: to assess for haemodynamic compromise and objectively measure oxygen saturations.
   - Spirometry: simple spirometry including peak expiratory flow rate (PEFR) and forced vital capacity (FVC) can be performed by the bedside.
   - Sputum MC&S: to allowing targeting of antibiotic therapy in acute infection.
   - Respiratory viral PCR: including COVID-19 and influenza testing.
   - ECG: to diagnose acute cardiac events.
   - Urinary pneumococcal/legionella antigen: to identify atypical respiratory pathogens.

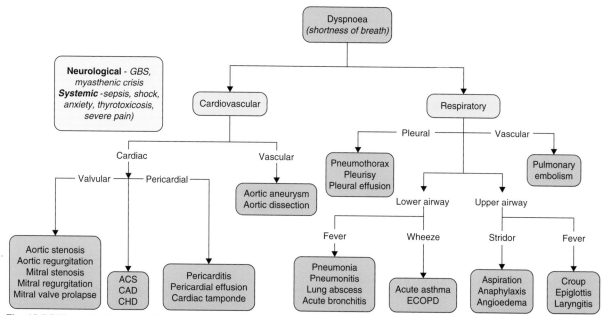

Fig. 10.7 Differential diagnosis of acute dyspnoea. Conditions which may require cardiothoracic intervention are highlighted in blue. *ACS*, Acute coronary syndrome; *CAD*, coronary artery disease; *CHD*, congenital heart disease; *ECOPD*, exacerbation of chronic obstructive pulmonary disease, which can be infective or noninfective; *GBS*, Guillain–Barré syndrome.

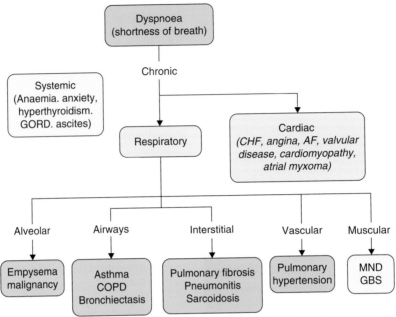

Fig. 10.8 Differential diagnosis of chronic dyspnoea. Conditions which may require cardiothoracic intervention are highlighted in blue. *AF*, Atrial fibrillation; *CHF*, congestive heart failure; *COPD*, chronic obstructive pulmonary disease; *GBS*, Guillain–Barré syndrome; *GORD*, gastro-oesophageal reflux disease; *MND*, motor neuron disease.

2. Bloods
   - ABG: to measure hypoxia and diagnose respiratory failure. ↓ pH and ↑ lactate suggest sepsis. ↑ bicarbonate indicates chronic metabolic compensation for respiratory acidosis.
   - FBC: ↓ Hb in anaemia is associated with dyspnoea. ↑ Hb suggests polycythaemia related to chronic hypoxic states (common in COPD).
   - CRP: ↑ in infective and inflammatory states.
   - Blood cultures: essential to diagnose sepsis in acute infection.
   - D-dimer: a sensitive but not specific marker, ↑ in systemic inflammatory states, infection and pulmonary embolism.
   - Troponins: rising serial troponins indicate acute ACS.
   - BNP: ↑ significantly in chronic heart failure.
   - U&Es: an AKI is a common finding in many acute causes of dyspnoea.
   - LFTs: ↑AST/ALT can be seen in ACS, liver failure and atypical pneumonia.
   - TSH: hyperthyroidism is commonly associated with dyspnoea.
3. Imaging
   - CXR: to diagnose pulmonary infection, effusion or malignancy, or demonstrate features of underlying cardiac disease.
   - TTE: to guide the diagnosis of chronic cardiac failure, valvular disease and pulmonary hypertension.
   - CTPA: the gold standard to diagnose or exclude PE.
   - High-resolution CT (HRCT): to evaluate for interstitial lung disease.

HINTS AND TIPS

- Acute dyspnoea is one of the earliest features of sepsis.
- Assess for signs of systemic infection and associated haemodynamic compromise.

Syncope

True syncope describes rapid onset, transient, loss of consciousness or short duration with spontaneous and complete recovery. It relates to global cerebral hypoperfusion (typically hypotension). Presyncope relates to the sensations a patient may experience indicating an imminent syncopal episode, including dizziness, nausea, visual disturbances and tinnitus (Fig. 10.9).

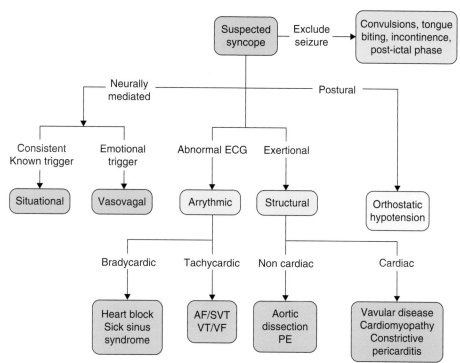

Fig. 10.9 Differential diagnosis of syncope. Conditions which may require cardiothoracic intervention are highlighted in blue. *AF*, Atrial fibrillation; *PE*, pulmonary embolism; *SVT*, supraventricular tachycardia; *VF*, ventricular fibrillation; *VT*, ventricular tachycardia.

HINTS AND TIPS

When diagnosing syncope, it is essential to differentiate it from other causes of transient loss of consciousness, including true and psychogenic seizures or transient ischaemic attacks. Key history questions to guide the differential diagnosis include the 5 **P**'s and 5 **C**'s:

- P - Precipitant
- P - Prodrome
- P - Position
- P - Palpitations
- P - Postevent phenomena
- C - Colour
- C - Convulsions
- C - Continence
- C - Cardiac problems
- C - Cardiac death family history

RED FLAG

- Syncope relating to underlying structural heart disease or arrhythmias is associated with a high risk of death.
- Red flag symptoms associated with life-threatening causes of syncope include chest or back pain, palpitations, haematemesis or melaena, and exertional syncope.
- Palpitations before a syncopal episode is a strong predictor of a cardiac cause.

Investigations for syncope

1. Bedside
   - Observations: a lying/standing blood pressure with a systolic ↓ of >20 mmHg on standing is diagnostic of orthostatic hypotension. Pulse rate and rhythm should be assessed to diagnose arrhythmias.
   - ECG: to rule out life-threatening arrhythmias. Abnormal ECG findings are a red flag for significant underlying pathology.

- CBG: hypoglycaemia may precipitate a syncopal episode or seizure.
2. Bloods
    - FBC: ↓ Hb indicates anaemia, which can worsen orthostatic hypotension, precipitate vasovagal syncopal episodes and cause arrhythmias if severe.
    - U&E: electrolyte abnormalities including hypo or hyperkalaemia can precipitate acute arrhythmias including AT and VF. Hyponatremia can result in seizures.
    - Serial troponins: serial elevation is suggestive of ACS.
    - Calcium/magnesium: hypocalcaemia and hypomagnesemia are known causes of seizures and should be ruled out in the patient with collapse.
3. Imaging
    - CXR: to exclude AD, PE and pericardial disease.
    - TTE: to detect structural heart disease in suspected cardiovascular pathology.
    - CT head: in suspected seizure or there is associated head injury.
    - CTPA: if PE is suspected as the likely diagnosis.

THE CARDIOVASCULAR EXAM

Features of the cardiovascular examination particularly relevant to cardiothoracic surgery are discussed below.

> **HINTS AND TIPS**
>
> The acronym **WIPER** can be used to prepare for the exam:
> - **W** – **W**ash your hands
> - **I** – **I**ntroduce yourself
> - **P** – **P**atient details
> - **E** – **E**xplain the procedure and **E**xpose appropriately
> - **R** – **R**eposition patient

Inspection

Inspect from the end of the bed for signs of cardiothoracic pathology:

- Cyanosis: a mottled, blue tinge to the skin that is common in congenital heart disease.
- Increased work of breathing: indicating underlying cardiovascular or respiratory disease.
- Finger clubbing: loss of the angle between the nail and nail bed, associated with congenital heart disease, and cardiac and lung malignancy.

- Malar flush: red discolouration of the cheeks, associated with severe mitral stenosis.
- Conjunctival pallor: severe anaemia is associated with malignancy and blood loss.

> **CLINICAL NOTES**
>
> - Marfan syndrome is a genetic CTD associated with arachnodactyly (long slender fingers), high arched palate and pectus excavatum.
> - It is a significant risk factor for AD and mitral valve prolapse.

Inspecting the precordium

Inspect the anterior and posterior chest wall to look for scars or deformities associated with cardiothoracic pathology (Fig. 10.10 and Table 10.2).

> **CLINICAL NOTES**
>
> - Minimally invasive surgery including video assisted thoracoscopic surgery (VATS) is increasingly used, due to the reduction in scarring, pain and recovery periods, and reduced risk of operative and postoperative complications.
> - Precordial scars will be increasingly less common with more widespread use of these approaches.

Palpation

Palpate the hands:

- Temperature: cool hands suggest poor peripheral perfusion, and sweaty, clammy hands may suggest ACS.
- Capillary refill time (CRT): CRT >2 s is associated with hypovolaemia, shock and sepsis.

Pulse

Palpate a peripheral and central pulse, assessing for the rate, rhythm and character:

- Pulse rate: assess the heart rate by measuring for 15 seconds and multiplying by 4. Tachycardia and bradycardia can be associated with acute haemodynamic compromise.
- Rhythm: irregular rhythms may relate to atrial fibrillation, ectopic beats and severe valvular lesions.

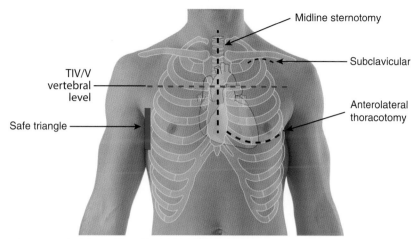

Fig. 10.10 Cardiothoracic surgery incisions. (From Vogl AW, Mitchell AWM, Drake R. *Gray's Basic Anatomy*. Churchill Livingstone, Elsevier Inc. 2013.)

- Character: a slow-rising pulse is associated with aortic stenosis, a bounding pulse severe aortic regurgitation and a weak pulse with hypovolemic states such as sepsis.
- Radio-radio delay: a loss of synchronicity between the radial pulses may be seen in AD and congenital aortic coarctation.
- Collapsing pulse: a pulse that rapidly increases then decreases, associated with severe valvular disease, congenital heart defects and high-output heart failure. Palpate the radial and brachial pulse on the same arm, then lift the patient's arm quickly. A tapping impulse felt through the arm muscle bulk indicates a collapsing pulse.

Blood pressure
Normal BP is around 120/80 mmHg. Abnormalities include:

- Hypertension: BP >140/0 mmHg. Chronic hypertension increases the risk of acute and chronic cardiac and vascular pathology.
- Hypotension: BP <90/60 mmHg. Indicates intravascular volume loss or severe haemodynamic compromise, seen in large-volume bleeding or cardiac arrest.
- Narrow pulse pressure: <25 mmHg difference between systolic and diastolic blood pressure. Seen in severe aortic stenosis and cardiac tamponade.
- Wide pulse pressure: >100 mmHg difference between systolic and diastolic blood pressure. Seen in severe aortic regurgitation and AD.
- Difference between arms: >20 mmHg difference in BP between arms suggests AD.

Table 10.2 Cardiothoracic incisions

Incision	Anatomy	Indications
Midline sternotomy	Substernal notch to xiphoid process	CABG Open valve surgery Cardiac transplant Congenital heart defects
Posterolateral thoracotomy	Mid-spinal line to anterior axillary line	Lobectomy Pneumonectomy Open lung biopsy Lung volume reduction/ bullectomy Single lung transplant
Anterolateral thoracotomy	Mid-axillary line to the lateral sternal border	
Clamshell	Bilateral anterolateral thoracotomy – extending between both mid-axillary lines	Widespread chest wall trauma Bilateral lung transplants
Sub-clavicular	4–5 cm incision in the left sub clavicular region	Pacemaker insertion
Safe triangle	The anterior border of latissimus dorsi, lateral border of pectoralis major, the base of the axilla and the 5th intercostal space	Chest drain insertions

Auscultation

The heart valves should be systematically auscultated using the diaphragm and the bell of the stethoscope while palpating a central pulse. The locations of the valves are:

- Mitral valve: 5th intercostal space, midclavicular line.
- Tricuspid valve: 4/5th intercostal space, lower left sternal edge.
- Aortic valve: 2nd intercostal space, right sternal edge.
- Pulmonary valve: 2nd intercostal space, left sternal edge.

Heart murmurs are produced due to turbulent blood through the heart valves. Carefully auscultate all heart valves to determine the timing and characteristics of murmurs (Figs 10.11-10.12).

HINTS AND TIPS

When auscultating the heart valves, remember RILEs:

- **R**ight-sided murmurs are loudest on **I**nspiration
- **L**eft sided murmurs loudest on **E**xpiration.

Perform accentuation manoeuvres to guide the likely diagnosis:

- Aortic stenosis: radiates to the carotid arteries when the patient holds their breath.
- Aortic regurgitation: loudest in the aortic area when sitting forward on expiration.

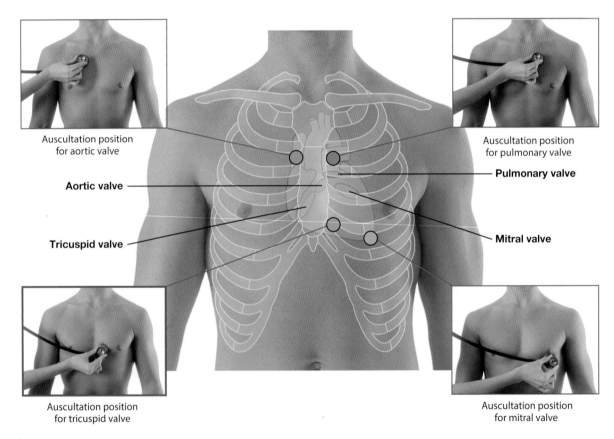

Auscultation position for aortic valve

Aortic valve

Tricuspid valve

Auscultation position for tricuspid valve

Auscultation position for pulmonary valve

Pulmonary valve

Mitral valve

Auscultation position for mitral valve

Fig. 10.11 Auscultation position of the heart valves. (From Vogl AW, Mitchell AWM, Drake R. *Gray's Basic Anatomy*. Churchill Livingstone, Elsevier Inc. 2013.)

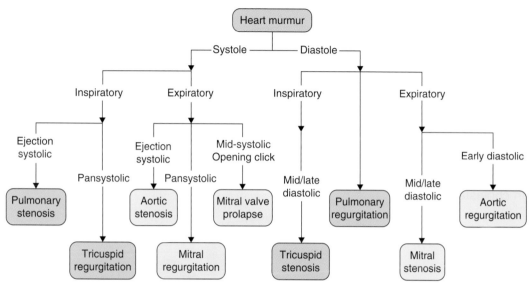

Fig. 10.12 Examination features of heart murmurs. Murmurs that are the most common in both exams and clinical practice, and additionally most likely to require cardiothoracic intervention, are highlighted in blue.

- Mitral regurgitation: loudest in the mitral area while lying on the left side during expiration, radiating to the axilla.
- Mitral stenosis: loudest in the mitral area using the bell of the stethoscope, while lying on the left side during expiration.

Completing the examination

Thank the patient, wash your hands and summarize your findings.

CARDIOTHORACIC SURGERY DISORDERS

Coronary artery disease

Coronary artery disease (CAD) is narrowing (stenosis) of the coronary vasculature. It most commonly arises due to atherosclerotic stiffening and stenosis of the coronary arteries (Fig. 10.13).

Stenosis results in insufficient myocardial blood supply to match oxygen demand, producing symptoms of angina when myocardial oxygen demand is increased, such as on exertion. Progressive, untreated ischaemia may result in ACS.

Treatment for CAD involves:

- Conservative management – lifestyle changes to target modifiable risk factors, including smoking cessation, weight reduction, dietary modifications, increased exercise and alcohol and stress reduction.
- Medical management – antianginals (beta-blockers, calcium channel blockers (CCBs) and nitrates), antiplatelets (aspirin or clopidogrel), antihypertensives (ace-inhibitors or angiotensin-receptor blockers) and statins.
- Surgical revascularization – with PCI or coronary artery bypass graft (CABG).

Coronary artery bypass graft

CABG is used to treat severe CAD of a main coronary artery. It involves revascularization of the myocardium using graft blood vessels to bypass obstructed coronary vasculature and re-establish blood supply to ischaemic areas.

Indications for CABG include:

- High-grade left main stem CAD.
- >70% stenosis of the proximal LAD.
- Symptomatic 2- or 3-vessel disease.
- Severe angina despite maximum medical therapy.
- Poor left ventricular function with viable myocardium upon revascularization.

Coronary angiography can be used to diagnose and locate the stenosis (Fig. 10.14).

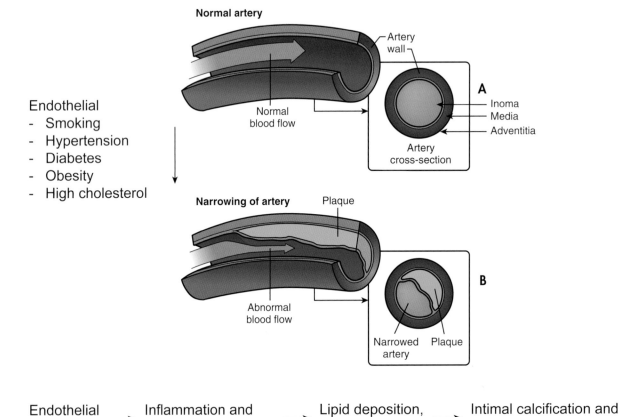

Normal artery

Artery wall

A
- Inoma
- Media
- Adventitia

Artery cross-section

Normal blood flow

Endothelial
- Smoking
- Hypertension
- Diabetes
- Obesity
- High cholesterol

Narrowing of artery   Plaque

B

Abnormal blood flow

Narrowed artery   Plaque

Endothelial dysfunction → Inflammation and immune cell invasion → Lipid deposition, plaque formation → Intimal calcification and stenosis

Fig. 10.13 Atherosclerosis and plaque formation. (A) Normal artery and blood flow. (B) Formation of an atheromatous plaque and arterial stenosis. (From Wilk MJ. *Sorrentino's Canadian Textbook for the Support Worker,* 5th Edition. Elsevier; 2022.)

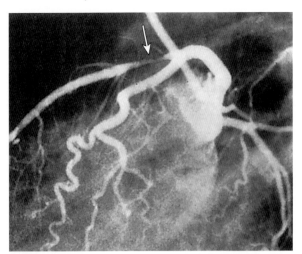

Fig. 10.14 Coronary angiography. Significant stenosis of the LAD on coronary angiography. (From Hubert R, VanMeter K. *Gould's Pathophysiology for the Health Professions,* 7th Edition. Saunders; 2023.)

Graft vessels

Both arterial and venous grafts can be used, depending on the suitability of available vessels and the number of grafts required. Venous grafts are anastomosed on either end to the coronary artery and the aorta, bypassing the stenosis. The great or short saphenous veins are typically used. Arterial grafts are pedicled grafts, which remain connected to their origin and are attached distally to the stenosis. The internal or left thoracic artery are typically used (Fig. 10.15).

CLINICAL NOTES

- The choice of arterial or venous donor vessels is dictated by the location of the stenosis and vessel availability.
- In severe vascular disease, there may be limited suitable options.

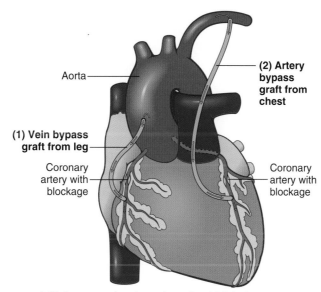

Aorta

(2) Artery bypass graft from chest

(1) Vein bypass graft from leg

Coronary artery with blockage

Coronary artery with blockage

Fig. 10.15 Coronary artery bypass graft (1) Anastomosis using vein graft, which is then anastomosed to the aorta. (2) Anastomosis using arterial graft, typically the internal thoracic artery, which is a pedicle graft, remaining connected to its origin. (From Chabner D-E. *The Language of Medicine,* 11th Edition. Elsevier; 2017.)

 HINTS AND TIPS

- Venous grafts become stenosed over time due to the high-pressure arterial circulation.
- Arterial grafts are preferred where possible to increase the lifespan of the graft.

The steps of a CABG involve:

1. Midline sternotomy: preferred for traditional CABG. Anterior or lateral thoracotomy may be used for minimally invasive procedures that do not use cardiopulmonary bypass.
2. Cardiopulmonary bypass: venous blood is taken from the vena cava and oxygenated using a gas-exchange machine before being returned to arterial circulation.
3. Cardioplegia: concentrated potassium citrate solution is administered via the coronary circulation resulting in a temporary, reversible cardiac arrest.
4. Anastomosis of bypass vessels: donor vessels are anastomosed to bypass stenosis.

Following this, cardioplegia is reversed, bypass suspended and the sternum reconstructed.

Complications

Complications of a CABG include:

- General surgical complications: pain, bleeding, infection.
- Postpericardiotomy syndrome: autoimmune pericarditis or pleuritis following cardiac surgery, presenting with fever, malaise, chest pain and dyspnoea. Treated with NSAIDs.
- Cardiac tamponade: postoperative acute pericardial effusion can result in cardiac tamponade and cardiogenic shock.
- Bypass occlusion: early graft occlusion can occur to inflammation and thromboembolic closure of the graft, typically prevented with postoperative antiplatelets.
- Arrhythmias: atrial fibrillation can develop postoperatively.
- Mediastinitis: mediastinal inflammation can occur postoperatively, presenting with fever, chest pain and surgical emphysema. Treatment is with surgical drainage, debridement and long-term antibiotics.
- Sternal wound complications: wound infection, dehiscence and osteomyelitis.

The prognosis is variable depending on the severity of stenosis, comorbidities, age and preoperative fitness. Successful grafts will last up to 15 years, and significantly improve mortality, particularly in patients with triple-vessel disease. However, without appropriate medical management and lifestyle changes, further atherosclerosis and further CAD may still develop.

Thoracic aortic aneurysm

A thoracic aortic aneurysm (TAA) is the abnormal dilation of the thoracic aorta. Dilation may affect the ascending or descending aorta, or the aortic arch. Risk factors include male sex, advancing age, connective tissue disease (CTD), smoking and uncontrolled systemic hypertension.

Symptoms and signs

TAAs are often asymptomatic and discovered incidentally. Large aneurysms may present with symptoms of obstruction or compression of surrounding structures:

- Chest pain: aneurysms exerting mass effect can result in chest and back pain.
- Oesophageal: dysphagia, odynophagia and weight loss.
- Superior vena cava (SVC): compression of the SVC can result in SVC syndrome, resulting in upper limb venous congestion, facial and upper limb flushing and oedema.
- Recurrent laryngeal nerve: hoarse voice, cough.
- Trachea: cough, wheeze or stridor and dyspnoea if severe.
- Sympathetic trunk: ipsilateral Horner syndrome (ptosis, miosis and anhidrosis).

HINTS AND TIPS

- A ruptured aneurysm results in acute haemodynamic compromise
- Urgent resuscitation and surgical repair are indicated to prevent major haemorrhage and death.

Investigations

Mediastinal imaging is the first-line diagnostic approach:

- CXR: will demonstrate a widened mediastinum.
- CTA: will demonstrate aortic dilation and associated dissection, perforation or rupture.
- TTE: a useful rapid bedside to evaluate aortic dilation, diagnose acute rupture and screen for concomitant cardiac disease (Fig. 10.16).

Management

Lifestyle measures include smoking cessation, BP control and reducing high cholesterol.

Surgical management depends on the size of the aneurysm and stability of the patient:

- Unstable patients: emergency TAA repair.
- Symptomatic patients: urgent TAA repair due to the high risk of rupture (days to weeks).

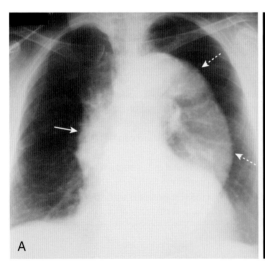
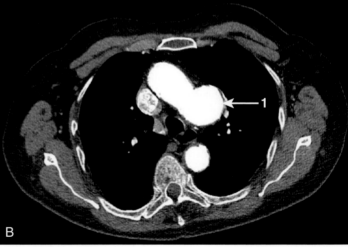

Fig. 10.16 Imaging findings in TAA. (A) CXR demonstrating significant widening of the mediastinum with an abnormally enlarged thoracic aorta. (B) CT Angiography of a TAA at the aortic arch. All the contrast is contained in one lumen, suggesting that there has been no dissection. (From A. Herring W. *Learning Radiology: Recognizing the Basics,* 5th Edition. Elsevier; 2024. B. Au-Yong I, Corne J. *Chest X-Ray Made Easy,* 5th Edition. Elsevier; 2023.)

- Asymptomatic patients: aneurysm surveillance may be appropriate if the aneurysm is small, involving 6 or 12-monthly CTA follow-up.

CLINICAL NOTES

- High-risk patients include large (>5.5 cm) and rapidly growing aneurysms (>0.5 cm/year)
- Patients with CTD, or comorbid cardiac pathology may have elective repair at smaller diameters due to the increased risk of rupture.

Surgical management

Surgical options include:

- Open surgical repair – for aneurysms of the ascending aorta or aortic arch. High associated mortality (10%) and morbidity (40%).
- TEVAR (thoracic endovascular aneurysm repair) – for aneurysms involving the descending aorta, where there is an appropriate site for graft placement and adequate vascular access (Fig. 10.17).

Annual postoperative surveillance is essential and involves monthly CTA for up to 1 year, with annual or biannual surveillance thereafter.

Complications

Complications include:

- TTA rupture: the most significant risk, with a mortality rate >50% due to massive haemorrhage and cardiac tamponade (Fig. 10.18). Those with large, rapidly enlarging aneurysms or those related to trauma are at the highest risk.
- Aortic valve regurgitation: due to aneurysms progressing to involve the aortic root.
- Aortic dissection: the weak aneurysm wall risks intimal injury and dissection.
- Embolism: stasis of blood flow results in thrombus formation and embolic ischemic.
- Surgical complications: including spinal cord injury, mesenteric or renal ischaemia, graft migration and endoleaks (continued blood flow into the aneurysm).

Aortic dissection

An aortic dissection (AD) is a tear in the intimal layer of the aorta, resulting in progressive haematoma formation in the

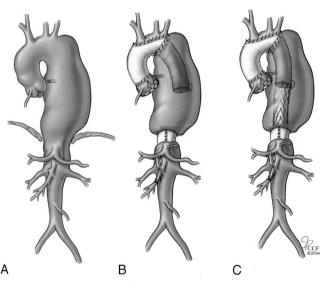

A   B   C

Fig. 10.17 Thoracic aortic aneurysm repair. (A) A significant TAA affecting the ascending aorta, aortic arch and descending aorta. (B) Replacement of the ascending aorta and arch with a graft sutured circumferentially to the aorta. The great vessels are resected and anastomosed to the graft and the distal end of the graft is placed within the descending aneurysm. (C) A stent is placed endovascularly into the descending aneurysm and sutured to the distal end of the graft. (From Sellke FW, Ruel M. *Atlas of Cardiac Surgical Techniques,* 2nd Edition. Elsevier; 2019.)

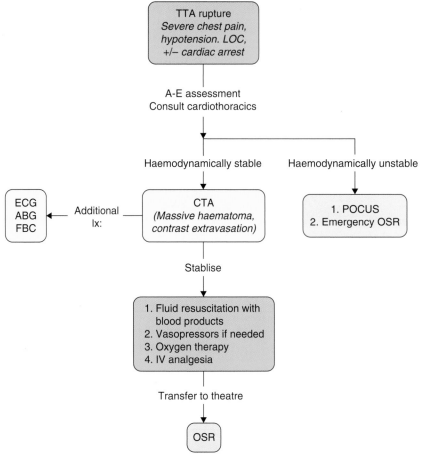

Fig. 10.18 Approach to the management of ruptured TAA. TEVAR can be considered in place of open surgical repair (OSR) for aneurysms involving the descending aorta only. *CTA*, CT angiography; *LOC*, loss of consciousness; *POCUS*, point of care ultrasound.

space between the intimal and medial layers. Risk factors include age, hypertension and CTD. It is classified based on the location of injury:

- Stanford type A – involving the ascending aorta (most common).
- Stanford type B – not involving the ascending aorta (Fig. 10.19).

Symptoms and signs

Features include:

- Chest pain: sudden onset, tearing central pain radiating to the neck or jaw.
- Syncope: relating to cerebral hypoperfusion.
- Blood pressure abnormalities: may include hypertension, hypotension, BP asymmetry between arms and a wide pulse pressure.

Investigations

Investigations include:

- All patients: ECG, FBC, G&S, D-dimer.
- Low-risk patients: screening imaging, including CXR and TTE. If positive, perform definitive imaging.
- High-risk patients: definitive imaging with CTA (gold standard), transoesophageal echocardiography (TOE) or Magnetic resonance angiography (MRA) (Fig. 10.20).

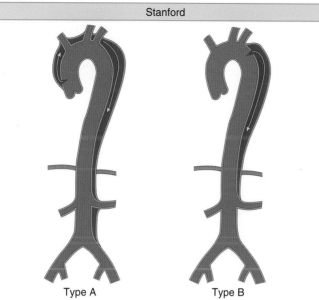

Fig. 10.19 Stanford classification of aortic dissection. Type A – involving the ascending aorta, which may spread to involve the aortic root, arch and descending aorta. Type B – involves the descending aorta only. (From Walls RM, Marill KA. *Rosen's Emergency Medicine: Concepts and Clinical Practice 2-Volume Set,* 10th Edition. Elsevier; 2023.)

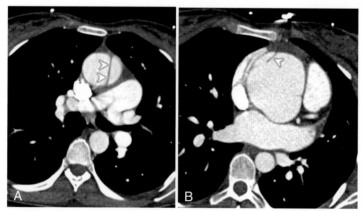

Fig. 10.20 CTA in aortic dissection. Dissection at the level of the (A) pulmonary artery and (B) aortic root. A false lumen is evident within the aorta, enlarging as it extends toward the aortic arch. (From Patlas MN. *Emergency Imaging of At-Risk Patients: General Principles.* Elsevier; 2023.)

CLINICAL NOTES

- In unstable patients, resuscitation and surgical repair are prioritized.
- Investigations are only performed if they do not delay operative management.
- In stable patients, determine the risk of dissection using an appropriate screening tool, e.g., the aortic dissection detection risk score (ADD-RS), before considering further investigations.

DIFFERENTIALS

Typical clinical features associated with a widened mediastinum on CXR is highly suggestive of dissection.

Management

Management depends on haemodynamic stability and classification of dissection (Fig. 10.21).

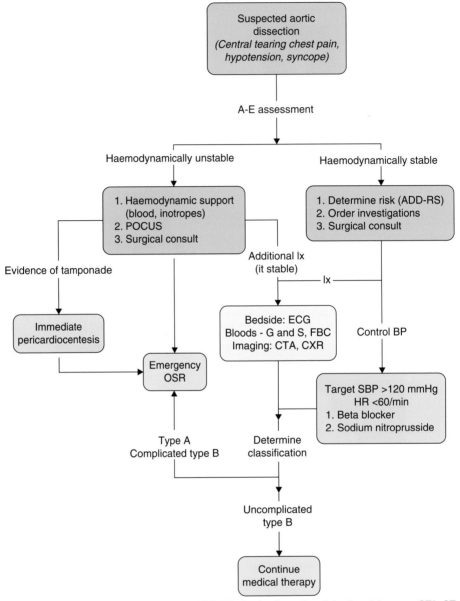

Fig. 10.21 Approach to the patient with aortic dissection. *ADD-RS,* Aortic dissection detection risk score; *CTA,* CT angiography; *G&S,* group and save; *OSR,* open surgical repair; *POCUS,* point of care ultrasound; *SBP,* systolic blood pressure.

- Medical: tight BP control, to within 100 to 120 mmHg, using beta-blockers, vasodilators (sodium nitroprusside) and calcium channel blockers.
- Surgical: indicated for all patients with Stanford A or complicated Stanford B dissection, involving open surgical repair and graft implantation, or endovascular stent implantation (Fig. 10.22).

HINTS AND TIPS

In Stanford B dissection, indications for surgery include organ ischaemia, hypotension, aortic rupture, aneurysmal expansion or severe symptoms.

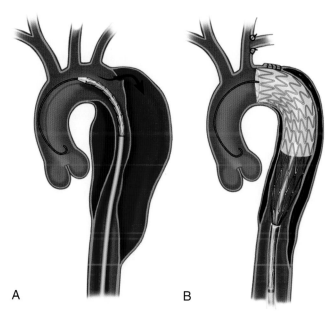

Fig. 10.22 Endovascular repair of type B aortic dissection. (A) The stent is positioned to cover the proximal entry tear via the femoral or iliac vessels. (B) Deployment of the stent graft to induce true lumen re-expansion and false lumen thrombosis. (From Conrad MF, Sidawy AN, Perler BA. *Rutherford's Vascular Surgery and Endovascular Therapy,* 10th Edition. Elsevier; 2023.)

Complications

Complications include:

- Myocardial infarction – with occlusion of the coronary artery supply.
- Stroke – if dissection extends into the carotids.
- Cardiac tamponade – haemopericardium progressing to cardiogenic shock.
- Aortic regurgitation – if dissection extends into the aortic root.
- Aortic rupture – rupture of the weakened aortic wall resulting in catastrophic blood loss, likely to result in death without emergency repair.
- Malperfusion syndrome – systemic organ ischaemia resulting from interruption of blood flow to major vascular beds resulting in acute organ failure or injury.

Prognosis relates to type and extent of injury, and speed of repair. Mortality can be up to 40%.

Pericardial effusion

Pericardial effusion describes the accumulation of fluid in the pericardial space. In chronic effusions, minimal pericardial stretch can occur, increasing fluid capacity short term. In acute

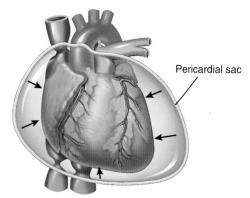

Fig. 10.23 Pericardial effusion and cardiac tamponade. Fluid-filled pericardial sac exerting pressure on the heart. (From *Mosby's Dictionary of Medicine, Nursing & Health Professions,* 11th Edition. Elsevier; 2022.)

effusions, capacity can be rapidly exceeded, resulting in compression of the heart, reduced CO, cardiac tamponade, obstructive shock and cardiac arrest. Haemopericardium results from trauma, myocardium rupture or AD. Serous effusion results from acute pericarditis, malignancy, autoimmune disease or right heart failure (Fig. 10.23).

Symptoms and signs

Chronic effusions may be asymptomatic initially. When symptoms develop, they include:

- Dyspnoea and orthopnoea.
- Retrosternal chest pain.
- Compressive symptoms, including nausea, dysphagia and hoarse voice.

Cardiac tamponade presents with Beck's triad:

- Hypotension: due to reduced cardiac output.
- Muffled heart sounds: fluid around the heart reduces sound transmission.
- Distended neck veins: due to elevated jugular venous pressures.

Further features include tachycardia, pulsus paradoxus (BP decrease >10 mmHg on inspiration) and signs of right heart failure.

Investigations

Unstable patients should be treated prior to diagnostic investigations. For stable patients, investigations include:

- ECG: to rule out ACS. In effusion and tamponade, sinus tachycardia, low voltage QRS complexes or electrical alternans may be evident.
- CXR: a useful initial screening tool, demonstrating the classical 'water bottle sign'.
- TTE: the gold standard to confirm the diagnosis.
- Pericardiocentesis: in chronic effusions, analysis of cell counts, glucose, protein and LDH can differentiate between transudative and exudative causes. Fluid can be sent for MC&S to evaluate for malignant and infectious aetiologies (Fig. 10.24 and Table 10.3).

CLINICAL NOTES

- Light's criteria suggest fluid is likely to be exudative if one of the following features are present:
- Pleural fluid protein/serum protein ratio >0.5
- Pleural fluid LDH/serum LDH ratio >0.6
- Pleural fluid LDH >⅔ the upper limit of serum LDH normal
- An isolated rise in LDH suggests malignant effusion

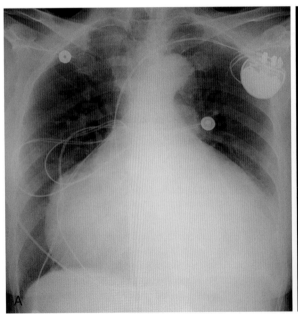
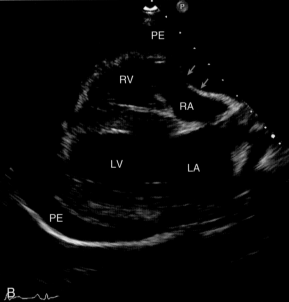

Fig. 10.24 Imaging findings in pericardial effusion and tamponade. (A) CXR findings in pericardial effusion, with a globular heart described as the water bottle sign. (B) TTE demonstrating anechoic space around the heart suggestive of large effusion. Collapse of the right atrial wall indicates development of tamponade. *LA,* Left atrium; *LV,* left ventricle; *PE,* pericardial effusion; *RA,* right atrium; *RV,* right ventricle. (From A. Herring W. *Learning Radiology: Recognizing the Basics,* 5th Edition. Elsevier; 2024. B. Silverstein DC, Hopper K. *Small Animal Critical Care Medicine,* 3rd Edition. Elsevier; 2023.)

Management

Management depends on the stability of the patient:

- Unstable patients: urgent therapeutic pericardiocentesis should be performed to drain the fluid and reduce cardiac compression.
- Stable patients: investigation and treatment of underlying disease. Pericardiocentesis can be performed diagnostically, or therapeutically in symptomatic effusions (Fig. 10.25).

Following stabilization, or for those with chronic or recurrent effusions, definitive surgical management should then be performed:

- Pericardiotomy: creation of a window to allow continuous drainage of pericardial fluid.

- Pericardiectomy: complete or partial removal of the pericardial sac, for definitive management of refractory effusions, constrictive pericarditis or purulent pericarditis.

> **RED FLAG**
>
> Haemopericardium resulting from penetrating injury should be managed with emergency surgery in preference to temporizing pericardiocentesis, to limit blood loss into the pericardial space.

Complications

Complications of pericardial effusions include:

- Cardiac tamponade: resulting in obstructive shock, and cardiac arrest.
- Large volume blood loss: in cases of traumatic haemopericardium.
- Venous thromboembolism: resulting in stroke or visceral ischaemia.
- Surgical complications: including bleeding, pneumomediastinum, pneumothorax, visceral/nerve injury and arrhythmias.

Table 10.3 Aetiology of pleural effusions

	Translate	Exudate
Appearance	Clear	Cloudy/chylous
Aetiology	Heart failure Kidney failure Liver failure Hypoalbuminemia	Infection – viral/ bacterial/tuberculosis Malignancy Autoimmune disease Systemic inflammation

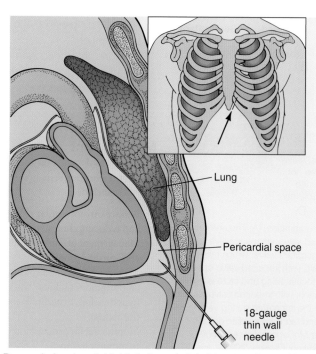

Fig. 10.25 Pericardiocentesis. Removal of pericardial fluid via the subxiphoid route using an 18-gauge needle. (From Pagana et al. *Mosby's® Manual of Diagnostic and Laboratory Tests,* 7th Edition. Elsevier; 2022.)

The prognosis is variable, depending on aetiology and extent of effusion, and associated complications.

Valvular disease

Valvular heart disease describes congenital or acquired conditions that impair valvular function, relating to stenosis or insufficiency (regurgitation). Acquired defects, typically degenerative aortic stenosis, are much more common. Stenosis results in systolic outflow obstruction, resulting in hypertrophic cardiomyopathy to maintain CO. Progressive hypertrophy reduces diastolic capacity, reducing CO, leading to heart failure. Regurgitation results in backflow of blood and dilated cardiomyopathy reducing contractility and CO, leading to heart failure (Figs 10.26-10.27).

Symptoms and signs

The symptoms of valvular disease relate to the pathology and valve affected (Table 10.4).

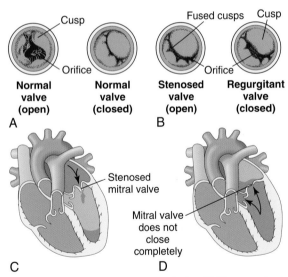

Fig. 10.26 Valvular stenosis and regurgitation. (A) The normal valve opening and closing. (B) A stenosed valve, via fused valve leaflets and impaired opening, and the regurgitant valve, which fails to close completely. (C) Mitral stenosis, with impaired valve opening during atrial systole, reducing ventricular filling and increasing atrial afterload. (D) Mitral regurgitation, with impaired valve closure, resulting in backflow of blood into the left atrium during ventricular systole, increasing atrial preload and reducing cardiac output. (From Power-Kean K. *Huether and McCance's Understanding Pathophysiology,* 2nd Canadian Edition. Elsevier; 2023.)

HINTS AND TIPS

- Tricuspid valve defects are rare.
- Risk factors include IVDU, rheumatic heart disease and CTD.
- Pulmonary valve defects are even rarer, typically relating to congenital heart disease.

Investigations

Investigations include:

- ECG: to assess heart rhythm and for evidence of heart strain.
- TTE: to characterize the valve pathology and effects on heart structure and CO. TOE can then be performed for a detailed assessment.
- CXR: to assess for pulmonary oedema or associated respiratory pathology.

Further investigations include CTA, coronary angiography and exercise stress testing.

CLINICAL NOTES

- AHA staging is used for valvular lesions, to monitor disease progression and determine need for intervention.
- Lesions are staged from A–D, by symptom severity, anatomical derangement and effects on cardiac structure and function.

Management

Management depends on the severity of pathology, associated symptoms and performance status of the patient. Supportive measures include:

- Reduce cardiovascular risk – stopping smoking, weight loss and reducing cholesterol.
- Management of complications – treatment of heart failure, endocarditis prophylaxis.
- Management of comorbidities – optimization of comorbidities that may worsen cardiac function, including hypertension, hyperlipidaemia, diabetes and atrial fibrillation.
- Monitoring for progression – regular cardiology follow-up to monitor lesions.

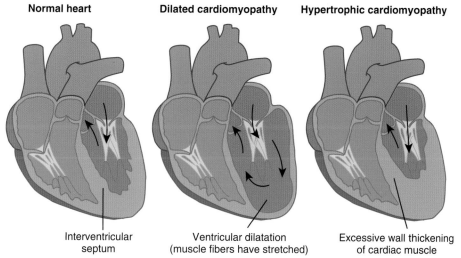

Normal heart   **Dilated cardiomyopathy**   **Hypertrophic cardiomyopathy**

Interventricular septum — Ventricular dilatation (muscle fibers have stretched) — Excessive wall thickening of cardiac muscle

Fig. 10.27 Dilated and hypertrophic cardiomyopathy. In dilated cardiomyopathy, the ventricles dilate to compensate for chronically increased preload, reducing contractility and systolic function. In hypertrophic cardiomyopathy, the ventricular wall hypertrophies to compensate for increased afterload, impairing diastolic filling. Both result in reduced cardiac output and eventual heart failure. (From Harding MM, Keegan P. *Lewis's Medical-Surgical Nursing: Assessment and Management of Clinical Problems,* 12th Edition. Elsevier; 2023.)

Table 10.4 Valvular pathology

Pathology	Aetiology	Clinical features
Aortic stenosis	Degenerative calcification Congenital defects – bicuspid aortic valve Rheumatic heart disease	Symptoms – SAD (syncope, angina, dyspnoea) Signs – decreased pulse pressure Murmur – ESM at 2nd intercostal space radiating to carotids,
Aortic regurgitation	Acute – IE, AD, trauma Chronic – CTD, rheumatic heart disease	Symptoms – SAD, palpitation, acute pulmonary oedema Signs – Water hammer pulse Murmur – Early diastolic murmur at left sternal edge
Mitral stenosis	Rheumatic heart disease	Symptoms – dyspnoea, fatigue, palpitations, PND Signs – malar flush, AF, peripheral/pulmonary oedema Murmur – diastolic murmur at apex, opening snap
Mitral regurgitation	Mitral valve prolapse Myocardial infarction Dilated cardiomyopathy Degenerative calcification IHD, rheumatic heart disease, IE	Symptoms – dyspnoea, pulmonary oedema, palpitations, fatigue, cough Signs – peripheral/pulmonary oedema, acute – cardiogenic shock Murmur – pansystolic murmur at apex, radiating to axilla

AD, Aortic dissection; *AF,* atrial fibrillation; *CTD,* connective tissue disease; *ESM,* ejection systolic murmur; *IE,* infective endocarditis; *IHD,* ischaemic heart disease; *PND,* paroxysmal nocturnal dyspnoea.

Acute valve regurgitation is a medical emergency, requiring urgent diagnosis, stabilization and management of acute complications and surgical repair. Following stabilization, investigation and treatment of the underlying cause can take place (Fig. 10.28).

Valve replacement surgery
Surgical valve replacement or repair is the definitive management option. The urgency of surgery depends on the severity of symptoms, associated complications and speed of progression. Symptomatic patients with severe lesions should undergo urgent surgery.

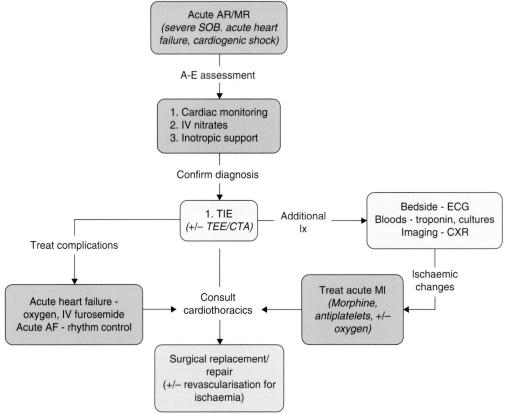

Fig. 10.28 Management of acute valve regurgitation. *AF*, Atrial fibrillation; *AR*, atrial regurgitation; *CTA*, CT angiography; *MI*, myocardial infarction; *MR*, mitral regurgitation; *TOE*, transoesophageal echocardiography; *TTE*, transthoracic echocardiography. Beta-blockers can be used in patients with acute AR relating to aortic dissection but should be avoided in other cases.

Surgical options include:

- Annuloplasty: reinforcement of regurgitant valves or leaflet repair.
- Valvuloplasty: to separate calcified or fused stenotic leaflets.
- Valve replacement: with mechanical or biological valves, via open surgery or endovascular transcatheter aortic valve insertion (TAVI) (Figs 10.29-10.30).

HINTS AND TIPS

- Mechanical valves are used in younger patients due to their longer lifespan.
- Lifelong anticoagulation with warfarin is required.
- Biological valves are preferred in older patients, those at high risk of bleeding, or those planning to conceive.
- DOACs are used for anticoagulation.

Complications

Complications include:

- Congestive heart failure: in severe and untreated valvular disease.
- Endocarditis: valvular pathology and valve surgery increase the risk of endocarditis and associated complications including embolic phenomena, abscesses and collections.
- Pulmonary congestion: leading to pulmonary oedema and pulmonary hypertension.
- Right heart failure: systemic symptoms including peripheral oedema, hepatosplenomegaly, liver failure and ascites and renal impairment.
- Arrhythmias: commonly atrial fibrillation, with associated thromboembolic risks.
- Surgical complications: prosthetic valves increase the risk of endocarditis, AF and VTE, and are at risk of dysfunction, including leakage, stenosis or regurgitation.

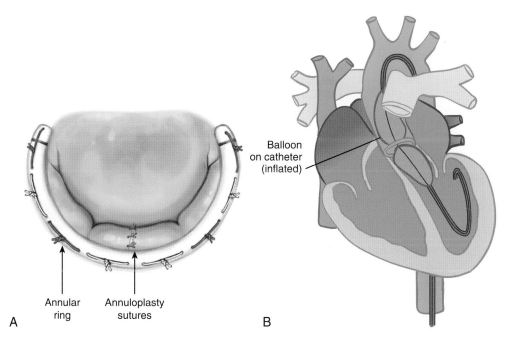

Fig. 10.29 Annuloplasty and valvuloplasty. (A) Sutures are placed around the annulus to correct the prolapse, before placing the ring to reinforce and restore the annular dimensions. (B) Balloon valvuloplasty of the aortic valve. A catheter is inserted endovascular, and a balloon is inflated to widen the stenotic valve. (From A. Bonow RO, Castillo JG, Otto CM, Adams DH. *Valvular Heart Disease: A Companion to Braunwald's Heart Disease,* 5th Edition. Elsevier; 2021. B. Malarvizhi S, Renuka K. *Black's Medical-Surgical Nursing: Clinical Management for Positive Outcomes*, First South Asia Edition. Elsevier; 2019.)

Pneumothorax

A pneumothorax is the abnormal presence of air in the pleural space. Increased intrapleural pressure results in loss of the negative pressure gradient between the pleural membranes, and partial or complete alveolar collapse. They can be spontaneous or related to trauma. Spontaneous trauma can be primary, or secondary, relating to underlying lung disease. Traumatic pneumothorax can be closed, typically following blunt trauma, or open, resulting from a chest wall lesion (Fig. 10.31).

HINTS AND TIPS

- Primary spontaneous pneumothorax is common in young, thin males, with a history of smoking.
- Secondary pneumothorax relates to underlying lung disease, including COPD, infection or malignancy.

RED FLAG

- Tension pneumothorax is a life-threatening condition resulting from progressive one-way entry of air into the pleural space.
- Increased intrapleural pressure results in lung collapse, midline shift and tracheal and cardiovascular compression.
- Life-threatening organ dysfunction and cardiorespiratory arrest will develop without urgent decompression with needle aspiration and definitive chest drain placement.

Symptoms and signs

Small pneumothoraxes may be asymptomatic initially. When symptoms develop, they include:

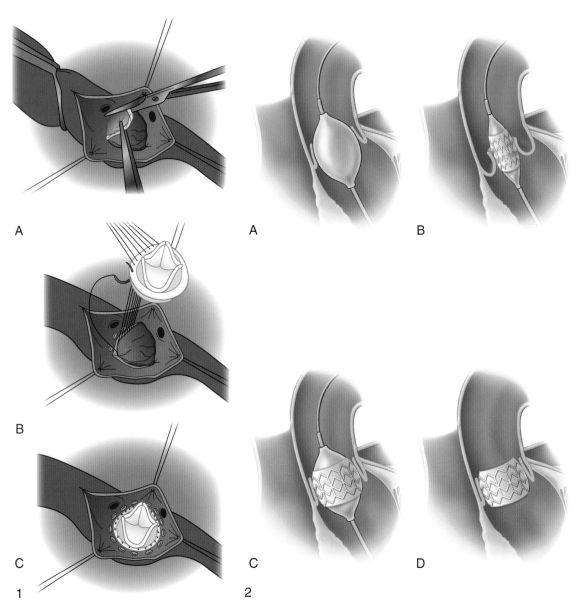

Fig. 10.30 Aortic valve replacement. (1) Aortic valve replacement surgery. An incision is made in the ascending aorta, exposing the valve and allowing for excision (A) before the replacement valve is implanted (B) and secured into palace (C). (2) Transcatheter Aortic Valve Insertion (TAVI). (A) A catheter is inserted via the femoral artery and balloon valvuloplasty is performed to expand the stenosed valve. (B) A collapsible replacement valve is inserted via the catheter and expanded (C) to replace the valve. (D) The catheter is removed, and the valve remains in situ. (From 1. Townsend CM et al. *Sabiston Textbook of Surgery: The Biological Basis of Modern Surgical Practice*, 21st Edition. Elsevier; 2022. 2. Ignatavicius DD, Rebar CR, Workman ML. *Medical-Surgical Nursing: Concepts for Interprofessional Collaborative Care*, 9th Edition. Elsevier; 2018.)

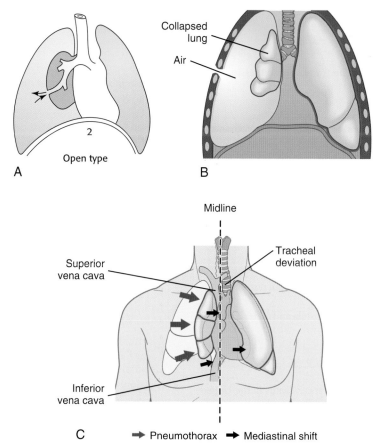

Fig. 10.31 Types of pneumothoraxes. (A) Spontaneous pneumothorax. (B) Open traumatic pneumothorax. (C) Tension pneumothorax with midline shift. (From Aggarwal AP, Mathew KG. *Medicine: Prep Manual for Undergraduates,* 7th Edition. Elsevier; 2023. B. Mondor EE, Harding MM *Lewis's Medical-Surgical Nursing: Assessment and Management of Clinical Problems,* 12th Edition. Elsevier; 2023. C. Seneviratne C, Cobbett SL, Mondor E, Tyerman J. *Lewis's Medical-Surgical Nursing in Canada: Assessment and Management of Clinical Problems,* 5th Edition. Elsevier; 2023.)

- Sudden onset dyspnoea.
- Sharp stabbing ipsilateral chest pain.
- Reduced breath sounds and chest expansion on the affected side.
- Hyper-resonant percussion node.
- Subcutaneous emphysema.
- Tracheal deviation.

HINTS AND TIPS

- In tension pneumothorax, tracheal deviation occurs away from the affected side.
- In non-tension pneumothorax, the trachea deviates toward the affected side.

CLINICAL NOTES

- Flail chest occurs following significant blunt chest wall trauma and fracture of three or more adjacent ribs in multiple places.
- Symptoms include paradoxical chest wall movement during respiration.
- It is a significant risk factor for pneumothorax.

Investigations

Tension pneumothorax is a clinical diagnosis, and if suspected, immediate treatment initiated in place of diagnostic investigations. Other variants can be diagnosed on CXR, which will show:

- Reduced lung markings on the affected side.
- Visible visceral pleural line parallel to the parietal pleura.

- Associated pulmonary disease, for example, hyper-expansion in COPD (Fig. 10.32).

Management

Acute management involves chest wall decompression and respiratory support (Fig. 10.33).

Surgical management

Patients with recurrent, bilateral or refractory pneumothoraxes or extensive underlying lung disease may be managed operatively, following stabilization. Operative approaches include:

- Lung repair – bullae resection or alveolar repair of the air leak.
- Pleurodesis – adhesion of the visceral and parietal pleural to prevent lung collapse, via surgical abrasion, pleurectomy or irritant administration including talcum powder.

Complications

Complications include:

- Acute cardiorespiratory arrest: resulting from respiratory failure and reduced CO.
- Surgical complications: persistent fistula and air leak and local injury or infection.

Lung cancer

Lung cancer is the leading cause of cancer deaths in the United Kingdom. Most cases are related to smoking. Other risk factors include environmental exposure to carcinogens, family history and chronic lung disease. Subtypes include small cell lung cancer (SCLC) and non-small cell lung cancer (NSCLC) which commonly relates to adenocarcinoma or squamous cell carcinoma.

> **HINTS AND TIPS**
>
> Adenocarcinoma is the most common lung malignancy in non-smokers.

Symptoms and signs

Patients are often asymptomatic initially. When symptoms develop, they include pulmonary and extrapulmonary symptoms, relating to the mass effect of the tumour. Many patients present late with features of metastatic disease (Table 10.5).

> **HINTS AND TIPS**
>
> - Constitutional features include **FLAWS**:
>   - **F** - **F**ever
>   - **L** - **L**ethargy
>   - **A** - **A**norexia
>   - **W** - **W**eight loss
>   - **S** - night **S**weats
> - Cervical lymphadenopathy is common.
> - Malignancy increases the risk of acute pulmonary disease including pneumonia, pleural effusion or pulmonary embolism.

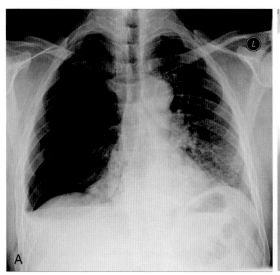
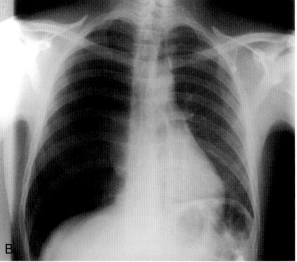

Fig. 10.32 CXR findings in pneumothorax. Loss of the lung markings on the affected side indicates lung collapse. (A) Traumatic pneumothorax relating to right-sided rib fractures. (B) Tension pneumothorax presents with tracheal deviation and mediastinal shift. (From A. Waldman SD. *The Chest Wall and Abdomen: Pain Medicine: A Case-Based Learning Series*. Elsevier; 2023. B. Hughes S, Randhawa G, Thomas C. *The Respiratory System: Basic Science and Clinical Conditions,* 3rd Edition. Elsevier; 2023.)

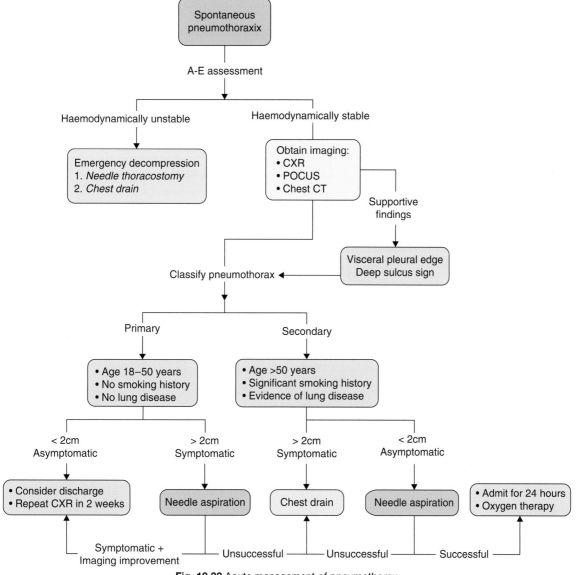

Fig. 10.33 Acute management of pneumothorax.

Investigations

Investigations include:

- Bloods: FBC may demonstrate anaemia. Hypercalcaemia is common. Deranged LFTs suggest metastatic disease.
- CXR: the first-line screening test.
- High-resolution CT (HRCT): performed following CXR suggestive of malignancy, or in high clinical suspicion (Fig. 10.34).

Table 10.5 Clinical features of lung cancer

	Symptoms	Signs
Pulmonary	Dyspnoea Cough +/- haemoptysis Wheeze Chest pain	↓ SpO$_2$ Clubbing Dull percussion note ↓ Air entry
Extrapulmonary (Typically related to apical NSCLC)	**Structure affected**	**Clinical features**
	Sympathetic ganglion	Horner syndrome (ptosis, miosis, anhidrosis)
	Brachial plexus	Neuralgia, focal neurological deficit
	Recurrent laryngeal nerve	Hoarse voice
	SVC	Upper limb swelling, SOB, Pemberton's sign
	Phrenic nerve	Hemidiaphragm paralysis, elevation on CXR
Metastatic	**Site**	**Clinical features**
	Lymphatics	Lymphangitic carcinomatosis (reticular erythema along the affected vessels)
	Brain	Seizures, focal neurological deficits, headaches and behavioural changes
	Liver	Posthepatic jaundice, nausea, ascites
	Bones	Bone pain, hypercalcaemia (constipation, polyuria, polydipsia, abdominal pain)

The diagnosis is confirmed with tumour biopsy and histology to confirm subtype. Staging can be done with CT/MRI imaging, or PET-CT to investigate for bony metastasis.

CLINICAL NOTES

Screening for lung cancer involves annual low-dose CT scan for current or ex-smokers aged 66-74.

Management

Management should take an MDT approach, depending on the patient's wishes and expected treatment goals. Many lung cancers are diagnosed late, and treatment is largely palliative. Surgical management is typically used for early-stage, nonmetastatic disease, for patients without significant comorbidities and adequate performance status. Options include:

- Sublobar resection: wedge resection or segmentectomy, for peripherally located, small tumours. Good preservation of lung function.
- Lobectomy: entire lobe resection for larger tumours with significant loss of lung function.
- Pneumonectomy: resection of an entire lung, for large, central tumours involving the main bronchi or hilum, associated with high morbidity and mortality (Figs 10.35-10.36).

Adjunctive measures include chemotherapy, immunotherapy and radiotherapy.

Complications

Complications include:

- Atelectasis: loss of lung volume relating to alveolar obstruction and collapse, presenting with SOB, dullness to percussion and reduced breath sounds.
- Pneumonia: recurrent chest infections should raise suspicion for underlying malignancy.
- Pleural effusion: large effusions, with high protein/LDH are suggestive of malignancy.
- Paraneoplastic phenomena: resulting from ectopic hormone release or stimulation of antibody production by the tumour (Table 10.6).

HINTS AND TIPS

SCLC is the most frequent neuroendocrine lung tumour, hence paraneoplastic phenomena are more common.

The prognosis relates to the extent of disease and the presence of metastasis. The overall 5-year survival rate is approximately 20%. Complete cessation of smoking is essential.

Mediastinal masses

The mediastinum is the space within the thoracic cavity containing the heart, trachea, oesophagus, thymus gland and neurovasculature. Benign or malignant masses may arise from any of the mediastinal structures. The location of the lesion can aid the differential diagnosis (Fig. 10.37 and Table 10.7).

HINTS AND TIPS

The 4 **T's** of mediastinal masses are:
- **T** - Thymoma
- **T** - Thyroid neoplasm
- **T** - Teratoma
- **T** - 'Terrible' lymphoma

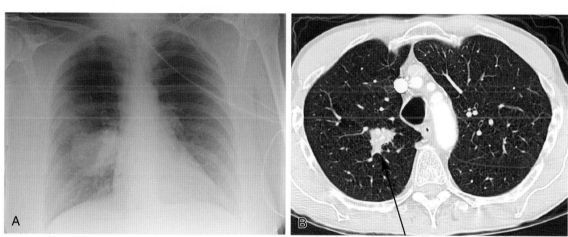

Fig. 10.34 Imaging findings in lung cancer. (A) Right hilar mass suspicious of lung cancer. Increased density and abnormal hilar contour are suggestive of a mass. Comparison with previous films is useful to detect changes and progression. (B) Axial CT chest, demonstrating an opacification within the right mid-zone suggestive of malignancy. (From A. Au-Yong I, Corne J. *Chest X-Ray Made Easy,* 5th Edition. Elsevier; 2023. B. Newell Jr. JD. *Developing the Digital Lung: From First Lung CT to Clinical AI: The Development of Quantitative X-Ray Computed Tomography of Diffuse Lung Disease Through the Use of Artificial Intelligence.* Elsevier; 2023.)

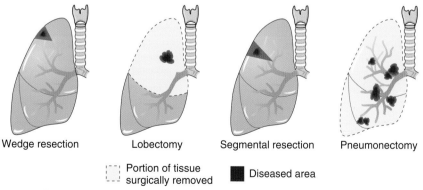

Fig. 10.35 Operative approaches to lung cancer. The amount of tissue resected depends on the extent and location of disease. (From Shiland BJ. *Mastering Healthcare Terminology,* 7th Edition. Mosby, Elsevier Inc. 2023.)

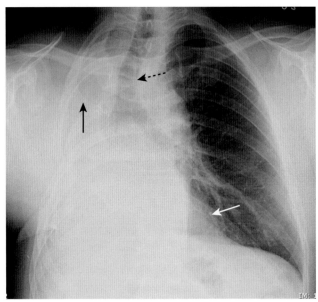

Fig. 10.36 CXR findings following pneumonectomy. Complete opacification of the right hemithorax, with mediastinal shift, and tracheal deviation, suggestive of large-scale lung volume loss. (From Herring W. *Learning Radiology: Recognizing the Basics,* 5th Edition. Elsevier; 2024.)

Table 10.6 Paraneoplastic manifestations of lung cancer

Syndrome	Secretion	Tumour	Clinical features
SIADH	Ectopic ADH	SCLC	Hyponatraemia (presenting with nausea, vomiting, muscle cramps/weakness, lethargy, confusion, seizures)
Cushing syndrome	Ectopic ACTH	SCLC	Hyperglycaemia, central weight gain, hypertension, gastric irritation, osteoporosis, muscle weakness, depression, psychosis, thin skin, easy bruising
Limbic encephalitis	Anti-Hu antibodies	SCLC	Short-term memory loss, confusion, hallucinations, seizures
Lambert-Eaton myasthenic syndrome	Anti-VGCC antibiotics	SCLC	Proximal muscle weakness, ptosis, slurred speech, dysphagia, autonomic dysfunction, posttetanic potentiation
Hypercalcemia	Ectopic PTH	NSCLC (predominantly squamous cell)	Bone, stones, groans, abdominal and psychiatric moans
Gynaecomastia	b-hCG	NSCLC	Gynaecomastia, mastodynia, galactorrhoea
Dermatomyositis	Anti-Mi-2, ANA	Both NSCLC and SCLC	Symmetrical progressive proximal muscle weakness, Gottron's papules, heliotrope rash

ACTH, Adrenocorticotropic hormone; ADH, antidiuretic hormone; ANA, antinuclear antibodies; PTH, parathyroid hormone; VGCC, voltage-gated calcium channels.

Symptoms and signs

Symptoms relate to the compression of regional structures:

- Airway: dyspnoea, cough, haemoptysis.
- Oesophagus: weight loss, dysphagia, odynophagia.
- SVC: facial and upper limb erythema and swelling, distended neck veins and headache.
- Sympathetic ganglia: ipsilateral Horner syndrome (ptosis, miosis, anhidrosis).

In malignant disease, constitutional features include fevers, lethargy, appetite and weight change, night sweats and lymphadenopathy.

> **CLINICAL NOTES**
>
> New myasthenic features (fatigability, ptosis, diplopia and dysarthria) should raise suspicion of a thymoma.

Investigations

Investigations typically relate to the suspected underlying aetiology:

- FBC and blood film: abnormalities suggest haematological malignancy.

- LDH: a nonspecific marker elevated in many malignancies.
- TFTs: derangement associated with mediastinal symptoms suggests a large goitre.
- Bone profile and PTH: if parathyroid disease is suspected.
- AFP/b-HCG: ↑ may suggest germ cell tumour.

Imaging studies include CXR and CT to assess the location and characteristics of the lesion. Further imaging studies depend on the likely diagnosis. Definitive pathological diagnosis with biopsy is often indicated before treatment can be initiated (Fig. 10.38).

Table 10.7 Structures in the mediastinum

Anterior	Middle	Posterior
Thymus gland	Heart	Intercostal vessels
Thyroid gland	Aorta and great	Spinal ganglia
Parathyroid gland	vessels	Sympathetic chain
Lymph nodes	Trachea and	Lymph nodes
	carina	
	Oesophagus	
	Lymph nodes	
	Vagus nerves	
	Thoracic duct	

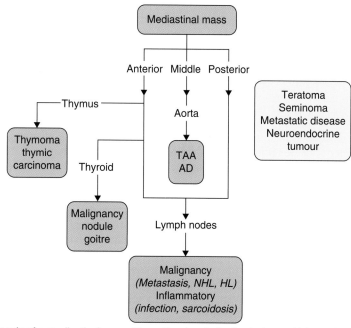

Fig. 10.37 Differential diagnosis of a mediastinal mass. The yellow box indicates lesions which can be found in any location. *AD*, Aortic dissection; *HL*, Hodgkin lymphoma; *NHL*, non-Hodgkin lymphoma; *TAA*, thoracic aortic aneurysm.

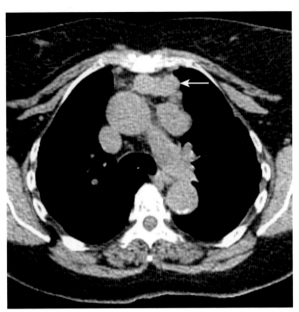

Fig. 10.38 CT imaging of mediastinal lesions. There is lobulated mass in the anterior mediastinum, suggestive of a thymoma. (From Mody DR et al. *Diagnostic Pathology: Cytopathology*, 3rd Edition. Elsevier; 2023.)

Management

Specific management relates to the underlying diagnosis. Surgical management may include:

- VATS: minimally invasive biopsy or excision evaluation for local metastasis.
- Sternotomy: for excision of large anterior lesions or treatment of vascular disease.
- Thoracotomy: preferred for excision of large middle or posterior lesions.

Complications

Complications relate to the underlying aetiology. General complications of a mediastinal mass include:

- SVC syndrome: compression of the SVC, presenting with acute dyspnoea, facial flushing and oedema. Urgent treatment with stenting or tumour debulking is required.
- Tracheal/bronchial obstruction: presenting with acute dyspnoea, relating to extrinsic compression or intrinsic compression. Requires urgent surgical decompression.

● Chapter Summary

- Indications for CABG include significant disease of the left main stem, proximal LAD or symptomatic 2- or 3-vessel disease
- True syncope is rapid in onset, of short duration, with spontaneous and complete recovery. Cardiac syncope requires urgent assessment and treatment, due to the life-threatening nature of the differentials.
- Aortic stenosis presents with syncope, angina, dyspnoea (SAD) and an ejection systolic murmur radiating to the carotids.
- Mitral regurgitation presents with dyspnoea, fatigue and palpitations, and a pansystolic murmur radiating to the axilla.
- Aortic dissection presents with sudden onset, central, tearing chest pain and haemodynamic instability. Surgical management includes open graft procedures or endovascular stenting.
- Acute, large pericardial effusions may cause cardiac tamponade, presenting with Beck's triad: hypotension, distended neck veins and muffled heart sounds.
- Aortic valve replacement may be performed via TAVI, endovascular aortic valvuloplasty and stent implantation, for those with limited life expectancy or high surgical risk.
- Recurrent pneumothorax can be managed with mechanical or chemical pleurodesis, to adhere the visceral and parietal pleura together and prevent lung collapse. Chemical options include talcum powder or tetracycline antibiotics.
- Lung cancer can be managed with wedge resection, segmentectomy, lobectomy or complete pneumonectomy, depending on the size and location of the lesion and associated metastatic disease.
- VATS is an increasingly preferred approach for cardiothoracic surgery, to reduce perioperative morbidity and mortality and improve surgical outcomes.

Chapter Summary—cont'd

UKMLA Conditions

Acute coronary syndromes
Aneurysms, ischaemic limb and occlusions
Aortic aneurysm
Aortic dissection
Aortic valve disease
Arrhythmias
Arterial thrombosis
Brain metastases
Cardiac arrest
Chronic obstructive pulmonary disease
Essential or secondary hypertension
Fibrotic lung disease
Hyperlipidemia
Infective endocarditis
Ischaemic heart disease
Lower respiratory tract infection
Lung cancer
Metastatic disease
Mitral valve disease
Myocardial infarction
Myocarditis
Patient on anticoagulant therapy
Patient on antiplatelet therapy
Pericardial disease
Peripheral oedema and ankle swelling
Pneumonia
Pneumothorax
Polycythaemia
Pulmonary embolism
Pulmonary hypertension
Respiratory arrest
Respiratory failure
Right heart valve disease
Shock
Stroke
Unstable angina
Vasovagal syncope

UKMLA Presentations

Blackouts and faints
Breathlessness
Cardiorespiratory arrest
Chest pain
Cough
Cyanosis
Decreased/loss of consciousness
Diplopia
Disease prevention/screening
Fever
Haemoptysis
Heart murmurs
Hypertension
Low blood pressure
Lower respiratory tract infection
Night sweats
Pain on inspiration
Palpitations
Peripheral oedema and ankle swelling
Pleural effusion
Shock
Weight loss

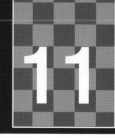

Perioperative management

PREOPERATIVE ASSESSMENT

A preoperative assessment involves a comprehensive history, examination and investigations to identify risk factors and comorbidities that may lead to perioperative complications.

> **CLINICAL NOTES**
>
> - Preoperative assessment typically happens 2-4 weeks before elective surgery.
> - For emergency surgery, a comprehensive assessment may not be possible.

History taking

History of presenting complaint (HPC)
Confirm the diagnosis and the scheduled procedure.

> **HINTS AND TIPS**
>
> Confirm the location of pathology and the side the procedure should be performed on if applicable!

Past medical history
A comprehensive past medical history should be taken to assess perioperative risk.

- Cardiovascular: hypertension, ischaemic heart disease (IHD), coronary artery disease (CAD), peripheral arterial disease (PAD), diabetes and obesity significantly increase the risk of perioperative complications.
- Respiratory: respiratory disease (particularly obstructive sleep apnoea) may lead to anaesthetic complications and necessitate ventilatory support postoperatively.
- Renal: a history of chronic kidney disease (CKD) or previous acute kidney injury (AKI) increases the risk of postoperative AKI.
- Gastrointestinal: liver disease risks bleeding postoperatively, and gastroesophageal reflux disease (GORD) or hiatal hernias can cause aspiration or airway difficulties.

- Neurological: surgery and anaesthesia may worsen symptoms or trigger crises of specific disorders, including myasthenia gravis. Cognitive disorders can influence capacity to consent for procedures.
- Blood borne viruses: it is essential to document HIV and hepatitis status prior to surgery.

Past surgical history
Enquire about previous operations, and any anaesthetic or perioperative complications.

Drug history
Take a full drug history, to screen for medications that need to be stopped on the day of surgery. Be sure to check allergy status.

> **CLINICAL NOTES**
>
> - Enquire specifically about previous reactions to anaesthesia, including dyspnoea, stridor, wheeze, rash or pruritus.
> - Intolerances or allergies to anaesthetic agents should be investigated thoroughly so alternatives can be identified if required.

Family history
A family history of anaesthetic complications may suggest hereditary sensitivities.

Social history
Relevant social history includes:

- Smoking history: to aid cardiovascular risk assessment.
- Alcohol intake: excess use can lead to postoperative complications and may require preoperative detox.
- Recreational drug use: stimulants can lead to anaesthetic complications. Intravenous use risks severe deep tissue and surgical site infections.
- Baseline functional status: to assess surgical risk and predict postoperative support needs.

Preoperative examination

A systematic physical examination is required, to screen for signs of underlying disease:

- Cardiovascular: assess for undiagnosed murmurs.
- Respiratory: screen of signs of heart failure or chronic respiratory disease.
- Abdominal: check for scars suggesting previous surgery, evidence of abdominal aneurysms and stigmata of chronic liver disease.

Airway assessment

Preoperative airway assessment involves a thorough history of airway complications, and specific examinations:

- Dental assessment: check for dental hardware, including dentures, crowns, bridges or loose teeth that may lead to airway difficulties and must be documented prior to surgery.
- Mallampati score: ask the patients to protrude their tongue, to visualize the faucial pillars (palatoglossal arches), soft palate and uvula, to predict ease of laryngoscopy (Fig. 11.1).
- Interincisal gap: the distance between the upper and lower incisors.
- Temporomandibular joint mobility: to assess ease of jaw thrust and mandible lift.
- Neck mobility: reduced neck flexion/extension may lead to difficult intubation.

Preoperative investigations

The exact investigations required relate to the patient comorbidities and nature of procedure.

1. Bedside
   - CBG : poor glycaemic control may need to be optimized prior to surgery.
   - ECG : to assess baseline cardiovascular risk and to compare with postoperatively if there are concerns of myocardial ischaemia perioperatively. cardiovascular risk and to compare with postoperatively if there are concerns for myocardial ischaemia.
   - Urinalysis + bHCG : to check for urinary tract infection (UTI) and exclude pregnancy in females of childbearing age.
   - MRSA swabs: to indicate need for decolonization preoperatively.
   - Spirometry: in chronic lung disease, to predict postoperative pulmonary complications.
   - Cardiopulmonary exercise testing: for high cardiac risk, to assess need for HDU/ITU postoperatively.
2. Bloods
   - FBC : to assess for anaemia or thrombocytopenia, and intraoperative bleeding risk. Blood transfusion may be required prior to surgery.
   - U&Es: to assess baseline renal function, inform fluid management and perioperative medication modifications.
   - LFTs: evidence of liver impairment informs anaesthetic medication choice.
   - Clotting screen: coagulopathy must be corrected preoperatively.
   - G&S: two samples must be sent for X-match and blood transfusion.
   - HbA1c: to assess long-term glycaemic control in diabetes.
   - TFTs : thyroid disease must be optimized preoperatively.
   - B_{12}/folate : deficiency causes anaemia and should be corrected preoperatively.

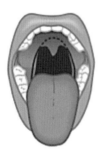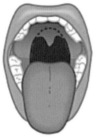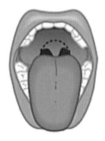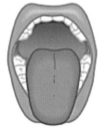

Class I: Soft palate, uvula, fauces, pillars visible	Class II: Soft palate, uvula, fauces visible	Class III: Soft palate, base of uvula visible	Class IV: Only hard palate visible
No difficulty	**No difficulty**	**Moderate difficulty**	**Severe difficulty**

Fig. 11.1 Mallampati score. Higher scores predict a more difficult airway for endotracheal intubation. (Whitten CE. *Anyone Can Intubate.* KW Publications; 1997.)

3. Imaging
   - CXR: to screen for heart failure or respiratory disease.
   - Echocardiogram: for risk stratification in those with evidence of underlying cardiac disease.

HINTS AND TIPS

- Specific imaging may be required preoperatively to aid procedure planning.
- Avoid ordering imaging without a specific indication, as incidental findings are common, and may result in unnecessary investigations and procedures.

PREOPERATIVE MANAGEMENT

Consent

Consent is the process of obtaining a patient's agreement to or authorization for a procedure. It must be obtained with adequate time, patience and clarity of explanation, with written information provided and language barriers addressed. Informed consent must be:

- Capacitous: patients must have documented capacity to make the decision.
- Voluntary: made without coercion or influence.
- Comprehensive: the patient must understand the diagnosis, prognosis, benefits and risk of both intervention and nonintervention, and likelihood of success.
- Full disclosure: relevant medical information must be shared by a person actively involved in care, who has clear knowledge of the procedure, risks and complications.

CLINICAL NOTES

Assess and document capacity using the principles of the mental capacity act – the patient must demonstrate ability to understand and retain information provided, weigh up the pros and cons, and make and communicate their decision.

Consent should be documented and signed by both the person obtaining consent and the patient. If a patient declines to consent, this should be clearly documented as well.

ETHICS

- Best interests decisions are made when consent cannot be obtained but withholding treatment would cause significant harm.
- Circumstances include when a patient lacks capacity, or in emergency situations.
- Be sure to involve seniors, and relatives where possible.

Medication

There are several medication modifications required perioperatively:

- Clopidogrel: typically stopped 7 days before surgery. Other antiplatelets may be continued.
- Hypoglycaemic agents: oral hypoglycaemics are typically stopped on the day of surgery.
- Insulin: long-acting insulins should be continued, with the dose reduced by 80% on the day before and day of surgery. Short-acting insulins should be stopped on the day of surgery, and a variable rate insulin infusion started, with concurrent potassium chloride with glucose and sodium chloride to prevent hypogycaemia.
- Oral contraceptive pill: stopped 4 weeks prior to surgery to reduce the risk of the risk of venous thromboembolism (VTE).
- Anticoagulation: the bleeding and thrombosis risk must be evaluated, and modifications made appropriately.
- Steroids: patients on long-term steroids will need their dose doubled perioperatively, to avoid adrenal crisis.
- Antibiotic prophylaxis: may be required for specific procedures.

Anticoagulation

Perioperative management of anticoagulation should be tailored to the patient and procedure, in consultation with the surgeon and anaesthetist. Surgery on patients receiving anticoagulation is associated with an increased bleeding risk; discontinuing anticoagulation increases thrombosis risk. A comprehensive risk assessment preoperatively is required to inform management.

Elective procedures
- 1 week before: assess bleeding and thrombotic risk.
- Low bleeding risk: consider continuing anticoagulation.
- High bleeding risk, low thrombotic risk: hold oral anticoagulants.
- High bleeding risk, moderate/high thrombotic risk: hold oral anticoagulation, consider bridging anticoagulation for warfarin.

Emergency procedures

- Low bleeding risk: consider continuing anticoagulation.
- Increased bleeding risk: consider anticoagulation reversal prior to procedure.
- Increased bleeding risk, high thrombotic risk: consider anticoagulation reversal, and need for bridging anticoagulation (Table 11.1).

> **CLINICAL NOTES**
>
> Make all perioperative medication decisions in consultation with seniors, including the surgeon and anaesthetist performing the procedure.

> **HINTS AND TIPS**
>
> Specific guidance on timings of anticoagulation cessation, management of INR and bridging anticoagulation will be available locally.

Postoperatively, anticoagulation can typically be restarted after 24 hours if there is no evidence of active bleeding and low bleeding risk. If there is a high bleeding risk, restarting anticoagulation may be delayed.

Table 11.1 Perioperative bleeding and thrombosis risk assessment

	Bleeding risk	Thrombosis risk
Patient factors	Age >65 Active cancer Abnormal renal/liver function History/predisposition to major bleeding Hypertension History of stroke Use of NSAIDs, anticoagulants, antiplatelets or steroids Excess alcohol use	History of stroke History of/risk factors for VTE Valvular heart disease Atrial fibrillation Cardiovascular disease Active cancer
Procedure factors	Cardiovascular surgery Total arthroplasty of major joint Spinal surgery Cancer surgery Surgery >60 minutes	Valve replacement Vascular surgery, i.e., aneurysm repair Total arthroplasty of major joint Endarterectomy Abdominal surgery

Many conditions and surgeries are associated with both increased bleeding and thrombosis risk, and perioperative anticoagulation management must be considered carefully.

> **CLINICAL NOTES**
>
> - Mechanical and/or pharmacological VTE prophylaxis is required for most hospital inpatients, particularly in the perioperative period.
> - Assess the thrombosis and bleeding risk appropriately to guide the choice, and the need for and timing of cessation and resumption pre- and postoperatively.
> - VTE prophylaxis is not required for day-case procedures.

INTRAOPERATIVE MANAGEMENT

Preparing for theatre

The WHO surgical safety is the standard of practice, and is completed at three key stages:

- Sign in: before induction of anaesthesia, the patient's identity and procedure are confirmed, allergies and airway issues are identified, and equipment is checked.
- Time out: before the operation starts, the whole team stops to confirm the patient's identity, check consent is in place, make introductions and discuss bleeding risk, antibiotic requirements and VTE prophylaxis.
- Sign out: before the patient leaves the theatre, the instrument count is confirmed, specimens are labelled and anticipated postoperative issues identified.

Other key preparation steps include:

- Patient position: as appropriate to allow adequate access to the operating area.
- Scrubbing, gloving and gowning: surgeons involved in the procedure should scrub thoroughly using aseptic nontouch techniques.
- Prepping the sterile field: cleaning the skin around the operating area, and placing sterile drapes to outline the surgical field.

Intraoperative monitoring

Intraoperative monitoring involves continued assessment of physiological variables during surgery to assess for patient deterioration and allow titration of anaesthetic medications. Variables that should be continually monitored include:

- Pulse oximetry: to assess oxygenation.

- Blood pressure: to assess haemodynamic status and the need for fluids.
- ECG: continuous ECG monitoring is required to detect arrhythmias.
- End-tidal carbon dioxide: to assess for respiratory depression and the development of type 2 respiratory failure.
- Temperature: to detect hypothermia or hyperthermia.
- Conscious level: the anaesthetist will monitor depth of sedation and adjust anaesthesia as required.
- Urine output: to assess intravascular fluid status and fluid requirements.

CLINICAL NOTES

Risk of transfusions include:
- ABO incompatibility
- Febrile transfusion reactions
- Haemolytic transfusion reactions
- Transfusion-related circulatory overload
- Transfusion-related lung injury
- Graft-versus-host disease

RED FLAG

- Malignant hyperthermia is a life-threatening anaesthetic complication, involving uncontrolled skeletal muscle contraction, hypermetabolism and increased body temperature.
- It is a hereditary response and often lethal.
- Treatment includes cessation of the triggering agent and dantrolene.

RED FLAG

- Perioperative blood loss and inflammation can cause cardiac complications
- ECGs should be monitored closely during the perioperative period for signs of acute arrhythmias and myocardial ischaemia.
- Ischaemic heart disease and atrial fibrillation are common postoperative complications.

Intraoperative fluid management

Normovolaemia must be achieved intraoperatively, to maintain adequate tissue perfusion. Both hypovolemia and hypervolemia are associated with significant morbidity and mortality. Intravascular volume status should be monitored, and fluid replacement given as required:

- Crystalloid solutions: including normal saline or Hartmann's, to replace losses and give boluses as required to maintain blood pressure.
- Transfusion: if transfusion thresholds (typically Hb <70/80 g/dL) are met, red blood cells (RBCs) can be given. Other blood products are used if there is evidence of coagulopathy.

POSTOPERATIVE MANAGEMENT

Fluids

Postoperative fluid prescribing should consider fluid status, indication, comorbidities, weight, and recent blood results. Sensible fluid losses describe quantifiable losses including urine, blood, diarrhoea or vomiting. Insensible losses describe unquantifiable losses, due to fever, tachypnoea or interstitial losses. Both should be considered when evaluating perioperative fluid requirements.

CLINICAL NOTES

A comprehensive fluid status assessment includes:
- Observations
- Mucous membranes
- Skin turgor
- Urine output
- JVP
- Peripheral and pulmonary oedema.

Fluid replacement

The indication for fluids guides the choice, rate and added components:

- Resuscitation: replacement of acute losses, typically boluses of 250/500 mL over 15 to 30 minutes depending on size and comorbidities.
- Maintenance: the daily requirements of a nil-by-mouth patient (Table 11.2).
- Replacement: if there are ongoing losses or a fluid deficit that exceeds maintenance requirements, additional fluids at modified rates can be given according to requirements.

Table 11.2 Maintenance fluids

Daily requirements	70 kg adult	Example regimen
Water – 25 mL/kg/day Na⁺ – 1 mmol/kg/day K⁺ – 1 mmol/kg/day Glucose – 50 g/day	Water – 1750 mL Na⁺ – 70 mmol K⁺ – 70 mmol Glucose – 50 g	1st bag (over 12 hours) 1L 0.9% NaCl + 40 mmol K⁺ 2nd bag (over 12 hours) 1L 5% dextrose + 20 mmol K⁺

Daily requirements do not have to be met exactly but should be targeted.

HINTS AND TIPS

Potassium should be given at a maximum rate of 10 mmol/hour, to prevent arrhythmias.

Analgesia

Postoperative pain should be managed according to the WHO analgesic ladder (Fig. 11.2).

RED FLAG

- Those on opiates must be monitored closely for toxicity.
- Signs include low respiratory rate, pinpoint pupils and reduced conscious level.
- Airway management and naloxone are required.

HINTS AND TIPS

- Side effects of opiates include urinary retention, constipation, nausea, delirium and sedation.
- Paralytic ileus (functional bowel obstruction) may also develop.
- If these occur, the analgesia regimen should be reviewed, and alternative (nonopiate) analgesia found.

Antibiotics

Antibiotics may be required for prophylaxis or treatment of infection postoperatively. Cultures of the relevant site should be taken, and antibiotics tailored according to sensitivities to more effectively treat infection and reduce the risk of antibiotic resistance.

Surgeries that require antibiotic prophylaxis include:

- Clean procedures involving prosthesis/implants: to reduce risk of periprosthetic sepsis.
- Clean-contaminated surgery: repair or removal of an internal organ, with no signs of active infection.
- Contaminated surgery: where the sterile field has been breached, there is gastrointestinal contamination, or where acute inflammation is detected.

Actively infected wounds require antibiotic treatment.

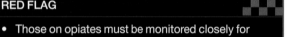
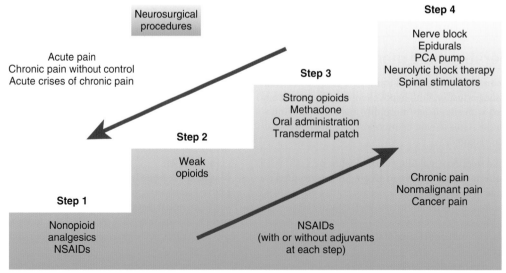

Fig. 11.2 WHO Analgesia ladder. Analgesia should be stepped up or down according to requirements. (From Bryant RA, Nix DP. *Acute & Chronic Wounds: Intraprofessionals from Novice to Expert*, 6th Edition. Elsevier Inc.; 2024.)

Nutrition

Perioperative malnutrition is common, relating to poor preoperative nutritional status, fasting periods, postoperative nausea or operative complications. Nutritional support is often required postoperatively, via enteral or parenteral routes. Options include:

- Enteral nutrition: nasogastric/nasojejunal feeding is typically sufficient postoperatively. If there are long-term nutritional requirements that cannot be met orally, percutaneous routes including gastrostomy or jejunostomy can be used.
- Total parenteral nutrition (TPN): delivery of complete nutritional requirements through central venous access. Used when enteral nutrition is not possible (Fig. 11.3).

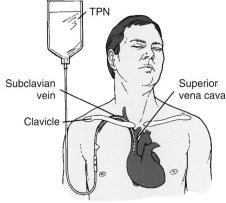

Fig. 11.3 Total parenteral nutrition. *TPN*, given via a tunnel central line. (From *Mosby's Dictionary of Medicine, Nursing & Health Professions*, 11th Edition. Elsevier; 2022.)

RED FLAG

Complications of TPN include:
- Line sepsis
- Refeeding syndrome
- Hepatic and biliary dysfunction
- VTE
- Pneumothorax.

Postoperative nausea is very common, and should be managed with appropriate antiemetics, and treatment of the underlying cause.

POSTOPERATIVE COMPLICATIONS

Postoperative pyrexia

Low-level pyrexia is common postoperatively due to the inflammatory response to surgical trauma. Prolonged (>24 hours) or significant pyrexia is abnormal (Fig. 11.4).

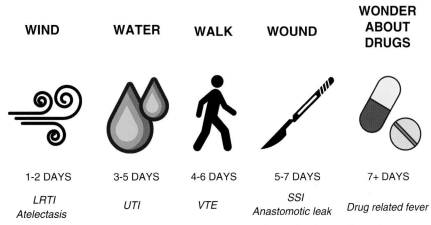

Fig. 11.4 The 5 W's can be used to predict the aetiology of infection in relation to the timing of pyrexia postoperatively.

Management

Patients with postoperative pyrexia should be managed with an A–E approach, with comprehensive assessment for haemodynamic instability and signs of infection.

The Sepsis 6 should be initiated:

- Blood cultures: to identify the aetiological organism.
- VBG: to assess for lactate, a marker of tissue hypoperfusion.
- Urine output: urine output <0.5 mg/kg/hour suggests hypovolaemia.
- Fluids: fluid resuscitation according to requirements.
- Oxygen: give high-flow oxygen and monitor SpO_2.
- Antibiotics: empiric antibiotics should be started and tailored to culture results.
- Bloods: for FBC, CRP, U&Es, LFTs, clotting, blood cultures and VBG.

RED FLAG

- Patients are at increased risk of infection postoperatively, due to hypovolaemia, malnutrition and inflammation, and a suppressed immune response.
- If there are signs of infection, prompt management with antibiotics and fluids is essential, to reduce the risk of multiorgan dysfunction, disseminated intravascular coagulation and death.

Bleeding

Perioperative haemorrhage can be classified based on the timing of bleeding:

- Primary bleeding: intraoperative bleeding, which should be resolved during surgery.
- Reactive bleeding: occurring within 24 hours of surgery, typically relating to a vasodilation of a blood vessel damaged intraoperatively.
- Secondary bleeding: occurring 7 to 10 days postoperatively, typically relating to infection, inflammation or vessel erosion.

Bleeding patients should be assessed with an A–E approach, to assess for signs of haemorrhagic shock and initiate resuscitation measures.

HINTS AND TIPS

- Signs of shock include tachycardia, tachypnoea, dizziness and decreased urine output.
- Hypotension is a late sign and should not be relied upon in isolation to assess intravascular volume status.

Blood transfusion should be given to replace losses (Table 11.3).

Table 11.3 Blood products

Product	Indications	Rate
Red blood cells (RBCs)	Acute blood loss Anaemia (Hb <70 g/L or symptomatic)	2–4 hours
Platelets	Haemorrhagic shock in trauma Thrombocytopenia <20 × 10^9/L Active bleeding with thrombocytopenia Preoperative platelets <50 × 10^9/L	30 minutes
Fresh frozen plasma* (FFP)	Disseminated intravascular coagulation (DIC) Haemorrhage relating to liver disease Massive haemorrhage (given after two units of RBCs)	30 minutes
Cryoprecipitate*	Massive haemorrhage DIC with fibrinogen <1 g/L Von Willebrand disease	Stat

*FFP and cryoprecipitate contain clotting factors, indicated in coagulopathy.

Chapter Summary

- Informed consent involves a comprehensive understanding of the procedure, risks, benefits and alternatives, made voluntarily, in a patient who has capacity.
- The components of capacity involve being able to understand and retain information and weigh up and communicate a decision.
- Hypoglycaemic agents must be stopped on the day of surgery, long-acting insulin continued with dose adjustments, and short-acting insulin changed to a variable rate infusion.
- Long-term steroids should be doubled perioperatively, to avoid adrenal crisis.
- Patients on anticoagulation must have their bleeding and thrombosis risk assessed prior to surgery to guide perioperative anticoagulation management.
- Completion of the WHO surgical safety checklist involves confirming the patient, surgeons and operation details, discussing perioperative management issues, and equipment checks before and after surgery.
- Postoperative fluid management involves maintenance fluids and replacement for ongoing losses.
- Antibiotic prophylaxis is indicated postoperatively for any nonclean surgeries, or those involving prosthesis.
- Postoperative malnutrition is common and should be identified and managed early, with enteral routes preferred.
- The aetiology of postoperative pyrexia in the order it develops postoperatively can be remembered by the 5 W's – wind, water, walk, wound and wonder about drugs.

UKMLA Conditions
Acid–base abnormality
Acute kidney injury
Adverse drug effects
Allergic disorder
Anaemia
Anaphylaxis
Arrhythmias
Breathlessness
Cardiac arrest
Cardiac failure
Chest pain
Chronic kidney disease
Chronic obstructive pulmonary disease
Cough
Cyanosis
Decreased/loss of consciousness
Deep vein thrombosis
Dehydration
Delirium
Deteriorating patient
Diabetes mellitus type 1 and 2
Diabetic nephropathy
Disseminated intravascular coagulation
Drug overdose
Fever
Hospital-acquired infections
Human immunodeficiency virus
Hyperthermia and hypothermia
Hypoglycaemia

UKMLA Presentations
Abnormal urinalysis
Acute and chronic pain management
Acute kidney injury
Acute rash
Allergies
Breathlessness
Cardiorespiratory arrest
Chest pain
Chronic kidney disease
Confusion
Cough
Cyanosis
Decreased appetite
Decreased/loss of consciousness
Dehydration
Deteriorating patient
Diabetes mellitus type 1 and 2
Disseminated intravascular coagulation
Dizziness
Driving advice
Drug overdose
Electrolyte abnormalities
Fatigue
Fever
Fit notes
Frailty
Haemoptysis
Hypoglycaemia Immobility
Intestinal obstruction and ileus

Continued

● Chapter Summary—cont'd

UKMLA Conditions

Incidental findings
Intestinal obstruction and ileus
Ischaemic heart disease
Lower respiratory tract infection
Malnutrition
Multiorgan dysfunction syndrome
Myasthenia gravis
Myocardial infarction
Obesity
Overdose
Pallor
Pancytopenia
Patient on anticoagulant therapy
Patient on antiplatelet therapy
Pulmonary embolism
Pulmonary hypertension
Respiratory arrest
Respiratory failure
Surgical site infection
Transfusion reactions
Urinary incontinence
Urinary symptoms
Urticaria
Vitamin B_{12} and/or folate deficiency
Vomiting
Wheeze

UKMLA Presentations

Low blood pressure
Lower respiratory tract infection
Malnutrition
Massive haemorrhage
Mental capacity concerns
Misplaced nasogastric tube
Nausea
Oliguria
Overdose
Pain on inspiration
Painful swollen leg
Pallor
Palpitations
Pleural effusion
Pneumonia
Postsurgical care and complications
Pruritus
Sepsis
Shock
Stridor
Trauma
Urinary incontinence
Urinary symptoms
Vomiting
Wheeze

Self-Assessment

UKMLA High Yield Association Table

Chapter 1 The upper gastrointestinal tract

Key findings	Diagnoses
Central tearing abdominal pain, hypotension	Ruptured AAA
Postprandial diffuse cramping abdominal pain	Mesenteric angina
Acute iliac fossa pain, positive pregnancy test	Ectopic pregnancy
Chest pain, dyspepsia nausea, acid brash, NSAID use	GORD
Chronic GORD, dysphagia	Oesophageal stricture
Barium swallow shows apple core lesion	Oesophageal adenocarcinoma
Progressive dysphagia, chest pain, weight loss, Hx of Barrett's oesophagus	Oesophageal adenocarcinoma
Dysphagia and weight loss, history of GORD	Oesophageal adenocarcinoma
Epigastric pain worse at night	Duodenal ulcer
Epigastric pain worse after meals	Gastric ulcer
Peptic ulcer disease, acute abdomen, fever	Perforated peptic ulcer
Melaena, epigastric pain, NSAIDs	Bleeding peptic ulcer
PUD, vomiting of undigested food, early satiety, weight loss	Gastric outlet obstruction
Anaemia, weight loss, dysphagia, Virchow's node	Gastric cancer
Corkscrew oesophagus	Diffuse oesophageal spasm
'Birds beak' oesophagus	Achalasia
Effortless regurgitation while lying flat	Achalasia
Double swallow and halitosis	Pharyngeal pouch
Small volume haematemesis, significant vomiting	Mallory Weiss tear
Significant vomiting, profuse haematemesis	Oesophageal rupture (Boerhaave syndrome)
Jaundice, pale urine, dark stools	Post hepatic jaundice
Raised AST/ALT	Hepatic LFTs
Raised ALP/y-GT	Cholestatic LFTs
Caput medusa, alcohol abuse	Portal hypertension
Large volume haematemesis and alcohol abuse	Variceal bleed
Cirrhosis, worsening abdominal pain, weight loss, night sweats	Hepatocellular carcinoma
Postprandial upper abdominal pain, flatulent dyspepsia	Biliary colic
RUQ pain after eating, middle-aged overweight female	Gallstones
Fever, RUQ pain, Murphy's sign, gallstones, middle-aged female	Acute cholecystitis
Fever, jaundice, right upper quadrant pain	Ascending cholangitis
Cholecystitis, subsequent small bowel obstruction	Gallstone ileus
ERCP shows 'beads on a string'	Primary sclerosing cholangitis

Continued

Key findings	Diagnoses
Acute epigastric pain radiating to the back, nausea, vomiting, raised amylase, alcohol use	Pancreatitis
Acute epigastric pain radiating to the back, nausea, vomiting, raised amylase, history of gallstones	Gallstone pancreatitis
Abdominal bruising (Cullen's/Grey-Turner's sign)	Haemorrhagic pancreatitis
Pancreatitis, acute dyspnoea, pulmonary infiltrates	Acute respiratory distress syndrome
Chronic epigastric pain, steatorrhoea, alcohol use, rapid onset/worsening diabetes	Chronic pancreatitis
Painless jaundice, palpable gallbladder	Pancreatic cancer (Courvoisier's law)

Chapter 2 The lower gastrointestinal tract

Key findings	Diagnoses
Causes of abdominal distention	Fat, Fluid, Flatus, Faeces, Foetus, Fulminant mass
Chronic malnutrition, seizures, arrhythmias, rhabdomyolysis	Refeeding syndrome
Generalised abdominal pain, rigidity, guarding, rebound tenderness	Peritonitis
Chronic liver disease, ascites, peritonitic signs	Spontaneous bacterial peritonitis
Abdominal pain migrating from the umbilicus to right iliac fossa, anorexia, low-grade fever	Appendicitis
Flushing, GI upset, valvular lesions, wheeze, hepatic involvement, pellagra	Carcinoid syndrome (appendiceal tumour)
Profuse bloody diarrhoea, dehydration, recent smoking cessation	Ulcerative colitis
Chronic diarrhoea, weight loss, ulcers, malabsorption	Crohn disease
Continuous colonic mucosal inflammation and surface erosions	Ulcerative colitis
Transmural noncontinuous (skip lesions) inflammation throughout the entire GIT, cobblestoning, ulceration	Crohn disease
Chronic diarrhoea, red painful eye	Inflammatory bowel disease, anterior uveitis
Abdominal distention, pain, obstipation, absent bowel sounds, coffee bean sign	Sigmoid volvulus
Profuse watery diarrhoea, recent antibiotic use	C. difficile, pseudomembranous colitis
Massive colonic dilation, profuse diarrhoea, rectal bleeding, haemodynamic instability, abdominal distention, absent bowel sounds	Toxic megacolon
Crohn disease, repeated bowel resection, steatorrhoea, weight loss, fatigue, malnutrition	Short bowel syndrome
Abdominal distention, pain, constipation, tinkling/hyperactive/absent bowel sounds	Bowel obstruction
Central dilated bowel loops, valvulae conniventes	Small bowel obstruction
Peripheral dilated bowel loops, haustra	Large bowel obstruction
CXR – air under diaphragm (pneumoperitoneum)	Bowel perforation
Postsurgery, constipation, abdominal pain, distention, absent bowel sounds	Paralytic ileus
Acute abdominal pain, bloody diarrhoea, atrial fibrillation	Acute mesenteric ischaemia
Postprandial pain, food aversion, abdominal bruit	Chronic mesenteric ischaemia
Sudden abdominal pain, bloody diarrhoea, history of atherosclerosis/vascular disease	Ischaemic colitis
Chronic constipation, left iliac fossa pain	Diverticulosis

Key findings	Diagnoses
Outpouchings of colonic mucosa on colonoscopy	Diverticular disease
Acute left iliac fossa pain, palpable mass, bright red rectal bleeding, history of constipation	Diverticulitis
Older adult, weight loss, change in bowel habit, unexplained anaemia	Colorectal carcinoma
Colonic polyposis, family history of colorectal cancer	Familial adenomatous polyposis
Bright red rectal bleeding, perianal mass, chronic constipation	Haemorrhoids
Severe perianal pain, pain on defecation, tender perianal mass	Thrombosed haemorrhoids
Severe anorectal pain, bright red rectal bleeding, perianal pruritis	Anal fissure
Anorectal pain, palpable subcutaneous mass, fevers, purulent anal discharge	Perianal abscess
Chronic anorectal pain, skin damage, anal discharge, Crohn's	Perianal fistula
Painless rectal mass, incontinence and perianal pruritus	Rectal prolapse
Rectal bleeding, palpable mass, HPV infection, anal intercourse	Anal carcinoma

Chapter 3 The anterior abdominal wall

Key findings	Diagnoses
Groin lump superomedial to the pubic tubercle, appearing after heavy lifting	Inguinal hernia
Groin lump inferolateral to the pubic tubercle, older multiparous woman	Femoral hernia
Groin lump, positive cough impulse	Direct inguinal hernia
Groin lump, negative cough impulse	Indirect inguinal hernia
Irreducible painful groin lump	Incarcerated hernia
Irreducible hernia, abdominal pain, obstipation	Obstructing hernia
Irreducible painful groin lump, systemic illness and sepsis	Strangulated hernia
Spouted stoma, green liquid stool	ileostomy
Spouted stoma, draining urine	Urostomy
Flat stoma, brown solid stool	Colostomy
Stoma output >1.5 L, dehydration	High output stoma
Stoma enlargement and reducible mass	Parastomal hernia
'Outie' belly button, palpable umbilical lump	Umbilical hernia
Palpable painful lump close to abdominal surgical incision	Incisional hernia
Chest trauma, respiratory distress, absent breath sounds, audible bowel sounds in chest	Diaphragmatic hernia

Chapter 4 Endocrine surgery

Key findings	Diagnoses
Fatigue, excessive urination, thirst, weight loss	Diabetes mellitus
Nontender mobile neck lump, moves on swallowing but not on tongue protrusion	Thyroid nodule
Nontender mobile neck lump, moves on swallowing and tongue protrusion	Thyroglossal duct cyst
Tender goitre, fever and flu-like symptoms, hyperthyroid then hypothyroid phase	Subacute thyroiditis (De Quervain's thyroiditis)
Slowly enlarging thyroid mass, female 30–50	Medullary thyroid carcinoma

Continued

Key findings	Diagnoses
Rapidly enlarging thyroid mass, hoarseness, dysphagia, dysphonia, smoking history	Anaplastic thyroid carcinoma
Loss of weight, increased appetite, agitation, heat intolerance	Hyperthyroidism
Weight gain, appetite loss, cold intolerance	Hypothyroidism
Waxy pretibial discolouration	Grave disease
Exophthalmos, oedema, ophthalmoplegia and lid lag	Thyroid eye disease
Midline semicircular ('half-moon') lower neck scar	Thyroidectomy
Laryngeal oedema, stridor and dyspnoea occurring hours after thyroid surgery	Immediate hematoma
Hoarse voice and cough, aspiration pneumonia, after thyroid surgery	Superior laryngeal nerve palsy
Perioral numbness, tetany and seizures after thyroid surgery	Hypoparathyroidism
Hypothermia, hypotension, ↓ GCS, following thyroid surgery	Myxoedema coma
Headache, diplopia, bitemporal hemianopia +/– hormone derangement	Pituitary macroadenoma
Severe headache, visual symptoms, acute adrenal insufficiency	Pituitary apoplexy
Galactorrhoea, amenorrhoea, reduced libido, gynaecomastia, infertility	Prolactinoma
Hands and feet growth, coarse facies, macroglossia	Acromegaly
Polyuria, polydipsia, concentration of urine following desmopressin	Cranial diabetes insipidus
Polyuria, polydipsia, no concentration of urine following desmopressin	Nephrogenic diabetes insipidus
Polyuria, polydipsia, water deprivation test – increased urine concentration	Primary polydipsia
Bone pain, renal stones, constipation, nausea, polyuria, polydipsia, depression	Hypercalcemia
↑ PTH, ↑ calcium	Primary hyperparathyroidism
↑ PTH, ↓ calcium, CKD	Secondary hyperparathyroidism
↑↑ PTH, ↑ calcium, CKD	Tertiary hyperparathyroidism
↑ Cortisol, ↑ ACTH	Pituitary adenoma (Cushing disease)
↑ Cortisol, ↓ ACTH	Adrenal adenoma
↑ Cortisol, ↑ ACTH, normal pituitary imaging	Ectopic ACTH secretion
Depression, hair loss, moon face, buffalo hump, osteoporosis, oesophagitis, hyperglycaemia, visceral obesity, decreased libido	Cushing syndrome
Fatigue, abdominal pain, anorexia, nausea and vomiting, hyperkalaemia, skin darkening	Adrenal insufficiency
ECG – tall, tented T waves, flattened P waves, broad QRS	Hyperkalaemia
Hypotension, shock, ↓ GCS, fever, vomiting, diarrhoea, abdominal pain, recent steroid cessation	Adrenal crisis
Hypokalaemia, ↓ aldosterone:renin ratio	Primary hyperaldosteronism
Hypertension, anxiety, sweating, paroxysmal atrial fibrillation, history of MEN2, ↑ urinary metanephrines	Pheochromocytoma
Episodic blood pressure crises with extreme hypertension, headaches, sweating, palpitations and pallor	Malignant hypertension
Painful, acute, soft mobile neck lump	Lymphadenitis (reactive lymphadenopathy)
Painless, progressively enlarging, firm, fixed, lymph nodes	Malignant lymphadenopathy
Unexplained weight loss, anorexia, fever, lethargy, malaise	Malignancy
Hoarseness, smoking history	Head and neck malignancy

Chapter 5 Breast surgery

Key findings	Diagnoses
Mastalgia, erythema, fever, pain while breastfeeding	Mastitis
Mastalgia, fluctuant mass, unilateral purulent nipple discharge	Breast abscess
Family history of breast cancer, new breast mass	Breast cancer, BRCA mutation
Painless, firm, irregular breast lump, skin thickening and dimpling (peau d'orange), nipple inversion, blood-stained discharge	Breast cancer
History of breast cancer, new first seizure	Brain metastasis
History of breast cancer, bone pain, ↑Ca	Bone metastasis
Breast trauma, painful breast lump	Fat necrosis
Milky nipple discharge, breast lump	Galactocele
Green nipple discharge, breast lump	Duct ectasia
Painless breast lump, skin erythema, rapid onset and progression	Inflammatory breast cancer
Breast lump, nipple eczema	Paget disease of the nipple
Painless mobile breast lump	Breast cyst
Cyclical breast pain/lumpiness	Fibrocystic change
Intermittent breast pain, premenstrual syndrome	Cyclical mastalgia
Gynaecomastia, testicular mass	Testicular cancer
Nontender, rubbery, mobile breast mass, age 20–30	Fibroadenoma
Palpable areolar lump, bloody/serous discharge, age 30–50	Intraductal papilloma

Chapter 6 Vascular surgery

Key findings	Diagnoses
Cramping muscle pain in the calves or thighs, worse on exertion, improved by rest	Intermittent claudication
Aching muscle pain relieved by leg elevation	Venous claudication
Cramping muscle pain relieved by leaning forward	Neurogenic claudication
Sudden onset severe limb pain, pallor, paraesthesia, and paralysis, pulselessness, cold, history of AF	Acute limb ischaemia
Aching, poorly localised abdominal pain, vascular risk factors	AAA
Sudden, severe abdominal pain, tachycardia hypotension and syncope	Ruptured AAA
History of AAA, sudden onset visceral and limb ischaemia and haemodynamic instability	Aortic dissection
ABPI <0.8, intermittent claudication	PAD
ABPI <0.5, rest pain, ulcers, gangrene	Critical limb ischaemia
ABPI >1.3	Arterial calcification – diabetes
Warm foot, loss of sensation, palpable pedal pulses, ulcers	Neuropathic diabetic foot
Diabetic ulcer, exposed bone, pus, erythema	Osteomyelitis
Recurrent foot trauma, deformity, loss of arch, loss of function	Charcot foot
Bilateral buttock/thigh claudication, erectile dysfunction and absent femoral pulses	Leriche syndrome
White, blue, red fingers upon cold exposure	Raynaud syndrome
Chronic limb ischaemia, black digital discolouration, skin breakdown	Gangrene
Red, itchy, crusted skin on lower legs	Venous eczema

Continued

Key findings	Diagnoses
Skin induration, swelling and thickening, inverted champagne bottle appearance	Lipodermatosclerosis
Lower limb hyperpigmentation, chronic venous disease	Hemosiderin deposition
Dilated tortuous superficial veins on lower legs	Varicose veins
Bilateral leg cramping, oedema, varicose veins, pruritus	Chronic venous insufficiency
Pain, erythema and induration of superficial vein	Superficial thrombophlebitis
Punchout, well-defined ulcer, severe pain	Arterial ulcers
Shallow, superficial, ulcer, irregular borders, medial malleoli	Venous ulcer
Ulcer over pressure point, deep, hyperkeratosis borders, surrounding callous	Neuropathic ulcer
Acute onset of dyspnoea, tachycardia and tachypnoea, pleuritic chest pain, cough and haemoptysis and low-grade fever	Pulmonary embolism
Acute calf erythema, swelling, tenderness, recent immobility, superficial vein dilation	Deep vein thrombosis
Venous stasis, endothelial injury, hypercoagulability	Virchow's triad
Aneurysmal sac enlargement post EVAR	Endoleak
Transient loss of sensory or motor function, amaurosis fugax, carotid bruit	Carotid artery stenosis
Aching, heavy legs, recurrent skin infections, hardening and tightening, warty growths and fluid leakage	Lymphoedema

Chapter 7 Urology

Key findings	Diagnoses
Discomfort, burning, stinging when passing urine	Urinary tract infection
Lower urinary tract symptoms, +ve nitrates/leukocytes	Urinary tract infection
Fever, loin pain, malaise, nausea and vomiting	Pyelonephritis
Severe, paroxysmal, unilateral loin to groin pain, LUTS	Renal stones
Acute urinary retention, tachycardia, visual impairment	Anticholinergic effects
Sudden inability to void, suprapubic pain, palpable bladder, agitation	Acute urinary retention
Progressive painless difficulty urinating, palpable bladder, overflow incontinence	Chronic urinary retention
High-volume urine output post catheterization	High-pressure chronic urinary retention
Nocturnal enuresis and LUTS, recent TWOC	Post obstructive diuresis
Involuntary urinary leakage upon ↑ intraabdominal pressure (coughing, sneezing, exercising)	Stress incontinence
Sudden urgency, involuntary urine leakage	Urge incontinence
Involuntary dribbling of urine, no urinary urge, postvoid residual volume	Overflow incontinence
Occupational exposure to rubber, plastics or dyes, painless haematuria	Bladder carcinoma
Painless testicular lump, male >60 years	Testicular seminoma
Painless testicular lump, young male, β-hCG positive	Nonseminoma testicular tumour
Haematuria, loin pain, palpable abdominal mass	Renal cell carcinoma
Frequency, urgency nocturia, older male DRE – symmetrically enlarged, smooth, non-tender prostate	Benign prostatic hyperplasia
Urinary retention, incontinence, haematuria, loin pain, sclerotic bony lesions	Prostate cancer
DRE with lobar asymmetry, hard, non-tender nodules	Prostate cancer
Unilateral scrotal pain, erythema, fever, dysuria, frequency	Epididymo-orchitis

Key findings	Diagnoses
Scrotal swelling, testicular and abdominal pain and scrotal elevation with a transverse lie	Testicular torsion
Sustained painful erection, not caused by sexual excitation or relieved by ejaculation	Priapism
Pain and erythema of the glans and foreskin, discharge, ulceration	Balanitis
Inability to retract the foreskin	Phimosis
Inability to return retracted foreskin to its original position	Paraphimosis
Sudden onset urinary retention/incontinence, back pain, saddle anaesthesia	Cauda equina syndrome
Reducible testicular mass ('bag of worms'), painless	Varicocele
Unilateral testicular swelling, transillumination	Hydrocele
Small firm, painless mass, palpable within the epididymis	Epididymal cyst
Irreducible, painful groin mass	Incarcerated hernia
Groin lump, painless, firm, rubbery, mobile	Malignant lymph node
Fever, acute dysuria, severe back and perineal pain and a tender, boggy warm prostate	Acute prostatitis
Fever, dysuria, tender prostate, >6 weeks	Chronic prostatitis
Graft pain, oedema, fever, ↑BP, AKI, <6 months of transplant	Acute graft rejection
Painful maculopapular rash, GI upset, jaundice, anaemia, <100 days of transplant	Graft versus host disease

Chapter 8 Ear, nose and throat

Key findings	Diagnoses
Hearing loss, use of cotton buds	Wax impaction
Otalgia, conductive hearing loss, otorrhoea, itch, history of swimming, erythema and swelling of EAC with sloughy discharge	Otitis externa
Otalgia, hearing loss, fever, TM erythema and effusion	Otitis media
Erythematous and swollen EAC with black spores	Fungal otitis externa
Severe otalgia, otorrhoea, hearing loss, CN palsy, history of diabetes, systemic illness	Malignant otitis externa
Otalgia, erythema and swelling of the mastoid, pinna protrusion	Mastoiditis
Painless, foul-smelling otorrhoea, hearing loss, aural fullness	Cholesteatoma
Progressive CHL, tinnitus, vertigo, middle-aged female following pregnancy	Otosclerosis
Exposure to cold weather, irregular subcutaneous pinna nodule	Chondrodermatitis nodularis helicis
Tinnitus, vertigo, aural fullness, facial droop. Neurofibromatosis type 2	Acoustic neuroma
Child, recurrent epistaxis, purpuric lesions on tongue and fingers	Hereditary haemorrhagic telangiectasia
Nasal congestion, anosmia, postnasal drip, recurrent rhinosinusitis	Nasal polyps
Smoker with facial pain, unilateral nasal polyps, posterior epistaxis	Nasopharyngeal carcinoma
Spreading erythema, confusion, >48 hours nasal packing	Toxic shock syndrome
Soft, fluctuant, transilluminates, anterior neck lump	Cystic hygroma
Halitosis, regurgitation, palpable neck lump	Pharyngeal pouch
Congenital neck swelling behind sternocleidomastoid	Branchial cyst
Submandibular/parotid pain and swelling when eating	Salivary duct calculi
Toxic child, drooling, stridor, unvaccinated	Epiglottis
Cervical lymphadenopathy, fever, malaise, testicular swelling	Mumps

Continued

Key findings	Diagnoses
Weber's lateralizes to the affected ear, Rinne's negative in the affected ear	Conductive hearing loss
Weber's lateralizes to unaffected ear, Rinne's positive in both ears	Sensorineural hearing loss
Dysphagia, dysarthria, diplopia, dysmetria and downbeat nystagmus	Central vertigo
Vertigo, postural instability, focal neurology, bidirectional nystagmus	Central vertigo
Vertigo, nausea, auditory symptoms, unilateral nystagmus	Peripheral vertigo
Negative head impulse, bidirectional nystagmus, vertical skew	Central vertigo
Positive head impulse, unidirectional nystagmus, absent skew	Peripheral vertigo
Sudden onset vertigo with changes in head position, seconds to minutes, spontaneously resolves, no hearing loss	BPPV
Sudden onset vertigo, minutes to hours, aural fullness, fluctuating hearing loss, tinnitus	Ménière disease
Sudden onset vertigo, hours to days, no hearing loss, preceding URTI	Vestibular neuritis
Sudden onset vertigo, hours to days, hearing loss, fever	Labyrinthitis
Sneezing, nasal congestion, rhinorrhoea, postnasal drip, hypertrophic turbinates, nasal polyps	Allergic rhinitis
Purulent rhinorrhoea, anosmia, facial pain	Rhinosinusitis
Sore throat, tonsillar exudate, pharyngeal erythema, inflamed tonsils	Bacterial tonsillitis
Sore throat, nasal congestion, rhinorrhoea, sneezing and cough. No fever	Viral tonsillitis
Unilateral tonsillar swelling and uvula deviation	Peritonsillar abscess
Pharyngitis, fever, lymphadenopathy, malaise, unwell intimate contact	Infectious mononucleosis
Daytime somnolence, snoring, apnoeic episodes, obesity male	Obstructive sleep apnoea
Vocal hoarseness, dry cough, stridor, fever	Laryngitis
Low-pitched vocal hoarseness, vocal overuse	Vocal cord nodule
Hoarseness >3 weeks in a smoker, dysphagia	Laryngeal cancer
Gradual painless unilateral parotid swelling	Pleomorphic adenoma
Unilateral complete facial droop, ptosis	Bell's palsy
Recent tonsillectomy, dyspnoea	Post tonsillectomy haemorrhage

Chapter 9 Plastics and skin surgery

Key findings	Diagnoses
Vesicular rash, dermatomal distribution	Herpes zoster (shingles)
Bilateral symmetrical flexural scaly lesions	Eczema
Salmon pink plaques on extensor surfaces	Psoriasis
Severe pain, skin erythema, black discolouration, tissue induration, skin emphysema, history of diabetes	Necrotizing fasciitis
Erythema, pain, non-blanching rash over the pressure area	Pressure ulcer
Pink nodule, surface sheen and crust, ulceration with a rolled edge, superficial telangiectasia History of sun exposure	Basal cell carcinoma
Inflamed lesion, everted edges, easy bleeding lesion, history of immunosuppression	Squamous cell carcinoma
Pigmented lesion, asymmetrical, border irregularity, large, recent changes, history of sun exposure	Malignant melanoma
Circumferential burn, severe limb pain, swelling	Compartment syndrome

Key findings	Diagnoses
Collagen deposition, proliferation of scar	Keloid scar
Scar thickening, tightening, reduced ROM	Scar contractures
Skin lump, central punctum, cheesy contents	Epidermal cyst
Subcutaneous lobulated fat mass	Lipoma
Raised, pigmented waxy lesion	Seborrheic keratosis
Hyperkeratotic scaly lesion on sun-exposed site	Actinic keratosis
Rapidly growing, locally destructive, ulcerating lesion, spontaneous regression	Keratoacanthoma
Rapid development of red mass after trauma, bleeds easily and excessively	Pyogenic granuloma
Blackening of the perineal skin, exudation, bullae	Fournier's gangrene
Burn with localized pain and erythema, blanching, rapid CRT	1st-degree burn
Burn with localized pain and erythema, blanching, blisters, slow CRT	2nd-degree burn, superficial partial thickness
Burn with minimal pain, mottled red/white skin, bullae, non-blanching	2nd-degree burn, deep partial thickness
Painless burn, tissue necrosis, black/grey eschar, non-blanching	3rd-degree burn

Chapter 10 Cardiothoracic surgery

Key findings	Diagnoses
Crushing central chest pain radiating to the left arm, neck and jaw	Acute coronary syndrome
Sharp pleuritic chest pain, dyspnoea, tachycardia	Pulmonary embolism
Syncope, angina, dyspnoea, ejection systolic murmur radiating to carotids	Aortic stenosis
Early diastolic murmur in the aortic area	Aortic regurgitation
Dyspnoea, fatigue, palpitations, pan systolic murmur in the mitral area, radiating to the axilla	Mitral regurgitation
Mid systolic murmur loudest in the mitral area	Mitral stenosis
Chest pain, dysphagia, hoarse voice, SVC syndrome	Thoracic aortic aneurysm
Upper limb venous congestion, facial and upper limb flushing and oedema	Superior vena cava syndrome
Ptosis, miosis and anhidrosis	Horner syndrome
Sudden onset, tearing central pain radiating to the neck or jaw, syncope, wide pulse pressure	Aortic dissection
Arachnodactyly, high-arched palate, pectus excavatum	Marfan syndrome
Dyspnoea and orthopnoea, retrosternal chest pain	Pericardial effusion
Hypotension, muffled heart, distended neck veins	Cardiac tamponade
Sudden dyspnoea, sharp stabbing ipsilateral chest pain, reduced breath sounds and chest expansion, hyper-resonant percussion	Pneumothorax
Dyspnoea, stabbing chest pain, haemodynamic instability and tracheal deviation	Tension pneumothorax
SOB, dull basal percussion and reduced breath sounds	Atelectasis
Dyspnoea, cough, weight loss, smoking history	Lung cancer
Lung cancer, nausea, vomiting, muscle cramps, seizures	Paraneoplastic SIADH
Lung cancer, bone stones, abdominal groans	Paraneoplastic PTH

Chapter 11 Perioperative management

Key findings	Diagnoses
Postoperative pyrexia day 1–2	LRTI, atelectasis
Postoperative pyrexia day 3–5	UTI
Postoperative pyrexia day 4–6	VTE
Postoperative pyrexia day 5–7	Surgical site infection

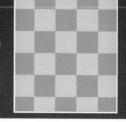

UKMLA Single Best Answer (SBA) questions

Chapter 1 The upper gastrointestinal tract

1. A 28-year-old man has recurrent burning central chest pain with nausea and a metallic taste in his mouth, worse at night or after a large meal. He has mild epigastric tenderness.

   Which is the most likely diagnosis?

   A Gastro-oesophageal reflux disease
   B Oesophageal cancer
   C Peptic ulcer disease
   D Pericarditis
   E Pulmonary embolism

2. A 52-year-old man has intermittent severe pain in his upper abdomen, relieved by eating but returning several hours afterwards and worse at night. He has hypertension and osteoarthritis, managed with ramipril and ibuprofen. There is marked epigastric tenderness.

   Which test is most likely to confirm the diagnosis?

   A Amylase
   B ECG
   C ERCP
   D OGD
   E Urea breath test

3. A 64-year-old man has 3 months of discomfort and pain when swallowing, with coughing, choking and regurgitation of food, and the feeling of food getting stuck. He is fatigued and has lost several kilos of weight without changing his diet. He has type 2 diabetes mellitus, hypercholesterolaemia and GORD, managed with metformin, atorvastatin and omeprazole, has smoked 20 cigarettes a day for 40 years, and drinks 2 bottles of wine a week.

   Which is the most likely diagnosis?

   A Achalasia
   B Hiatus hernia
   C Oesophageal carcinoma
   D Oesophageal stricture
   E Pharyngeal pouch

4. A 32-year-old man has vomited a large volume of fresh red blood three times over the past hour. He feels dizzy and nauseated and appears confused. He is pale, clammy, tender in the epigastrium with marked yellowing of the sclera and cachexic. Digital rectal examination reveals black, tarry stool.

   Which is the most likely diagnosis?

   A Boerhaave syndrome
   B Gastric cancer
   C Mallory Weiss tear
   D Oesophageal varices
   E Peptic ulcer disease

5. A 45-year-old woman has sudden, sharp abdominal pain for 6 hours, that radiates to her right shoulder. She feels nauseated and has vomited twice. Her temperature is 38.1°C, pulse 112 bpm and BP 125/87 mmHg. She has right upper quadrant tenderness, worse on inspiration during palpation.

   Which is the most appropriate initial investigation?

   A Amylase
   B Abdominal CT scan
   C Abdominal ultrasound
   D Endoscopic retrograde cholangiopancreatography
   E Liver function tests

6. A 48-year-old woman has sudden severe upper abdominal pain and nausea, after intermittent sharp pains in her right upper abdomen for 3 weeks. Her temperature is 38.3°C, pulse 119 bpm and BP 105/82 mmHg. She is exquisitely tender in the right upper quadrant, with marked yellowing of the sclera.

   Which is the most likely diagnosis?

   A Ascending cholangitis
   B Acute cholecystitis
   C Biliary colic
   D Hepatitis
   E Pancreatitis

7. A 44-year-old man has sudden, severe pain in his upper abdomen that radiates to the back, with nausea and vomiting. He drinks a bottle of vodka a week. His temperature is 37.8°C, pulse 121 bpm, BP 118/83 mmHg, respiratory rate 32 breaths per minute and oxygen saturation 92% on breathing air. He has diffuse abdominal tenderness with guarding in the epigastrium.

   Which is the most appropriate management?

   A Intravenous antibiotics
   B Intravenous fluids
   C Endoscopic retrograde cholangiopancreatography
   D Oesophagogastroduodenoscopy
   E Terlipressin

8. A 72-year-old man has increased stool frequency for 3 months, with multiple episodes per day, of loose pale stools, with darkening of his urine, fatigue and 5 kilos of unintentional weight loss. He drinks several bottles of wine a week. He appears underweight, with marked yellowing of the sclera, mild epigastric tenderness and a palpable epigastric mass.

   Which is the most likely diagnosis?

   A Cholangiocarcinoma
   B Chronic hepatitis
   C Gallstones
   D Pancreatic cancer
   E Pancreatitis

9. A 31-year-old woman has 3 months of discomfort when swallowing and the feeling of food getting stuck, with involuntary regurgitation of food when she lies down. She has lost over a stone in weight in this period and has had several chest infections recently, treated with oral antibiotics (Fig. 1).

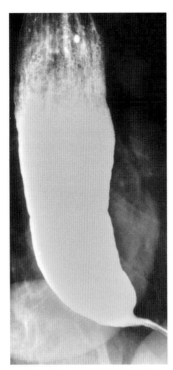

Fig. 1 Barium swallow (From Flint PW et al., *Cummings otolaryngology, head and neck surgery*, 7th Edition. Philadelphia, Elsevier; 2021.)

   Which is the most likely diagnosis?

   A Achalasia
   B Gastroesophageal reflux disease
   C Oesophageal stricture
   D Pharyngeal pouch
   E Plummer-Vinson syndrome

10. A 22-year-old woman has 2 months of burning pain in her upper abdomen that radiates to her chest, with nausea and a metallic taste, worse when eating or lying down. She has mild epigastric tenderness.

    Which is the most appropriate management?

    A Amoxicillin, clarithromycin and omeprazole
    B Bismuth salts
    C Famotidine
    D Lansoprazole
    E Peptac liquid

11. A 44-year-old woman has 6 months of upper abdominal cramping after meals, which can last hours, with nausea. Her abdomen is soft and nontender (Fig. 2).

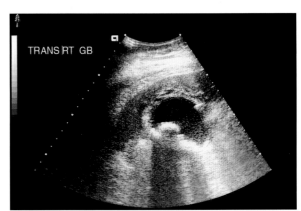

Fig. 2 Abdominal ultrasound (From Acher AW, Kelly KJ, Jarnagin, Weber SM. *Blumgart's Surgery of the Liver, Biliary Tract and Pancreas, 7th Edition*. Elsevier; 2023.)

    Which is the most appropriate treatment?

    A Cholecystectomy
    B Cholecystostomy
    C Endoscopic retrograde cholangiopancreatography
    D Intravenous antibiotics
    E Intravenous fluids

12. A 48-year-old woman has sudden severe pain in her upper abdomen for 6 hours, which radiates to the back, with nausea, vomiting and diarrhoea. She has biliary colic,

managed with over-the-counter analgesia. Her temperature is 38.2°C, pulse 127 bpm and BP 112/86 mmHg. She has exquisite tenderness and guarding in the epigastrium.

Which is the most likely diagnosis?

A Ascending cholangitis
B Acute cholecystitis
C Pancreatitis
D Perforated peptic ulcer
E Pyelonephritis

13. A 48-year-old man has years of constant upper abdominal discomfort, with several episodes of intense, severe pain, with nausea, vomiting and diarrhoea. He has foul diarrhoea up to eight times per day, with fatigue, extreme thirst and a constant need to pass urine. He drinks a bottle of vodka a day. He is unkempt and cachectic, appears jaundiced, with excoriations over his arms and legs. He has diffuse abdominal pain, worse in the epigastrium (Fig. 3).

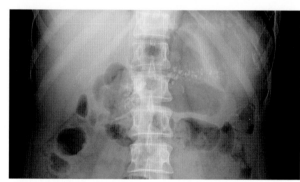

Fig. 3 Abdominal X-ray (From Ravindran R. Chronic pancreatitis. *MPSUR* 2019.)

Which is the most likely diagnosis?

A Biliary colic
B Chronic pancreatitis
C Coeliac disease
D Inflammatory bowel disease
E Irritable bowel syndrome

14. A 42-year-old man has 3 months of burning upper abdominal pain after meals, which lasts for several hours. He has passed several large, foul, black stools in the last few days. He takes over-the-counter ibuprofen for lower back pain, has smoked 20 cigarettes a day for 25 years and drinks a bottle of wine a day. His pulse is 118 bpm and BP 98/62 mmHg. There is exquisite epigastric tenderness, with black stool in the rectum.

Which is the most likely diagnosis?

A Bleeding peptic ulcer
B Dieulafoy lesion
C Gastric cancer
D Mallory Weiss tear
E Oesophageal varices

15. A 48-year-old woman has cramping pain in her upper abdomen after heavy meals which lasts for several hours, with flatulence and indigestion. She has mild right upper quadrant tenderness.

Which is the most likely diagnosis?

A Acute cholecystitis
B Ascending cholangitis
C Biliary colic
D Pancreatitis
E Peptic ulcer disease

16. A 32-year-old man has 4 weeks of burning chest pain radiating to the upper abdomen, with nausea, vomiting and a foul taste, which is worse after meals, when he drinks alcohol, and at night. He has mild epigastric tenderness.

Which is the most appropriate immediate investigation?

A Amylase
B Barium swallow
C Oesophageal manometry
D Oesophagogastroduodenoscopy
E Urea breath test

17. A 52-year-old man has severe upper abdominal pain, fever and malaise, after several months of intermittent colicky pain in his right upper abdomen after meals, with nausea and indigestion. His temperature is 38.3°C, pulse 127 bpm and BP 105/81 mmHg. There is exquisite tenderness in the right upper quadrant and yellowing of the sclera.

Which is the most appropriate treatment?

A Cholecystectomy
B Endoscopic retrograde cholangiopancreatography
C Extracorporeal shockwave lithotripsy
D Oesophagogastroduodenoscopy
E Percutaneous transhepatic cholangiogram

18. A 42-year-old man has sudden severe upper abdominal pain after an alcoholic binge, which radiates to the back, with severe nausea and vomiting. He drinks several bottles of whiskey a week. His temperature is 37.9°C, pulse 115 bpm and BP 109/72 mmHg. He has severe epigastric

tenderness, jaundice and excoriations over the abdomen and upper arms.

Which test is most likely to confirm the diagnosis?

A Abdominal ultrasound
B Amylase
C Endoscopic retrograde cholangiopancreatography
D Lipase
E Oesophagogastroduodenoscopy

19. A 62-year-old woman has 1 month of discomfort when swallowing, with several episodes of choking and regurgitation, following many years of intermittent heartburn and nausea after meals. She has lost several kilos of weight in the past month due to her symptoms.

Which is the most likely diagnosis?

A Achalasia
B Diffuse oesophageal spasm
C Gastroesophageal reflux disease
D Oesophageal carcinoma
E Oesophageal stricture

20. A 22-year-old man has nausea, vomiting and diarrhoea for 1 day, with over 20 episodes of vomiting, and streaks of bright red blood in the most recent vomit. He feels fatigued and feverish. Several members of his family are also unwell. His temperature is 38.2°C, pulse 82 bpm and BP 123/82 mmHg.

Which is the most likely diagnosis?

A Boerhaave syndrome
B Bleeding peptic ulcer
C Mallory Weiss tear
D Oesophagitis
E Oesophageal varices

21. A 42-year-old woman has 2 months of intermittent upper abdominal cramping after meals, which lasts several hours, with nausea, heartburn, increased stool frequency and darkening of her urine. She has mild right upper quadrant tenderness, yellowing of the sclera and excoriations over the upper arms (Fig. 4).

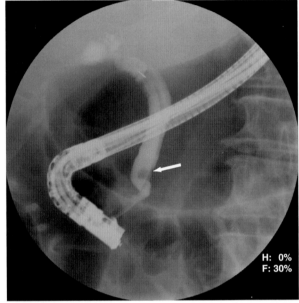

H: 0%
F: 30%

Fig. 4 Endoscopic retrograde cholangiopancreatography (From Townsend CM et al., *Sabiston textbook of surgery*. 21st Edition. St Louis, Elsevier; 2022.)

Which is the most likely diagnosis?

A Acute cholecystitis
B Ascending cholangitis
C Biliary colic
D Cholelithiasis
E Choledocholithiasis

22. A 42-year-old man vomited a large volume of fresh blood 30 minutes ago and has vomited 3 times since, with approximately two cups of bright red blood each time. His temperature is 37.2°C, pulse 128 bpm and BP 82/61 mmHg. He is disorientated, cachectic, has yellow skin discolouration and excoriations and dilated tortuous veins over the abdomen, with diffuse abdominal guarding and tenderness.

Which is the most appropriate next step?

A Intravenous antibiotics
B Intravenous fluids
C Intravenous PPI
D Oesophagogastroduodenoscopy
E Terlipressin

23. A 52-year-old man has intermittent, sudden chest pain while eating, with the feeling of food getting stuck, and occasional regurgitation. He has GORD, managed with omeprazole (Fig. 5).

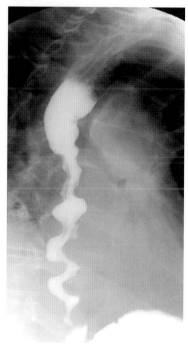

Fig. 5 Barium swallow (From Maher M et al., *Grainger & Allison's Diagnostic Radiology: Abdominal Imaging,* 6th Edition. Elsevier; 2016.)

Which is the most appropriate treatment?

A Heller's cardiomyotomy
B High dose PPI
C Metoclopramide
D Surgical resection
E Verapamil

24. A 48-year-old woman has sudden severe upper abdominal pain, with nausea and indigestion, after several months of intermittent upper abdominal discomfort after meals. She has type 2 diabetes mellitus, managed with metformin. Her temperature is 38.2°C, pulse 115 bpm and BP 92/73 mmHg. She has right upper quadrant tenderness, worse on inspiration during palpation.

Which is the most appropriate next step?

A Cholecystectomy
B Cholecystostomy
C Endoscopic retrograde cholangiopancreatography

D Intravenous antibiotics
E Intravenous fluids

25. A 72-year-old woman has 2 episodes of brown, granular vomit, after several days of intermittent epigastric discomfort and passing several large, foul, black stools. She has osteoarthritis, managed with ibuprofen. She appears pale and slightly disoriented. Her pulse is 119 bpm and BP 92/62 mmHg. She has epigastric tenderness.

Which is the most appropriate definitive treatment?

A Endoscopic retrograde cholangiopancreatography
B Intravenous antibiotics
C Intravenous omeprazole
D Oesophagogastroduodenoscopy
E Terlipressin

Chapter 2 The lower gastrointestinal tract

1. A 14-year-old girl has central aching abdominal pain for 12 hours which has progressed to stabbing, severe pain on the lower right-hand side, with nausea, vomiting and loss of appetite. Her temperature is 37.8°C.

Which is most likely to confirm the diagnosis?

A Abdominal ultrasound
B Faecal calprotectin
C Laparoscopic appendectomy
D Pregnancy test
E Transvaginal ultrasound

2. A 54-year-old man has sudden, severe, generalized abdominal pain for 2 hours, with nausea, vomiting, fever and rigors. He has chronic liver disease and chronic pancreatitis and is currently drinking two bottles of vodka a week. He has abdominal rigidity, distension and rebound tenderness and marked yellowing of the sclera.

Which is the most likely diagnosis?

A Appendicitis
B Ascending cholangitis
C Bowel perforation
D Pancreatitis
E Spontaneous bacterial peritonitis

3. A 32-year-old woman has cramping abdominal pain and increased stool frequency for 3 days, which has progressed to severe, generalized abdominal pain, profuse diarrhoea, nausea and vomiting and fever. She has Crohn disease, managed with azathioprine. Her temperature is 37.9°C, pulse 113 bpm and BP 105/85 mmHg. She has

abdominal distention, guarding and diffuse abdominal tenderness.

Which is the most appropriate next step?

A Buscopan
B Intravenous antibiotics
C Intravenous hydrocortisone
D Laparoscopic bowel resection
E Oral mesalazine

4. An 84-year-old woman has 72 hours of generalized abdominal pain, with nausea, vomiting and loss of appetite. She cannot remember the last time she opened her bowels. Her pulse is 98 bpm and BP 105/86 mmHg. She has dry mucous membranes and reduced skin turgor, with diffuse abdominal distention and tenderness and hyperactive, high-pitched bowel sounds.

Which is most likely to confirm the diagnosis?

A Abdominal X-ray
B Barium swallow
C Chest X-ray
D Colonoscopy
E CT abdomen/pelvis

5. A 62-year-old man has sudden severe abdominal pain, with profuse bloody diarrhoea, fever, nausea and vomiting. His temperature is 38.1°C, pulse 102 bpm and irregularly irregular and BP 90/65 mmHg. His abdomen is distended, rigid, with rebound tenderness.

Which is the most likely diagnosis?

A Acute mesenteric ischaemia
B Angiodysplasia
C Diverticular bleed
D Inflammatory bowel disease
E Ruptured abdominal aortic aneurysm

6. A 64-year-old woman has 6 months of intermittent left lower abdominal pain, with mild nausea. She typically opens her bowels once or twice a week. She has hypertension, managed with amlodipine, and has smoked 10 cigarettes a day for 30 years. She has mild tenderness in the left lower quadrant (Fig. 6).

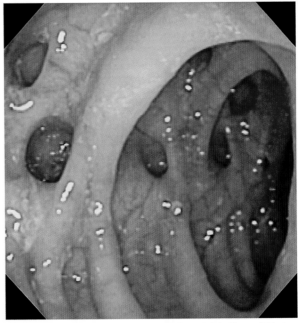

Fig. 6 Colonoscopy (From Rubin DT, Brandt LJ, Chung RT, et al., *Sleisenger y Fordtran. Enfermedades digestivas y hepáticas: Fisiopatología, diagnóstico y tratamiento*, 11.ª Edición. Elsevier; 2022.)

Which is the most appropriate management?

A Bowel rest
B Corticosteroids
C Elective colectomy
D Oral antibiotics
E Lifestyle advice

7. A 28-year-old man has 1 month of increased stool frequency up to 8 times a day of loose, watery stool, with urgency and fresh red blood in the stool. He has generalized abdominal pain relieved on opening his bowels. He has recently stopped smoking.

Which test is most likely to confirm the diagnosis?

A Antitissue-transglutaminase antibodies
B Colonoscopy
C ESR
D Faecal calprotectin
E Stool MC&S

8. A 35-year-old woman has 1 week of bright red blood when she wipes after opening her bowels and anal itch (Fig. 7). She typically opens her bowels twice a week.

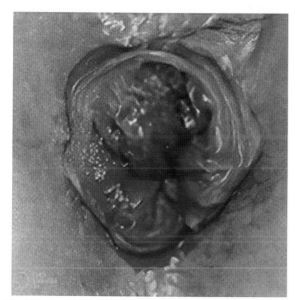

Fig. 7 Perineal exam (From Abrahams PH et al., *Abrahams' and McMinn's Clinical Atlas of Human Anatomy*, 8th Edition. Elsevier; 2020.)

Which is the most likely diagnosis?

A   Anal fissures
B   Anal fistula
C   Haemorrhoids
D   Rectal prolapse
E   Ulcerative colitis

9. A 65-year-old man has 3 months of fatigue, dizziness, occasional breathlessness and chest tightness. He has occasional mild abdominal discomfort and episodes of loose stool. He has hypercholesterolaemia, managed with atorvastatin. He has conjunctival pallor.

Investigations:

Hb 97 g/dL (130–180)

Which is the most appropriate next step?

A   Chest X-ray
B   Colonoscopy
C   FIT test
D   Stool MC&S
E   Thyroid function tests

10. A 28-year-old woman has 3 days of severe anal pain and pruritis, with bloody anal discharge, malaise, fever and rigors. She has Crohn's disease, managed with azathioprine. She has perianal discharge, erythema of the anal skin and a palpable perianal mass.

Which is the most appropriate management?

A   Analgesia

B   Fistulotomy
C   Incision and drainage
D   Laxatives
E   Topical hydrocortisone

11. A 32-year-old man has 3 days of bloody diarrhoea, up to 8 episodes a day, with abdominal pain, nausea and vomiting and malaise. He has ulcerative colitis, managed with mesalazine. His temperature is 38.1°C, pulse 112 bpm and BP 98/64 mmHg. He has dry mucous membranes and reduced skin turgor. His abdomen is distended, with hyperactive bowel sounds (Fig. 8).

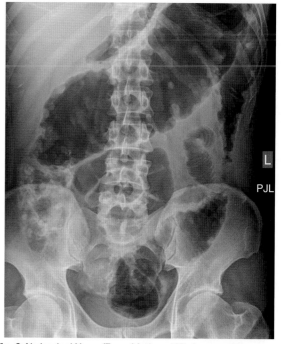

Fig. 8 Abdominal X-ray (From Mathew KG, Aggarwal P. *Medicine: Prep Manual for Undergraduates*, 7th Edition. Elsevier; 2023.)

Which is the most likely diagnosis?

A   Diverticulitis
B   Large bowel obstruction
C   Mesenteric ischaemia
D   Paralytic ileus
E   Toxic megacolon

12. A 54-year-old man has 4 months of abdominal pain after eating, that lasts several hours, with nausea, bloating and occasional episodes of diarrhoea, with 5 kilos of weight loss. He has hypertension and high cholesterol, managed

with ramipril and atorvastatin. He has smoked 20 cigarettes a day for 30 years.

Which is the most likely diagnosis?

A   Chronic mesenteric ischaemia
B   Coeliac disease
C   Diverticular disease
D   Gallstones
E   Gastric ulcer

13. A 72-year-old woman has colicky abdominal pain for 4 days, with nausea, abdominal distention and constipation. She has had several similar, milder episodes of abdominal pain for the last 3 months which have resolved. Her pulse is 105 bpm and BP 115/87 mmHg. She has diffuse abdominal tenderness, with tympanic percussion, and absent bowel sounds (Fig. 9).

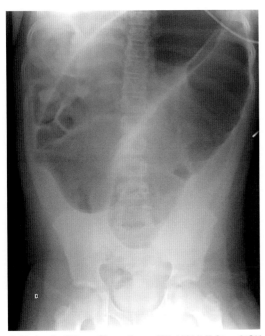

Fig. 9 Abdominal X-ray (From Omar AM. *USMLE Step 2 CK Plus*. Elsevier; 2023.)

Which is the most appropriate next step?

A   Emergency laparotomy
B   Intravenous antibiotics
C   Laxatives
D   Nasogastric tube and IV fluids
E   Rigid sigmoidoscopy

14. A 67-year-old woman has passed 3 large stools over the past 3 hours, which are black, foul and tarry in

consistency. She has aortic stenosis and atrial fibrillation, managed with bisoprolol and apixaban. Her pulse is 102 bpm and BP 115/85 mmHg. She has dark red blood per rectum.

Which test is most likely to confirm the diagnosis?

A   Abdominal X-ray
B   Anoscopy
C   Colonoscopy
D   CT angiography
E   Endoscopy

15. A 23-year-old woman has 6 months of crampy abdominal pain relieved by opening her bowels, with abdominal bloating, flatulent dyspepsia, with intermittent diarrhoea and constipation. She has anxiety, managed with sertraline. Her abdomen is soft and nontender.

What is the most likely diagnosis?

A   Coeliac disease
B   Crohn's disease
C   Hyperthyroidism
D   Irritable bowel syndrome
E   Pancreatic insufficiency

16. A 62-year-old man has a positive FIT test. He feels otherwise well. He has high cholesterol, managed with atorvastatin. His abdomen is soft and non-tender.

Which is the most appropriate next step?

A   Abdominal X-ray
B   Digital rectal exam
C   Full blood count
D   Colonoscopy
E   CT abdomen

17. A 62-year-old woman has gradually worsening left abdominal pain for 24 hours, with nausea, vomiting and fever. She typically opens her bowels once a week. She has hypothyroidism, managed with levothyroxine. Her temperature is 37.8°C, pulse 87 bpm and BP 107/79 mmHg. She has mild tenderness in the left lower quadrant, with a palpable mass.

Which test is most likely to confirm the diagnosis?

A   Abdominal ultrasound
B   Abdominal X-ray
C   Colonoscopy
D   CT abdomen and pelvis
E   Stool MC&S

18. A 52-year-old man has sudden severe abdominal pain and profuse bloody diarrhoea, with nausea and vomiting. He has atrial fibrillation, managed with apixaban and bisoprolol. His temperature is 38.1°C, pulse 127 bpm and

BP 90/65 mmHg. He has diffuse abdominal tenderness, guarding and rigidity (Fig. 10).

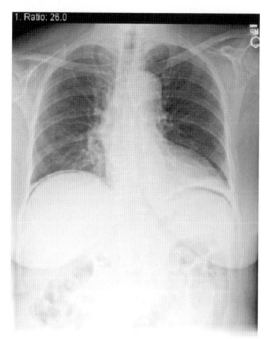

Fig. 10 Chest X-ray (From Brakenridge S et al., *Textbook of Critical Care*, 8th Edition. Elsevier; 2024.)

Which is the most appropriate definitive management?

A Angioplasty and stenting
B Bowel rest
C Intravenous antibiotics
D Intravenous fluids and nasogastric tube
E Urgent laparotomy

19. A 37-year-old woman has diarrhoea up to 8 times a day, with pale, greasy stools, nausea and vomiting and loss of appetite. She was discharged from hospital 3 weeks previously following partial small bowel resection for a Crohn's flare. She takes regular infliximab to maintain remission. She appears underweight, with conjunctival pallor and dry mucous membranes.

    Which is the most likely diagnosis?

    A Chronic mesenteric ischaemia
    B Coeliac disease
    C Lactose intolerance
    D Pancreatic insufficiency
    E Short bowel syndrome

20. A 28-year-old man has sudden intense pain, with redness and watery discharge and blurring of his vision (Fig. 11). He has ulcerative colitis, managed with sulphasalazine.

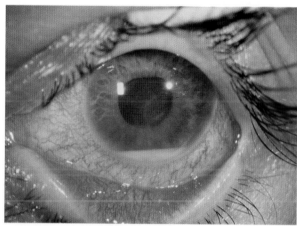

Fig. 11 Left eye (From Duker JS, Read RW, Yanoff M. *Ophthalmology*, 6th Edition. Elsevier; 2023.)

Which is the most likely diagnosis?

A Angle-closure glaucoma
B Anterior uveitis
C Blepharitis
D Episcleritis
E Scleritis

Chapter 3 The anterior abdominal wall

1. A 28-year-old man has a painless right groin lump which appeared suddenly after moving some heavy boxes. There is a soft groin swelling superomedial to the pubic tubercle, which is reducible, does not transilluminate and enlarges on coughing.

    Which is the likely diagnosis?

    A Direct inguinal hernia
    B Femoral hernia
    C Hydrocele
    D Indirect inguinal hernia
    E Testicular torsion

2. A 54-year-old man has 2 days of worsening lower abdominal pain, which is now severe and constant with nausea, vomiting and inability to open his bowels, after 1 month of a painless left groin lump. He has diffuse abdominal tenderness and distention, with a tender mass in the left lower quadrant and absent bowel sounds.

Which is the most appropriate definitive management?

A   Elective surgical repair

B   Emergency surgical repair

C   Endoscopic decompression

D   Nasogastric tube and intravenous fluids

E   Watchful waiting

3. A 42-year-old man has severe upper abdominal pain and bruising across the chest and abdomen after a road traffic accident. His pulse is 130 bpm, BP 128/78 mmHg, respiratory rate 42 breaths per minute and oxygen saturation 86% on breathing air. He has absent breath sounds on the left chest with audible bowel sounds in the left lower zone (Fig. 12).

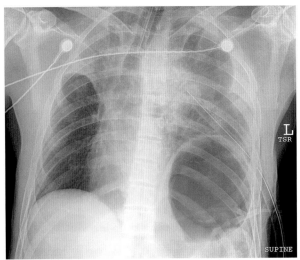

Fig. 12 Chest X-ray (From Evers BM, Carmichael SP II, Mattox KL. *Sabiston Textbook of Surgery: The Biological Basis of Modern Surgical Practice*, 21st Edition. Elsevier; 2022.)

Which is the most likely diagnosis?

A   Acute respiratory distress syndrome

B   Diaphragmatic hernia

C   Fat emboli

D   Pleural effusion

E   Tension pneumothorax

4. An 84-year-old man is admitted following a fall. A stoma bag is present in the left iliac fossa (Fig. 13).

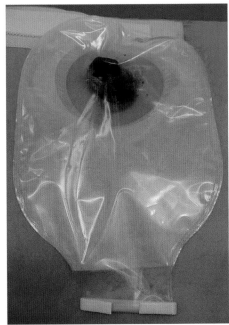

Fig. 13 (From Biers SM, Arulampalam THA, Quick CRG. *Essential Surgery: Problems, Diagnosis and Management*, 6th Edition. Elsevier; 2020.)

Which is the most likely stoma type?

A   Colostomy

B   Gastrostomy

C   Ileostomy

D   Nephrostomy

E   Urostomy

5. An 82-year-old woman has intermittent left-sided groin swelling for several weeks, with mild lower abdominal pain and urinary frequency. She has COPD and stress incontinence, managed with salbutamol inhalers and duloxetine. She had a previous hysterectomy (Fig. 14).

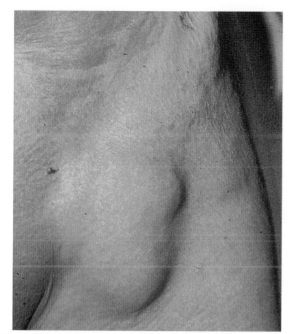

Fig. 14 Groin exam (From Hagen-Ansert SL *Textbook of Diagnostic Sonography*, 7th Edition. Elsevier; 2012.)

Which is the most likely diagnosis?

A Femoral hernia
B Inguinal hernia
C Lymphadenopathy
D Psoas abscess
E Saphena varix

Chapter 4 Endocrine surgery

1. A 60-year-old man has a small, painless neck lump for 1 week. There is a 4 × 2 cm lump to the left of the midline in the lower neck, that is firm, smooth and nontender, which moves on swallowing, but not on tongue protrusion.

    Which is the most likely diagnosis?

    A Branchial cyst
    B Carotid artery aneurysm
    C Reactive lymphadenopathy
    D Thyroglossal cyst
    E Thyroid nodule

2. A 28-year-old man has several weeks of insatiable thirst and increased urinary frequency, with fatigue, weakness and episodes of dizziness. He had a minor head injury after a road traffic accident 3 weeks ago. He appears dehydrated, with dry mucous membranes and reduced skin turgor.

Which test is most likely to confirm the diagnosis?

A Capillary blood glucose
B Paired urine and serum osmolality
C Parathyroid hormone
D Urinary 5-HIAA
E Water deprivation test

3. A 23-year-old woman has 2 weeks of frequent intense muscle cramps in her limbs, with pins and needles and muscle twitching after a subtotal thyroidectomy for Grave disease. She has widespread fasciculations at rest and perioral numbness.

    Which is the most appropriate treatment?

    A Insulin and dextrose
    B Intravenous bisphosphonates
    C Intravenous calcium gluconate
    D Intravenous fluids
    E Oral calcium and vitamin D

4. A 65-year-old man has 3 months of increasing difficulty swallowing with nausea, dyspepsia, painful regurgitation and 5 kilos of weight loss, after several years of indigestion symptoms managed with over-the-counter antacids. He is pale, with a firm swelling in the left supraclavicular fossa and mild epigastric tenderness.

    Which is the most likely diagnosis?

    A Gastric cancer
    B Lymphoma
    C Pharyngeal pouch
    D Subclavian aneurysm
    E Thymoma

5. A 70-year-old woman has 2 months of an enlarging lump in the front and middle of her neck, with a hoarse voice, difficulty swallowing, cough productive of blood-stained sputum, with fatigue and appetite loss. She appears cachectic, with audible stridor and a large hard mass in the lower anterior aspect of the neck.

    Which is the most appropriate next step?

    A Thyroid biopsy
    B Thyroid function test
    C Thyroid ultrasound
    D Two-week wait referral
    E Urgent hospital referral

6. A 38-year-old woman 2 hours post total thyroidectomy for papillary thyroid cancer becomes breathless. Her respiratory rate is 32 breaths per minute and oxygen saturation 88% on breathing air. There is an audible stridor and marked swelling around the surgical wound.

Which is the most likely diagnosis?

A   Anaphylaxis

B   Immediate haematoma

C   Laryngospasm

D   Postextubation stridor

E   Recurrent laryngeal nerve injury

7. A 28-year-old man has 1 month of severe daily headaches, with nausea, blurred vision, fatigue, widespread muscle weakness and cramps, and increased muscle weakness and cramps and increased urinary frequency and thirst. His pulse is 87 bpm and BP 220/135 mmHg (Fig. 15).

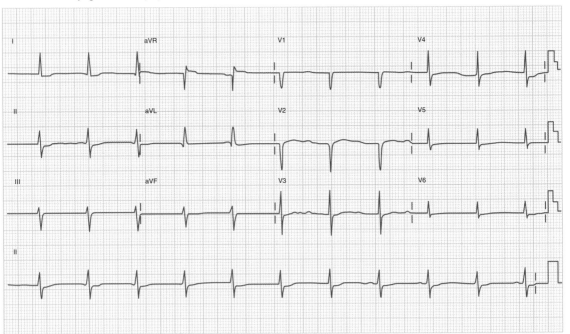

Fig. 15 ECG (With permission from Hammond K., Wilson M, Sanche S, Wilson TW. *Cocktail paralysis. The American Journal of Medicine.* Elsevier; 2009.)

Which is the most appropriate next step?

A   Intravenous potassium chloride

B   Percutaneous renal artery angioplasty

C   Pituitary surgery

D   Spironolactone

E   Unilateral adrenalectomy

8. A 32-year-old woman has 3 months of nausea, with constipation, increased urinary frequency and fatigue. She has dry mucous membranes and reduced skin turgor, with abdominal distention and hard stool in the rectum.

Which is the most likely cause?

A   Adrenal insufficiency

B   Hypercalcaemia of malignancy

C   Osteomalacia

D   Parathyroid adenoma

E   Renal osteodystrophy

9. A 64-year-old woman has 1 month of increasing discomfort when swallowing, with a persistent cough, breathlessness, hoarse voice, occasional central chest pain, fatigue and 5 kilos of unintentional weight loss. She has myasthenia gravis, managed with pyridostigmine. There is swelling of the upper limbs and face, and distended veins over the neck and chest.

What is the most likely diagnosis?

A   Laryngeal carcinoma

B   Lymphoma

C   Sarcoidosis

D   Thymoma

E   Thyroid carcinoma

10. A 28-year-old man has 3 days of a constant, severe headache, with nausea, vomiting, blurred vision and palpitations. His temperature is 37.8°C, pulse 137 bpm and BP 223/147 mmHg. He is sweaty and tremulous (Fig. 16).

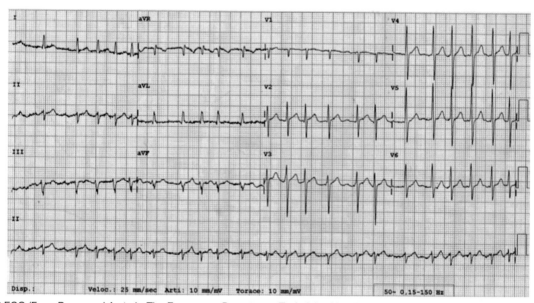

Fig. 16 ECG (From Pourmand A et al., *The Emergency Department Technician Handbook*. Elsevier; 2024.)

Which test is most likely to confirm the diagnosis?

A 24-hour urinary catecholamines
B Blood renin/aldosterone ratio
C Thyroid function tests
D Urinary 5-HIAA
E Urinary free cortisol

Chapter 5 Breast surgery

1. A 32-year-old woman 3 weeks postpartum has 2 days of left breast pain, with redness, swelling and pain when breastfeeding. Both she and her baby have been well thus far. Her temperature is 37.7°C. The left breast is tender and warm to touch, with milky nipple discharge.

   Which is the most likely diagnosis?

   A Breast abscess
   B Cyclical mastalgia
   C Duct ectasia
   D Inflammatory breast cancer
   E Mastitis

2. A 54-year-old woman has 2 weeks of painless right breast lump. There is a 3 cm lump in the upper outer quadrant of the right breast, which is firm and nonmobile, with mild puckering of the surrounding skin.

   Which is the most appropriate next step?

   A Breast biopsy
   B Breast MRI
   C Breast ultrasound

D Fine needle aspiration
E Mammogram

3. A 72-year-old woman is drowsy after sudden loss of consciousness with symmetrical twitching of the upper limbs and loss of continence for 2 minutes, which spontaneously terminated. She had a mastectomy 2 years ago for breast cancer.

   Which is the most likely diagnosis?

   A Alcohol withdrawal
   B Brain metastasis
   C Epilepsy
   D Hypoglycaemia
   E Meningitis

4. An 84-year-old woman has a right breast lump.

   Investigations:

   Core needle biopsy: ER/PR –ve, HER2+ve adenocarcinoma

   Following mastectomy with sentinel lymph node biopsy her tumour is staged as T2N0M0.

   Which medication should be added to her management?

   A Fulvestrant
   B Goserelin
   C Herceptin
   D Tamoxifen
   E Letrozole

5. A 62-year-old woman has 1 week of worsening right breast pain, with skin redness and dimpling, and blood-stained nipple discharge. The right breast is erythematous, swollen and tender (Fig. 17).

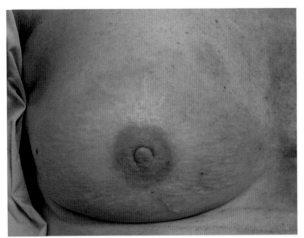

Fig. 17 Breast exam (From Dundas K et al., *Macleod's Clinical Examination*, 15th Edition. Elsevier; 2024.)

Which is the most likely diagnosis?

A Breast abscess
B Cellulitis
C Inflammatory breast cancer
D Mastitis
E Paget's disease of the breast

6. A 23-year-old woman has 6 months of bilateral breast aching every month, with breast swelling and fatigue, which lasts for several days before resolving, with mood fluctuations and headaches. Both breasts are mildly tender in the upper outer quadrant.

Which is the most appropriate treatment?

A Analgesia and supportive bra
B Breast aspiration
C Duct excision
D Flucloxacillin
E Oral contraceptives

7. A 28-year-old woman 6 weeks postpartum has 1 week of right breast pain and inability to breast feed. Both she and her baby are otherwise well. Her temperature is 38.1°C, pulse 101 bpm and BP 105/86 mmHg. The right breast is exquisitely tender, with a fluctuant mass in the periareolar area, and purulent nipple discharge.

Which is the most appropriate treatment?

A Antipyretics and analgesia
B Duct excision

C Evening primrose oil
D Fine needle aspiration
E Warm and cold compresses

8. A 54-year-old woman has 3 weeks of a painless rash on the right nipple which is spreading across her breast, with itch and blood-tinged nipple discharge (Fig. 18).

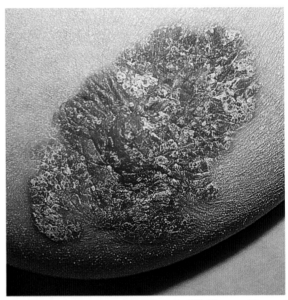

Fig. 18 Breast exam (From Habif T et al., *Skin Disease: Diagnosis and Treatment,* 1st South Asia Edition. Elsevier; 2018.)

Which is the most likely diagnosis?

A Inflammatory breast cancer
B Mastitis
C Mamillary eczema
D Nipple candidiasis
E Paget disease of the breast

9. A 27-year-old woman has 2 weeks of mildly tender multiple lumps in both breasts, with clear nipple discharge. There are two lumps in the right breast and three in the left, all 2 to 3 cm in diameter, which are mobile and mild tender.

Which is the most appropriate treatment?

A Analgesia and supportive bra
B Antibiotics
C Evening primrose oil
D Lump excision
E Warm and cold compresses

10. A 27-year-old woman has 1 week of a mildly tender small lump in her right breast. There is a 3 cm soft lump in the lower right quadrant of the right breast, that is fluctuant and mobile.

Which is the most appropriate investigation?

A Breast ultrasound
B Excisional biopsy
C Fine needle aspiration
D Mammogram
E Punch biopsy

Chapter 6 Vascular surgery

1. A 63-year-old woman has 2 days of worsening right calf pain, with swelling, heaviness and redness and warmth to the skin after a long-haul flight (Fig. 19). She is having increasing difficulty mobilizing due to the pain. She has smoked 10 cigarettes a day for 30 years.

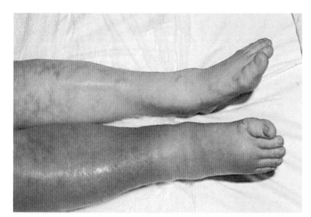

Fig. 19 Lower limbs (From Lewis SM. *Medical-surgical nursing: assessment and management of clinical problems*, 8th Edition. St. Louis, Mosby; 2011.)

Which is the most appropriate treatment?

A Analgesia
B Apixaban
C Cetraben cream
D Flucloxacillin
E Heparin infusion

2. A 68-year-old man has 1 month of constant aching pain in his lower back. He has hypertension and high cholesterol, managed with amlodipine and atorvastatin, and has smoked 30 cigarettes a day for 40 years. He has central lower back pain and mild umbilical tenderness, with an audible abdominal bruit.

Which test is most likely to confirm the diagnosis?

A Abdominal ultrasound
B Abdominal X-ray
C Bladder scan
D CT KUB
E Lumbosacral MRI

3. An 82-year-old woman is delirious following a fall. Her pulse is 56 bpm and BP 98/72 mmHg. She is cachexic and unkempt. She has a painless sloughy lesion on the lateral aspect of the left ankle, with surrounding erythema (Fig. 20).

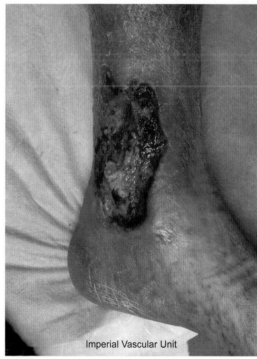

Imperial Vascular Unit

Fig. 20 (From Kinross J, Rasheed S, Chaudry MA. *Clinical Surgery*, 4th Edition. Elsevier; 2023.)

Which is the most likely diagnosis?

A Arterial ulcer
B Diabetic ulcer
C Neuropathic ulcer
D Pressure ulcer
E Venous ulcer

4. A 74-year-old man has 2 years of worsening right calf pain, initially on exertion but now a constant aching pain, worse at night. He has smoked 30 cigarettes a day for 50 years. There is a large, well-defined deep ulcer at the base of the first metatarsal, with grey-black discolouration of the toes and foot and absent pedal pulses.

Which is the most appropriate treatment?

A Amputation

B Fasciotomy

C Intravenous antibiotics

D Surgical debridement

E Thrombolysis

5. A 54-year-old man has 6 months of cramping pain in his right calf when walking, which is worse uphill, and relieved by rest. The right leg is unaffected. He has type 2 diabetes mellitus, managed with metformin, and has smoked 20 cigarettes a day for 30 years. His calves are soft, with palpable pedal pulses.

Which is the most likely diagnosis?

A Chronic compartment syndrome

B Chronic venous insufficiency

C Critical limb ischaemia

D Intermittent claudication

E Spinal stenosis

6. A 64-year-old man has sudden severe abdominal pain and collapses. His pulse is 120 bpm and BP 80/65 mmHg. There is severe abdominal tenderness with a pulsatile abdominal mass.

Which is the most appropriate next step?

A Endovascular aneurysm repair

B High-flow nasal oxygen

C Intravenous antibiotics

D Intravenous fluids

E Open surgical repair

7. A 63-year-old man has bilateral cramping leg pain when walking, relieved by rest. He has hypertension, managed with amlodipine and losartan, drinks a bottle of wine a week, and has smoked 10 cigarettes a day for 40 years. His legs are soft, with palpable pedal pulses.

Investigations:

ABPI: 0.8 in the left leg and 0.7 in the right.

Which medication should be added to his management?

A Apixaban

B Aspirin

C Clopidogrel

D Dabigatran

E Unfractionated heparin

8. A 62-year-old man has sudden severe pain in his right leg, with pins and needles and inability to weight bear. He has atrial fibrillation, managed with apixaban and bisoprolol. His right calf is pale and cold, with absent pedal pulses.

Which is the most likely diagnosis?

A Acute limb ischaemia

B Critical limb ischaemia

C Deep vein thrombosis

D Intermittent claudication

E Venous claudication

9. A 68-year-old man has abdominal aortic aneurysm screening. He has smoked 20 cigarettes a day for 20 years. His abdomen is soft, with no masses or audible bruits.

Investigations:

ABPI 0.9 in both legs.

Abdominal ultrasound: aortic diameter of 5.8 cm, with no evidence of thrombus or dissection.

Which is the most appropriate treatment?

A Discharge without follow-up.

B Endovascular aneurysm repair

C Open surgical repair

D Structured exercise therapy

E Surveillance US in 6 months

10. A 52-year-old woman has 2 hours of sharp right chest pain, worse on inspiration, with breathlessness, nonproductive cough and palpitations. Her pulse is 110 bpm and BP 125/82 mmHg. Her chest is clear and calves are soft and non-tender.

Which test is most likely to confirm the diagnosis?

A Chest X-ray

B CTPA

C D-dimer

D ECG

E VQ scan

11. A 64-year-old woman has 6 months of bilateral lower leg cramping, itching and swelling, worse in heat and after long periods of standing, relieved by rest and leg elevation (Fig. 21).

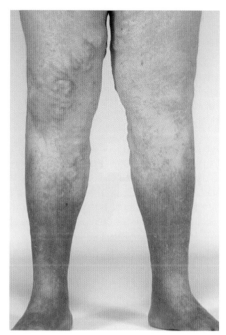

Fig. 21 Lower limbs (From Loscalzo J, et al., *Vascular Medicine: A Companion to Braunwald's Heart Disease*, 2nd Edition. Elsevier; 2013.)

Which is the most likely diagnosis?

A Cellulitis
B Chronic venous insufficiency
C Lymphoedema
D Superficial thrombophlebitis
E Telangiectasis

12. A 63-year-old man has 6 months of cramping pain in his left calf, initially on exertion but now constant, worst at night. He has hypertension and high cholesterol, managed with amlodipine, ramipril and atorvastatin, and has smoked 20 cigarettes a day for 40 years. His left leg is tender, cool and pale. The posterior tibial pulse is diminished and the dorsalis pedis pulse is absent.

    Which is the most appropriate next step?

    A CT angiography
    B Digital subtraction angiography
    C Duplex ultrasound
    D MR angiography
    E Transcutaneous oximetry

13. A 54-year-old woman has 3 months of worsening lower limb swelling, with aching, itching and difficulty mobilizing due to the weight of her legs. She had a hysterectomy with radical lymph node dissection for endometrial cancer 6 months ago. There is bilateral firm swelling of the lower legs (Fig. 22).

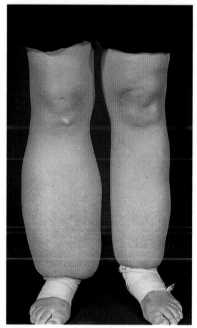

Fig. 22 Swelling of the lower legs (From Shiland BJ, Zenith. *Medical Assistant: Cardiopulmonary Systems, Vital Signs, Electrocardiography and CPR—Module D*, 2nd Edition. Elsevier; 2016.)

Which is the most likely diagnosis?

A Cellulitis
B Chronic venous insufficiency
C Deep vein thrombosis
D Lipoedema
E Lymphoedema

14. A 64-year-old woman has 1 year of leg swelling, with aching pain and itch. She has hypertension, managed with amlodipine. She has bilateral oedema to the knees, with brown calf discolouration and dilated superficial veins.

    Which is the most appropriate treatment?

    A Compression bandages
    B Emollients
    C Phlebotonic supplements
    D Topical steroids
    E Vein ligation

15. A 63-year-old man is referred for structured exercise therapy following an ABPI of 0.6. He has type 2 diabetes mellitus and peripheral arterial disease, managed with metformin, clopidogrel and atorvastatin, drinks a crate of beers a week, and has smoked 20 cigarettes a day for the past 30 years. His BMI is 38 kg/m^2.

Which is the most important additional treatment step?

A Alcohol reduction

B Compression bandaging

C Smoking cessation

D Supportive footwear

E Weight loss

Chapter 7 Urology

1. A 70-year-old man has several months of difficulty initiating his urinary stream, poor flow and terminal dribbling, with nocturia and a feeling of incomplete emptying. He has type 2 diabetes mellitus and hypertension, managed with metformin, gliclazide and ramipril. His abdomen is soft and nontender. He has an enlarged, firm, smooth prostate.

   Which is the most appropriate treatment?

   A Levofloxacin

   B Mirabegron

   C Oxybutynin

   D Tamsulosin

   E Trimethoprim

2. A 72-year-old man has 1 month of intermittent blood in his urine, with increased urinary frequency, urgency and nocturia, with fatigue and 3 kilos of weight loss. He has hypertension and atrial fibrillation, managed with amlodipine, bisoprolol and apixaban, and has smoked 30 cigarettes a day for 40 years. He appears pale. He has a distended but soft abdomen, with pitting oedema to the shins.

   Which is the most likely diagnosis?

   A Bladder cancer

   B Kidney stones

   C Prostatitis

   D Urethral clot

   E Urinary tract infection

3. A 40-year-old woman has 3 months of involuntary urinary leakage when coughing or sneezing, with urinary frequency and nocturia. She has had 3 vaginal deliveries with a second-degree perineal tear after the third delivery.

   Which is the most appropriate next step?

   A Bladder retraining

   B Colposuspension

   C Duloxetine

   D Oxybutynin

   E Pelvic floor muscle training

4. A 25-year-old woman has 2 days of increased urinary frequency and burning discomfort when urinating, with lower back pain, nausea and vomiting and visible blood in her urine. Her temperature is 38.3°C, pulse 108 bpm and BP 92/71 mmHg. She is exquisitely tender in the right flank.

   Which is the most likely diagnosis?

   A Ectopic pregnancy

   B Pyelonephritis

   C Renal colic

   D Ureteral clot

   E Urinary tract infection

5. A 16-year-old boy has sudden severe groin pain and swelling, with lower abdominal pain, nausea and vomiting, after 3 days of intermittent episodes of mild pain that resolved. His pulse is 125 bpm and BP 119/82 mmHg. His scrotum is red, the left testis is tender and fixed in a high horizontal position, and the cremasteric reflex is absent.

   Which is the most appropriate treatment?

   A Incision and drainage

   B Oral antibiotics

   C Manual reduction

   D Urgent scrotal exploration

   E Routine urological referral

6. A 38-year-old man has 1 month of difficulty initiating and maintaining an erection before engaging in sexual intercourse. His libido has decreased, and he feels anxious about his sexual performance. He can achieve an erection alone.

   Which is the most appropriate immediate investigation?

   A Echocardiogram

   B FSH and LH

   C HbA1c

   D Prolactin

   E PSA

7. A 40-year-old man has a sudden inability to pass urine, with back pain, lower abdominal pain and swelling. He uses regular over-the-counter analgesia for lower back pain. He has lower abdominal tenderness and marked distention, with a palpable bladder.

   Investigations:

   Postvoid residual bladder scan: 600 mL

   Which is the most likely cause?

   A Benign prostatic hypertrophy

   B Constipation

   C Prolapsed intervertebral disc

   D Ureteric calculi

   E Urethral stricture

8. A 19-year-old man has a firm, non-tender lump in his right testicle, which he noticed 3 days ago. There is a firm, non-

fluctuant 2 cm mass on the right testicle, that is irregular, does not transilluminate and cannot be reduced.

Which is the most likely diagnosis?

A Epididymal cyst
B Hydrocele
C Inguinal hernia
D Testicular seminoma
E Varicocele

9. A 23-year-old woman has sudden severe left abdominal pain, radiating to the groin, with nausea and vomiting, increased urinary frequency, dysuria and visible blood in the urine. Her temperature is 37.1°C, pulse 115 bpm and BP 110/78 mmHg. She has exquisite tenderness in the left flank (Fig. 23).

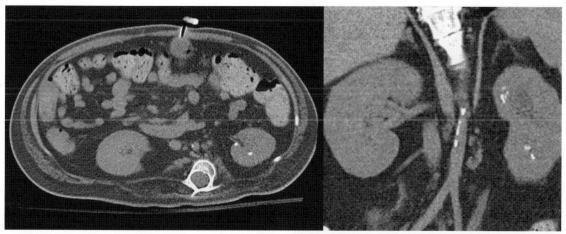

Fig. 23 CT abdomen (From Walters MM et al., *Pediatric Radiology: The Requisites*, 4th Edition. Elsevier; 2017.)

Which is the most appropriate treatment?

A Catheterization
B Extracorporeal shock wave lithotripsy
C Intravenous antibiotics
D Percutaneous nephrostomy
E PR diclofenac

10. A 68-year-old man has 3 days of increased urinary frequency and nocturia, with a gradual onset of left testicular pain and swelling. He has benign prostatic hyperplasia, managed with tamsulosin. He has left testicular tenderness and swelling.

Investigations.

Urinalysis: 2+ blood, 2+ leukocytes and 2+ nitrites.

Which is the most likely diagnosis?

A Epididymitis
B Lower urinary tract infection
C Orchitis
D Prostatitis
E Pyelonephritis

Chapter 8 Ear, nose and throat

1. A 24-year-old woman has worsening left ear pain, hearing loss, itching and discharge since returning from holiday 3 days ago (Fig. 24).

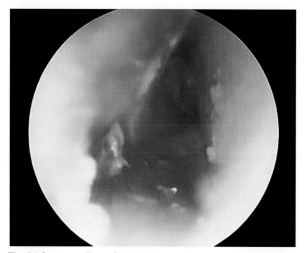

Fig. 24 Otoscopy (From Chi DH, Tobey A. Otolaryngology. In: Zitelli BJ, McIntire SC, Nowalk AJ, Garrison J, eds. Zitelli and Davis' Atlas of Pediatric Physical Diagnosis. 8th Edition. Elsevier; 2018:868–915.)

Which is the most likely diagnosis?

A Impacted ear wax
B Mastoiditis
C Otitis externa
D Otitis media
E Otitis media with effusion

2. A 6-year-old boy has 2 days of severe right-sided headache and fever, with right-sided hearing loss, after 1 week of coryzal symptoms (Fig. 25). His temperature is 38.2°C.

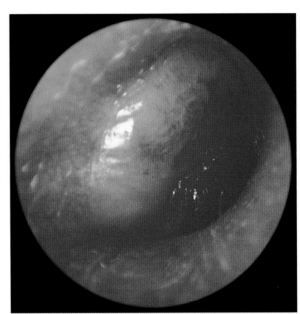

Fig. 25 Otoscopy (From Shiland BJ, Zenith. *Medical Assistant: Integumentary, Sensory Systems, Patient Care and Communication—Module A.* Elsevier; 2010.)

Which is the most appropriate treatment?

A ENT referral
B Gentamicin and hydrocortisone topical drops
C Olive oil topical drops
D Oral antibiotics
E Regular analgesia

3. A 33-year-old woman has 2 months of episodes of severe dizziness, with the room spinning around her, nausea, hearing loss and ringing in her ears. These are debilitating, and last several hours, before spontaneously resolving. The external auditory canal is clear and there is no effusion behind the tympanic membrane.

Which is the most appropriate treatment?

A Betahistine
B Epley manoeuvre
C Olive oil drops
D Prochlorperazine
E Vestibular rehabilitation

4. A 24-year-old woman has frequent dizziness when she stands up, with the room spinning around her, which spontaneously resolves within minutes. She has no hearing loss or ringing in her ears. She has migraines, managed with propranolol. Her dizziness is reproducible on changing of the head position.

Which is the most likely diagnosis?

A Acoustic neuroma
B Benign paroxysmal positional vertigo
C Labyrinthitis
D Meniere's disease
E Vestibular migraine

5. A 53-year-old man has 3 months of nasal congestion and increased nasal discharge from the right nostril, which is occasionally blood-stained, with absent sense of smell on the right (Fig. 26). He has had repeated sinus infections over this period. He has high cholesterol and peripheral vascular disease, managed with atorvastatin and clopidogrel, and has smoked 20 cigarettes a day for 30 years.

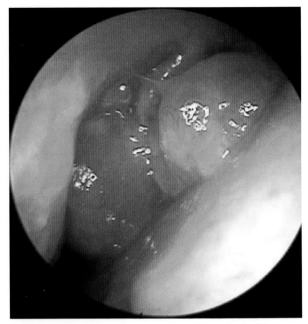

Fig. 26 Anterior rhinoscopy (From Leung DYM, Akdis CA, Bacharier LB, et al. (eds). *Pediatric Allergy Principles and Practice* 4th Edition. Philadelphia: Elsevier; 2021. Figure 24-1)

Which is the most appropriate next step?

A Nasal decongestants
B Nasal corticosteroids
C Oral antihistamines
D Reassurance and safety netting
E Urgent ENT referral

6. A 22-year-old man has 6 months of worsening nasal congestion, clear nasal discharge and a reduced sense of smell, a persistent cough and feeling of a need to clear his throat constantly. He has asthma, managed with salbutamol and beclomethasone inhalers, and takes over-the-counter antihistamines for allergic rhinitis. He has profuse, clear nasal discharge and mild bilateral inflammation of the nasal turbinates.

    Which is the most likely diagnosis?

    A Allergic rhinitis
    B Chronic rhinosinusitis
    C Nasopharyngeal carcinoma
    D Nasal polyps
    E Postnasal drip

7. A 16-year-old girl has 5 days of worsening sore throat, fever and general malaise, with reduced oral intake due to pain. Her temperature is 38.7ºC, pulse 112 bpm and BP 98/63 mmHg. She is speaking with a muffled, thick voice, has difficulty opening her mouth and tender cervical lymphadenopathy (Fig. 27).

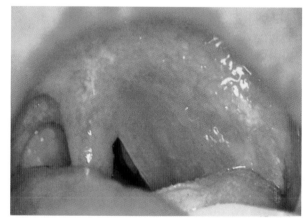

Fig. 27 Throat examination (From Vardaxis N, Nagy S, Harris P. *Mosby's Dictionary of Medicine, Nursing & Health Professions*, 3rd Revised Edition. Elsevier; 2019.)

    Which is the most likely diagnosis?

    A Epiglottis
    B Infectious mononucleosis
    C Peritonsillar abscess
    D Retropharyngeal abscesses
    E Tonsillitis

8. A 17-year-old boy has 10 days of a worsening sore throat, headache and fever. He feels generally unwell, is fatigued, and has lost his appetite. His girlfriend is also unwell with similar symptoms. His temperature is 37.8ºC, pulse 102 bpm and BP 115/87 mmHg. He has bilateral tender cervical lymphadenopathy, mild yellowing of the sclera and mild tenderness in the left upper quadrant (Fig. 28).

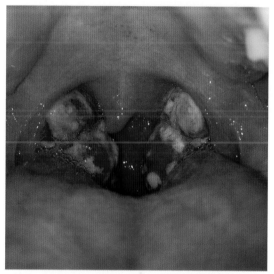

Fig. 28 Throat examination (Courtesy Dr. Lauren Kjolhede, Baylor College of Medicine, Children's Hospital of San Antonio, San Antonio, TX. In Hoffman R et al: Hematology, basic principles and practice, ed 7, Philadelphia, 2018, Elsevier.)

    Which is the most appropriate treatment?

    A Delayed antibiotic prescription
    B Incision and drainage
    C Oral amoxicillin
    D Oral phenoxymethylpenicillin
    E Reassurance and safety netting

9. A 73-year-old man has a sore throat and difficulty swallowing for 4 weeks, with a new raspy quality to his voice. He is an ex-smoker of 50-pack years. He has mild diffuse neck tenderness.

    Which is the most likely diagnosis?

    A Laryngitis
    B Thyroiditis
    C Vocal cord nodule
    D Laryngeal carcinoma
    E Laryngeal papillomatosis

10. A 52-year-old man has 6 months of fatigue, despite sleeping for over 9 hours a night, and feels unrefreshed when he wakes up in the morning. He has type 2 diabetes mellitus, managed with daily insulin injections, has smoked 20 cigarettes a day for 30 years, and drinks two bottles of wine a week. His BMI is 39 kg/m^2.

Which test is most likely to confirm the diagnosis?

A Capillary blood glucose
B Chest X-ray
C Full blood count
D Polysomnography
E Thyroid function tests

Chapter 9 Plastics and skin surgery

1. A 54-year-old man has 2 months of a small, pigmented lesion on his left forearm, that has grown and become slightly raised (Fig. 29). He works on building sites and goes on several foreign holidays a year.

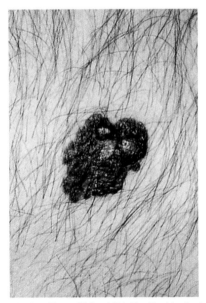

Fig. 29 Skin lesion (From Shiland BJ, Zenith. *Medical Assistant: Integumentary, Sensory Systems, Patient Care and Communication—Module A*. Elsevier; 2010.)

Which is the most likely diagnosis?

A Basal cell carcinoma
B Dysplastic nevus
C Malignant melanoma
D Squamous cell carcinoma
E Seborrheic keratosis

2. An 82-year-old woman is admitted following a fall. She was on the floor for 3 days. She is delirious, cachectic and unkempt (Fig. 30).

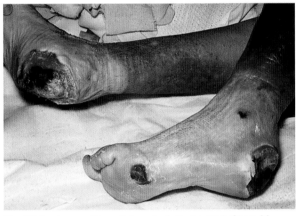

Fig. 30 Foot exam (From Edwards A, Drake WM, Glynn M. *Hutchison's Clinical Methods: An Integrated Approach to Clinical Practice*, 25th Edition. Elsevier; 2023.)

Which is the most likely diagnosis?

A Arterial ulcer
B Dry gangrene
C Necrotizing fasciitis
D Neuropathic ulcer
E Pressure ulcer

3. A 54-year-old man has worsening pain and swelling in his right calf after a superficial graze while gardening, with inability to weight bear. He has type 2 diabetes mellitus and high cholesterol, managed with metformin and dapagliflozin. There is a large area of dusky red and purple discolouration on the right calf, and the skin is firm, with palpable subcutaneous crepitus.

Which is the most appropriate treatment?

A Amputation
B Apixaban
C Intravenous antibiotics
D Revascularization
E Surgical debridement

4. A 64-year-old woman has 6 months of a painless lesion on her chest, that has grown, and occasionally bleeds (Fig. 31).

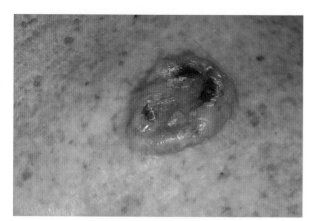

Fig. 31 Skin lesion (From Micheletti R et al., *Andrews' Diseases of the Skin Clinical Atlas*, 2nd Edition. Elsevier; 2023.)

Which is the most likely diagnosis?

A Basal cell carcinoma
B Bowen disease
C Keratoacanthoma
D Marjolin's ulcer
E Squamous cell carcinoma

5. A 76-year-old man has a raised lesion on his neck for 3 months that is slowly growing (Fig. 32). The lesion is painless but has bled on several occasions. He has type 1 diabetes mellitus managed with insulin and takes tacrolimus following renal transplant for end-stage renal failure 6 months ago.

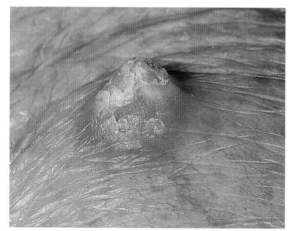

Fig. 32 Skin lesion (From Habif T et al., Skin disease: Diagnosis and treatment, 3rd Edition. Elsevier; 2011.)

Which is the most appropriate treatment?

A 5-fluorouracil
B Cryotherapy
C Radiotherapy
D Reassure and discharge
E Wide local excision

6. A 28-year-old man has 3 days of severe pain in his lower right leg and foot, which is rapidly worsening, with skin discolouration and sensory loss (Fig. 33). He is an intravenous drug user. His temperature is 38.1°C, pulse 127 bpm and BP 125/82 mmHg. His leg is severely tender, with induration of the underlying tissues, and palpable crepitus.

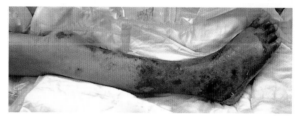

Fig. 33 Left leg (With permission from Endo, A., Matsuoka, R., Mizuno Y., Doi, A, & Nishioka, H. (2016). Sequential necrotizing fasciitis caused by the monomicrobial pathogens Streptococcus equisimilis and extended-spectrum beta-lactamase-producing Escherichia coli. Journal of Infection and Chemotherapy. Elsevier. © 2016 Japanese Society of Chemotherapy and The Japanese Association for Infectious Diseases. Published by Elsevier Ltd. All rights reserved.)

Which test is most likely to confirm the diagnosis?

A Blood cultures
B CT angiography
C Deep tissue biopsy
D Lower limb MRI
E Wound swab

7. A 32-year-old woman has a dark lesion on her back for 2 months that has doubled in size, that is painless and does not itch or bleed (Fig. 34).

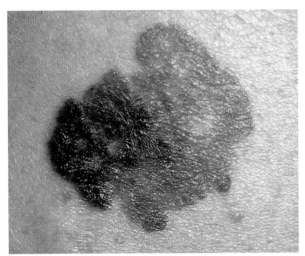

Fig. 34 Skin lesion (Courtesy of Habif T. Nevi and malignant melanoma. In: Habif T, ed. Clinical Dermatology. 5th Edition. St Louis, Missouri: Mosby; 2010.)

Which is the most appropriate investigation?

A Fine needle aspiration
B Full-thickness excisional biopsy
C Incisional biopsy
D Punch biopsy
E Skin scrape

8. A 32-year-old man has severe leg pain and inability to weight bear following a fall while hiking, with a large shin laceration. There is no sensory loss and pedal pulses are palpable.

Investigations:

Leg X-ray: compound tibiofibular fracture.

Which is the most appropriate immediate management?

A Analgesia
B Antiemetics
C Intravenous antibiotics
D Intravenous fluids
E Tetanus vaccine

9. A 28-year-old man has circumferential burns over his lower legs after a house fire. Following resuscitation, he develops severe leg pain and swelling, with firm shiny skin and absent pedal pulses.

Which is the most appropriate treatment?

A Amputation
B Escharotomy
C Revascularization
D Split-thickness skin graft
E Surgical debridement

10. An 82-year-old woman has worsening hip pain 3 days post left hemiarthroplasty for a fractured neck of femur. She has rheumatoid arthritis, managed with methotrexate. Her temperature is 38.2°C, pulse 110 bpm and BP 105/82 mmHg. Her hip is extremely tender, with black skin discolouration, exudate and palpable subcutaneous crepitus (Fig. 35).

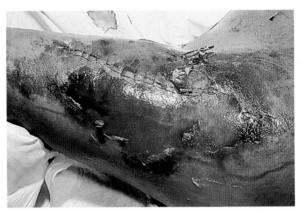

Fig. 35 Left hip (From Spicer WJ. *Clinical Microbiology and Infectious Diseases: An Illustrated Colour Text*, 2nd Edition. Elsevier; 2008.)

Which is the most likely diagnosis?

A Cellulitis
B Erysipelas
C Necrotizing fasciitis
D Osteomyelitis
E Pressure ulcer

Chapter 10 Cardiothoracic surgery

1. A 72-year-old man has 3 months of central chest tightness on exertion, with nausea, shortness of breath and light-headedness, which resolves within minutes of activity stopping. He has high cholesterol and hypertension, managed with atorvastatin and losartan, and has smoked 20 cigarettes a day for 40 years.

Investigations:

Echocardiogram: triple vessel coronary disease and impaired left ventricular function.

Which is the most appropriate treatment?

A Coronary artery bypass graft
B Endovascular thrombectomy
C GTN spray
D High dose atorvastatin
E Percutaneous Coronary Intervention

2. A 36-year-old woman suddenly becomes severely breathless, lightheaded and collapses. Her pulse is 132

bpm and BP 80/62 mmHg. She has a loud pansystolic murmur radiating to the axilla.

Investigations:

Echocardiogram: severe mitral regurgitation

Valve replacement surgery is planned.

Which is the most appropriate postoperative anticoagulation?

A Aspirin
B Clopidogrel
C Low-molecular-weight heparin
D Rivaroxaban
E Warfarin

3. A 72-year-old man has a 20-minute episode of left facial weakness and numbness, with blurring of the vision in his left eye, and slurred speech, which spontaneously resolved. He has hypertension and hypercholesterolaemia, managed with amlodipine, losartan and atorvastatin, and has smoked 20 cigarettes a day for 40 years. His pulse is 92 bpm and BP 142/97 mmHg. He has a left carotid bruit.

Which test is most likely to confirm the diagnosis?

A Carotid ultrasound
B CT head
C Echocardiogram
D Lipid levels
E MRI angiogram

4. A 24-year-old man has sudden central tearing chest pain that radiates to the back, with dizziness, nausea and several episodes of blood-stained vomit. He has Marfan's syndrome. His pulse is 145 bpm and BP 86/54 mmHg (Fig. 36).

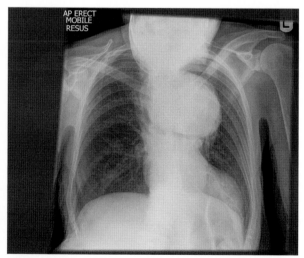

Fig. 36 Chest X-ray (From Au-Yong I, Corne J. *Chest X-Ray Made Easy*, 5th Edition. Elsevier; 2023.)

Which is the most appropriate treatment?

A Chest drain
B Open thoracic aneurysm repair
C Percutaneous coronary intervention
D Pericardiocentesis
E Thoracic endovascular aortic repair

5. A 77-year-old man has worsening severe breathlessness and cough productive of clear sputum. He has chronic congestive heart failure, managed with ramipril, bisoprolol, spironolactone, dapagliflozin, atorvastatin and isosorbide mononitrate. His pulse is 86 bpm, BP 138/76 mmHg, respiratory rate 32 breaths per minute and oxygen saturation 91% on breathing air. He has widespread chest wheeze and coarse bibasal crepitations, with pitting oedema up to the thighs.

Investigations:

Echocardiogram: left ventricular ejection fraction of 33% and uncoordinated ventricular contraction.

Which is the most appropriate next step?

A Cardiac resynchronization therapy
B Implantable cardiac defibrillator
C Heart transplant
D Left ventricular assist device
E Sacubitril-valsartan

6. A 74-year-old woman has a fall after sudden loss of consciousness while standing. She has had intermittent chest pains and breathlessness for 1 month. She has hypertension, managed with amlodipine. Her pulse is 85 bpm and BP 145/121 mmHg. She has a slow-rising pulse and an ejection systolic murmur that radiates to the carotids.

Which is the most appropriate investigation?

A 24-hour blood pressure monitoring
B Cardiac MRI
C Coronary angiogram
D ECG
E Echocardiogram

7. A 28-year-old man has sudden sharp pain in his right chest while playing sports, worse on inspiration. His pulse is 87 bpm, BP 121/89 mmHg and oxygen saturations 92% on breathing air (Fig. 37).

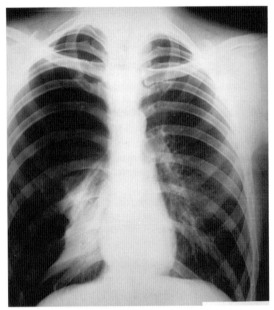

Fig. 37 Chest X-ray (From Kowalczyk, N. Radiographic pathology for technologists. Elsevier; 2021.)

Which is the most appropriate next step?

A   Chest drain
B   Discharge with follow-up
C   Finger thoracostomy
D   Intubation and ventilation
E   Needle aspiration

8.   A 32-year-old woman has 2 weeks of breathlessness and chest discomfort, worse lying flat or on exertion, with discomfort while swallowing, and the feeling of food getting stuck. She has systemic lupus erythematosus, managed with hydroxychloroquine. She has quiet heart sounds and a JVP 5 cm above the sternal angle (Fig. 38).

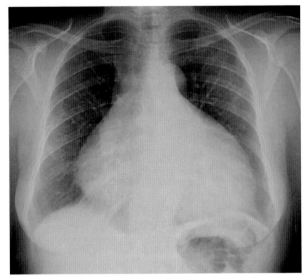

Fig. 38 Chest X-ray (From Herring W. *Learning Radiology: Recognizing the Basics*, 5th Edition. Elsevier; 2024.)

Which is the most likely diagnosis?

A   Atelectasis
B   Dilated cardiomyopathy
C   Heart failure
D   Pericardial effusion
E   Pleural effusion

9.   A 65-year-old man has 3 months of increasing chest discomfort, a persistent cough and shortness of breath, with difficulty swallowing and frequent regurgitation and hiccups. He has hypertension and hypercholesterolaemia, managed with amlodipine and atorvastatin. His pulse is 96 bpm and BP 160/85 mmHg. He has a diastolic murmur and pitting oedema to mid-shin.

Which is the most likely diagnosis?

A   Heart failure
B   Hiatus hernia
C   Gastro-oesophageal reflux disease
D   Lung cancer
E   Thoracic aortic aneurysm

10. A 28-year-old man has severe bruising over the chest wall after a road traffic accident. His pulse is 128 bpm, BP 90/65 mmHg respiratory rate 41 breaths per minute and oxygen saturation 87% on breathing air. He has right tracheal deviation, with reduced air entry and hyperressonant percussion on the left chest.

    Which is the most appropriate next step?

    A Chest drain
    B Chest X-ray
    C Fluid resuscitation
    D High-flow oxygen
    E Needle aspiration

Chapter 11 Perioperative management

1. A 52-year-old man is nil by mouth awaiting cholecystectomy for cholecystitis. He weighs 95 kg.

    Which is the most appropriate fluid regimen?

    A 1 L 0.9% NaCl + 20 mmol KCl over 12 hours, 1 L 5% dextrose and 40 mmol KCl over 12 hours
    B 1 L 0.9% NaCl + 40 mmol KCl over 8 hours, 1 L 5% dextrose and 40 mmol KCl over 8 hours, 500 mL 5% dextrose and 20 mmol KCl over 8 hours
    C 1 L 0.9% NaCl + 40 mmol KCl over 8 hours, 1 L 5% dextrose and 40 mmol KCl over 8 hours, 500 mL 5% dextrose and 20 mmol KCl over 1 hour
    D 1 L 0.9% NaCl + 40 mmol KCl over 8 hours, 1 L 5% dextrose over 6 hours, 500 mL 5% dextrose and 20 mmol KCl over 10 hours
    E 1 L 0.9% NaCl + 40 mmol KCl over 12 hours, 1 L 0.9% NaCl and 40 mmol KCl over 10 hours, 500 mL 5% dextrose and 20 mmol KCl over 6 hours

2. A 64-year-old man is awaiting elective total knee replacement. He has type 2 diabetes mellitus, high cholesterol, hypertension and osteoarthritis, managed with metformin, gliclazide, atorvastatin, ramipril and paracetamol.

    Which medication must be stopped on the day of surgery?

    A Atorvastatin
    B Gliclazide
    C Metformin
    D Paracetamol
    E Ramipril

3. A 72-year-old man is five days post right hemicolectomy with colostomy formation for caecal carcinoma. He is having total parenteral nutrition due to nausea and vomiting and has several rigors when the nurses are changing his feed. His temperature is 38.2°C, pulse 121 bpm and BP 105/86 mmHg.

    What is the likely diagnosis?

    A Anastomotic leak
    B Atelectasis
    C Central line sepsis
    D Pulmonary embolism
    E Urinary tract infection

4. A 72-year-old woman becomes drowsy 2 days post left mastectomy for breast cancer. Her pain is being managed with intravenous morphine. Her respiratory rate is 8 breaths per minute and oxygen saturation 91% on breathing air. She is unrousable to pain, with visible twitching of the upper and lower limbs, and pinpoint pupils.

    Which is the most appropriate next step?

    A Intramuscular lorazepam
    B Intravenous antibiotics
    C Intravenous fluids
    D Intubation and ventilation
    E Naloxone

5. An 82-year-old woman becomes delirious 3 days post left hemiarthroplasty for fractured neck of femur fracture. Her temperature is 37.8°C, pulse 110 bpm and BP 125/82 mmHg. Her catheter is draining dark, malodorous urine.

    Which is the most appropriate next step?

    A Apixaban
    B Catheter removal
    C Intravenous antibiotics
    D Intravenous fluids
    E Intravenous paracetamolUKMLA Single Best Answer (SBA) questions

Chapter 1 The upper gastrointestinal tract

1. A. Burning or stabbing central chest pain, with nausea and acid brash, worse lying down or after eating, are typical features of GORD. PUD is less commonly associated with heartburn and nausea. There are no red flag features of malignancy.

2. D. Epigastric pain, which is constant, severe, wakes a patient from sleep, relieved by eating, likely relates to a duodenal ulcer. NSAID use is a key risk factor. Gastric ulcers cause pain while eating but are less troublesome at night. An OGD would confirm the diagnosis and allow instant CLO testing for *H. pylori*, which can then be eradicated if present.

3. B. Oesophageal carcinoma presents with progressive dysphagia and weight loss. Chronic poorly controlled GORD triggers metaplasia of oesophageal to premalignant Barrett's oesophagus, which then undergoes dysplastic change to carcinoma. Smoking, alcohol use and obesity increase the risk. Achalasia presents with progressive dysphagia and weight loss, but regurgitation occurs while lying flat and is effortless.

4. D. Bleeding oesophageal varices present with frank, large-volume haematemesis, with extensive blood loss causing dizziness, confusion and pallor. Abdominal tenderness, jaundice and malnourishment suggest chronic liver disease, which can result in varices, which are prone to bleeding. Boerhaave syndrome and Mallory-Weiss tears also present with frank haematemesis, although after a period of intense retching or vomiting, and bleeding, and peptic ulcers more commonly present with melaena or coffee-ground vomit.

5. C. Acute cholecystitis presents with sudden onset right upper quadrant pain that radiates to the shoulder, nausea, vomiting, fever and tachycardia. A positive Murphy's sign (inspiratory pain on palpation) is highly suggestive of cholecystitis. Abdominal US should be the initial investigation and will show a thickened gallbladder wall, stones or sludge in the gallbladder and oedema.

6. A. Charcot's triad of fever, jaundice and right upper quadrant pain is pathognomonic for ascending cholangitis. The history of intermittent right upper quadrant pain indicates biliary colic, with likely obstruction of the common bile duct with a gallstone, and subsequent inflammation and infection. Acute cholecystitis does not cause jaundice, as there is no biliary obstruction.

7. B. Acute epigastric pain radiating through to the back, nausea and vomiting, fever, tachycardia and respiratory distress, with a history of alcohol abuse, is highly suggestive of acute pancreatitis. Intravenous fluids, along with adequate analgesia and early nutrition are the mainstays of treatment. Antibiotics are reserved for complications including abscesses or necrosis. ERCP would be indicated in gallstone pancreatitis.

8. D. Courvoisier's law states that a palpable gallbladder with jaundice is unlikely to relate to gallstones. It typically relates to malignancy, with cancer of the head of the pancreas the most common cause. Cholangiocarcinoma presents similarly, though it is less common, and associated with conditions such as ulcerative colitis and primary sclerosing cholangitis.

9. A. Progressive dysphagia, weight loss and recurrent aspiration pneumonia are typical for achalasia. It is common in young women. Regurgitation occurs lying flat and is effortless. The barium swallow shows the characteristic 'bird's beak' appearance of the lower oesophagus, with proximal dilation and constriction at the lower oesophageal sphincter.

10. D. She has typical features of GORD. A PPI or *H. pylori* testing and treatment are appropriate first-line steps, then switching to the alternative strategy if treatment fails. If she tested positive for *H. pylori*, then eradication therapy can be used, with two antibiotics and a PPI, but this should not be given without a positive test. Bismuth salts, H2 antagonists and Peptac liquid can be used as adjunctive or alternative measures for symptomatic relief.

11. A. She has features of biliary colic, with intermittent upper abdominal pain and nausea after meals. The US shows the gallstones within the gallbladder. For symptomatic gallstones, the definitive management is cholecystectomy.

12. C. Epigastric pain, nausea, vomiting and diarrhoea, with a history of gallstones, suggests pancreatitis. Acute cholecystitis presents with RUQ pain, that radiates to the shoulder. There are no urinary symptoms of pyelonephritis. A perforated ulcer would present with peritonitic features.

13. B. Chronic abdominal pain with a history of alcohol abuse and repeated episodes of acute pancreatitis, suggests chronic pancreatitis. Continued inflammation results in pancreatic calcification, which can be seen on X-ray.

Steatorrhoea and osmotic symptoms indicate impaired pancreatic exocrine and endocrine functions. Jaundice and pruritus occur when the calcified pancreas compresses the terminal portion of the common bile duct.

14. A. Melaena suggests UGIB. A history of heavy alcohol use, smoking and NSAIDs increases the risk of a peptic ulcer, suggested by chronic abdominal pain. Oesophageal varices are more commonly present with frank haematemesis and haemodynamic compromise. Dieulafoy lesions are rare vascular abnormalities.

15. C. Intermittent right upper quadrant pain, worse with heavy meals, with flatulence and indigestion suggests gallstones. The absence of fever rules out acute biliary infection. Pancreatitis presents with severe pain, nausea and vomiting and systemic compromise.

16. E. The management of GORD involves full dose PPI or testing and treatment of *H. pylori*, with a urea breath test. OGD is reserved for refractory cases. Barium swallows and oesophageal manometry can be used to exclude differentials such as achalasia, diffuse oesophageal spasm or oesophageal cancer.

17. B. The patient presents with Charcot triad: fever, jaundice, right upper quadrant pain, suggesting ascending cholangitis. ERCP is required to remove the stones obstructing the common bile duct. PTC accesses the bile tracts through the skin and liver and is used if ERCP fails or is not suitable. Lithotripsy can be used to fragment gallstones if they are large or inaccessible during ERCP.

18. A. Severe upper abdominal pain, nausea and vomiting after an alcoholic binge suggest acute pancreatitis. Abdominal US demonstrating pancreatic inflammation will confirm the likely diagnosis. Lipase and amylase are both raised in acute pancreatitis; however, lipase is more sensitive and specific. ERCP is used to diagnose and treat biliary pathology, which can cause pancreatitis – however, alcohol abuse is the more likely aetiology in this case.

19. E. Benign oesophageal strictures are common in those with a long history of poorly managed GORD. Oesophagitis results from irritation of the oesophageal lining by stomach acid, and when the inflammation heals, the tissue becomes fibrotic, resulting in strictures. Weight loss can occur due to difficulty swallowing and food avoidance. The absence of appetite change, signs of anaemia or chest pain makes oesophageal carcinoma less likely.

20. C. Small-volume haematemesis after repeated vomiting suggests a Mallory Weiss tear. Varices and Boerhaave syndrome present with large-volume haematemesis and haemodynamic compromise, and peptic ulcers more commonly present with melaena or coffee-ground vomit.

Oesophagitis can rarely present with small-volume haematemesis, but there would likely be a history of reflux symptoms.

21. E. The ERCP shows a gallstone partially obstructing the common bile duct, known as choledocholithiasis. Symptoms of jaundice, abdominal pain, pale stools and pruritus occur due to partial obstruction of biliary flow. There is no fever to indicate acute infection. Cholelithiasis simply refers to the presence of gallstones in the gallbladder.

22. B. The priority in acute hypotension is restoration of intravascular volume with fluids. Blood should then be replaced where lost if possible. Antibiotics and terlipressin should then be given, given the likely diagnosis of bleeding oesophageal varices, suggested by the volume of haematemesis and signs of chronic liver disease. Following this endoscopic haemostasis is required. PPIs may be given before or after endoscopy.

23. E. This is a typical history of diffuse oesophageal spasm. The corkscrew oesophagus on barium swallow confirms the diagnosis. Management includes calcium channel blockers to relax the uncoordinated oesophageal contractions. Heller's cardiomyotomy is used in achalasia, surgical resection for tumours, and PPIs and prokinetic agents such as metoclopramide can improve nausea in GORD or hiatus hernia.

24. D. Acute cholecystitis presents with fever and RUQ pain and is suggested by the history of biliary colic. The initial treatment is antibiotic therapy. Early cholecystectomy is then typically required. Cholecystostomy is used to drain a gallbladder empyema and ERCP to remove stones obstructing the bile ducts.

25. D. A bleeding peptic ulcer is suggested by coffee-ground vomit, melaena and a history of NSAID use. Endoscopic haemostasis is indicated to control the bleeding. Terlipressin and intravenous antibiotics are used in variceal bleeds. PPIs may be used before or after OGD.

Chapter 2 The lower gastrointestinal tract

1. C. Migratory abdominal pain, nausea and vomiting and low-grade fever are classic symptoms of appendicitis, which is definitively diagnosed and treated with laparoscopic appendectomy. US is used prior to laparoscopy if there is diagnostic uncertainty. Pregnancy should be excluded in females of childbearing age.

2. E. SBP presents with peritonitis, suggested by abdominal rigidity, rebound tenderness, fevers and rigors. Underlying ascites can be complicated by the spontaneous infection of ascitic fluid. Pancreatitis typically presents with

epigastric pain radiating to the back. Bowel perforation can cause peritonitis but there are no features in the history to suggest this.

3. C. An acute IBD flare is suggested by abdominal pain, diarrhoea, nausea and vomiting and fever. Management involves admission, resuscitation and intravenous steroids. Bowel resection can be considered if steroids fail to control symptoms. Antibiotics may be used if there is an associated abscess or perforation. Oral mesalazine is indicated for the long-term treatment of ulcerative colitis.

4. E. Bowel obstruction is suggested by obstipation, abdominal pain, vomiting and dehydration. CT is used to confirm the diagnosis, transition point, and complications including perforation. Abdominal X-rays may demonstrate dilated bowel loops and free intraperitoneal air but cannot confirm the diagnosis.

5. A. Acute abdominal pain, bloody diarrhoea and atrial fibrillation is the triad of acute mesenteric ischaemia. Peritonitic features are often present. Angiodysplasia and diverticular bleeds are typically painful. A ruptured AAA would be associated with profound haemodynamic instability.

6. E. Diverticular disease is suggested by mild abdominal pain in the left lower quadrant, a history of chronic constipation and colonic outpouchings on colonoscopy. Diverticular disease should be managed with lifestyle advice including dietary modifications and smoking cessation, to reduce progression. Antibiotics and bowel rest may be used in acute diverticulitis. Elective colectomy is reserved for those with frequent diverticular complications.

7. B. Ulcerative colitis is suggested by profuse, bloody diarrhoea, abdominal pain and faecal urgency, in a young male who recently stopped smoking. Faecal calprotectin and ESR will be elevated, but colonoscopy is required for definitive diagnosis, with a characteristic 'starry sky' appearance of the colon suggesting multiple shallow ulcerations. Stool MC&S should be ordered to exclude infectious colitis. Anti-TTG antibodies are used to diagnose coeliac disease.

8. C. Haemorrhoids are suggested by painless, bright red rectal bleeding and anal itch, relating to chronic constipation and straining, with a visible haemorrhoid prolapse on examination. Anal fissures are extremely painful, and fistulas are associated with IBD and mucopurulent anal discharge. A rectal prolapse typically affects older individuals and presents with incontinence and a large rectal mass. Ulcerative colitis presents with bloody diarrhoea.

9. B. Red flags features for colorectal carcinoma, include new, unexplained anaemia, fatigue, change in bowel habit and abdominal pain. NICE guidance indicates that adults >60 with these features should be referred for an urgent colonoscopy to excuse malignancy. FIT testing is used for screening for microscopic blood in the stool in asymptomatic patients. The cause of diarrhoea is unlikely to be infectious, given the time course. Thyroid hormone derangement can be associated with anaemia, fatigue and diarrhoea; however, other red flag features should be investigated first.

10. C. Anal pain, bloody discharge and fevers with a history of Crohn's disease suggest a perianal abscess formation, a complication of an anal fistula. Analgesia and laxatives are appropriate supportive measures; however, abscesses require incision and drainage to ensure resolution and avoid worsening of infection. Topical hydrocortisone is used in haemorrhoids.

11. E. Profuse bloody diarrhoea, vomiting, abdominal pain and distention, with haemodynamic instability with a history of UC suggests fulminant colitis. Toxic megacolon is suggested by the gross dilation of the large bowel on X-ray.

12. A. Chronic mesenteric ischaemia presents with postprandial pain and weight loss due to food aversion. Vascular risk factors, including hypertension, high cholesterol and smoking, place him at high risk. Gallstones and gastric ulcers are associated with postprandial pain, though typically present with dyspepsia. Diverticular disease is associated with chronic constipation, and coeliac disease malabsorption and failure to thrive in children.

13. D. A sigmoid volvulus is suggested by abdominal pain, nausea, distention and constipation, with the X-ray features of a 'coffee-bean' resulting from twisting of the bowel on the mesentery and dilation of the proximal and distal segments. Previous episodes of colicky abdominal pain which resolve are common. The definitive management is with endoscopic decompression; however, the initial resuscitation involves IV fluids and nasogastric tube placement ('drip and suck').

14. C. Sudden painless melaena suggests angiodysplasia, which is associated with aortic stenosis, and best diagnosed on colonoscopy which will visualize arterial malformations and allow for endoscopic cautery. CT angiography can be used if colonoscopy is not possible.

15. D. The A, B and Cs of IBS are abdominal pain, bloating and change in bowel habit. It is common in those with anxiety. The abdominal examination will be normal. There are no features to suggest IBD, pancreatic insufficiency or coeliac disease.

16. D. A positive FIT test indicates the passage of occult blood in the stool. All patients with a positive test should be

referred for colonoscopy to exclude colorectal cancer. Digital rectal exam would be useful, but it is likely to be normal, given the lack of bowel symptoms. FBC may demonstrate anaemia but will not determine the source of bleeding.

17. D. Diverticulitis is suggested by left-sided abdominal pain and mass, and low-grade fever, with a history of chronic constipation. CT will demonstrate colonic outpouchings, signs of inflammation and bowel wall thickening and mesenteric fat stranding. Complications including abscesses and perforation can also be identified. Point-of-care ultrasound can be performed in acutely unstable patients.

18. E. Bowel perforation is suggested by pneumoperitoneum on chest X-ray. The history suggests acute mesenteric ischaemia, with abdominal pain, bloody diarrhoea and a past medical history of atrial fibrillation. IV antibiotics, IV fluids and bowel rest are all appropriate supportive measures – however, the definitive management is with urgent laparotomy. Angioplasty and stenting can be considered in cases without perforation.

19. E. All these diagnoses can result in malabsorptive symptoms including steatorrhoea and weight loss, evidence of anaemia and dehydration. The history of small bowel resection suggests short bowel syndrome, a common complication of repeated operative management of Crohn's.

20. B. A red, painful eye, photophobia, visual changes and evidence of hypopyon and posterior synechiae on examination suggests anterior uveitis. Anterior uveitis is associated with HLA-B27 conditions, including inflammatory bowel disease. Scleritis presents with a painful red eye, however, it is more commonly associated with rheumatoid arthritis.

Chapter 3 The anterior abdominal wall

1. A. A groin lump superomedial to the pubic tubercle suggests an inguinal hernia. The enlargement on coughing suggests it is a direct hernia. Inguinal hernias are common in adults and often related to heavy lifting. Testicular torsion presents with an acute history of severe pain, scrotal swelling and abnormal testicular lie.

2. B. Acute bowel obstruction is suggested by abdominal pain, nausea and vomiting and constipation. A tender mass in the left lower quadrant with a previous painless groin lump suggests an inguinal hernia, which can become incarcerated and result in bowel obstruction. Initial resuscitation includes nasogastric tube and intravenous fluids; however, the definitive management is emergency hernia repair.

3. B. Respiratory distress following blunt force chest trauma, with absent ipsilateral breath sounds, chest X-ray demonstrating mediastinal shift and audible bowel sounds in the chest suggest a diaphragmatic hernia. The chest X-ray demonstrates the air-filled bowel in the chest.

4. C. An ileostomy is formed from exterioration of the ileum after bowel resection. They are spouted, as the enzymes in the small bowel can irritate the skin. Faeces drains into the bag and is typically paler and softer than the contents of a colostomy. They are typically located in the right iliac fossa, but location should not be relied upon to determine stoma type.

5. A. Femoral hernias are common in older, multiparous women. A chronic cough is a risk factor. Femoral hernias present with a groin lump inferolateral to the pubic tubercle. Inguinal hernias are more common in younger men, and present with a groin lump superomedial to the pubic tubercle.

Chapter 4 Endocrine surgery

1. E. A firm, painless mass that moves on swallowing, not tongue protrusion suggests a thyroid nodule. Thyroglossal duct cysts move on tongue protrusion and swallowing. Branchial cysts are large and posterior. Reactive lymphadenopathy is typically tender and associated with infection.

2. E. The water deprivation test is used to diagnose diabetes insipidus. Head injuries can result in cranial diabetes insipidus, resulting in low urine osmolality after water deprivation, and a high urine osmolality after synthetic ADH is given. Diabetes mellitus is the main differential but typically presents with weight loss associated with osmotic symptoms.

3. C. Hypocalcaemia can occur as a complication of thyroidectomy, and damage to the parathyroid glands. Symptoms can develop if severe and include muscle cramps, paraesthesia and perioral numbness. Hypocalcaemia is a medical emergency and should be managed with intravenous calcium gluconate. Oral calcium and vitamin D can follow if the response is insufficient.

4. A. A palpable node in the left supraclavicular fossa is known as Trosier's sign, which is the finding of an enlarged, hardened Virchow's node. This is likely to represent gastric cancer. Dysphagia, weight loss and vomiting can occur with a pharyngeal pouch, however, this produces a soft swelling in the left side of the neck. Thymomas can present with swallowing difficulties and cough but are not associated with Virchow's node.

5. E. Evidence of upper airway obstruction warrants urgent referral to secure the airway before further investigations. A rapidly enlarging neck lump associated with hoarseness, weight loss and fatigue suggests malignancy; in this case, anaplastic carcinoma of the thyroid is most likely given the speed of growth. Biopsy will confirm the diagnosis.

6. B. Immediate haematoma is a surgical emergency that can occur in the hours following an operation. In thyroid surgery, haematoma results in laryngeal oedema, stridor and dyspnoea. It requires an immediate return to the theatre to control the haemorrhage and secure the airway. Postextubation stridor occurs following difficult intubation or extubation and is typically mild and self-limiting. Laryngospasm is a transient vocal cord spasm that can occur immediately following extubation, and results in stridor and dyspnoea.

7. A. Malignant hypertension and evidence of hypokalaemia, indicated by symptoms of muscle weakness and cramping, and the ECG findings of T wave inversion, ST depression, QT prolongation and a visible U wave suggest hyperaldosteronism. Excessive aldosterone release results in increased salt and water reabsorption in the distal tubule of the kidney, leading to hypokalaemia, hypernatraemia and hypertension. The priority in the first instance is to treat hypokalaemia, which is a medical emergency, with intravenous potassium chloride. Definitive management relates to the underlying cause.

8. D. Symptoms of hypercalcaemia include bone pain, abdominal pain and constipation, nausea and vomiting, polyuria and polydipsia and fatigue. The most common cause is a solitary parathyroid adenoma, otherwise known as primary hyperparathyroidism.

9. D. Swallowing difficulties, hoarseness, cough and chest pain are compressive features of a mediastinal mass. Swelling of the upper extremities and distended veins over the chest indicate superior vena cava obstruction. Patients with myasthenia gravis are at risk of thymomas, tumours of the thymus gland in the mediastinum.

10. A. These are the signs and symptoms of a pheochromocytoma. High levels of catecholamines including adrenaline and noradrenaline released from the tumour cause malignant hypertension, anxiety, tremor, sweating and paroxysmal atrial fibrillation. Pheochromocytomas are associated with the multiple endocrine neoplasia conditions and are diagnosed by high levels of catecholamines or metanephrines in the urine.

Chapter 5 Breast surgery

1. E. Mastitis is suggested by mastalgia, breast erythema and fever. Mastitis is common in lactating mothers. There is no mass or purulent nipple discharge to suggest breast abscess. Inflammatory breast cancer presents similarly to mastitis, however, an acute history of mastalgia in a breastfeeding mother more likely relates to infection. Duct ectasia presents with cream, green or grey nipple discharge. Cyclical mastalgia relates to menstruation.

2. E. Any unexplained breast lump should have a triple assessment, involving clinical assessment, imaging and breast biopsy. Mammogram is preferred in women >35 and should be performed before biopsy so the lump can be accurately located and assessed to determine biopsy method. Breast US is used in women <35.

3. B. A first-episode seizure with a history of breast cancer suggests recurrence with brain metastatic disease. Breast cancer commonly metastasizes to the brain, bone, liver or lung.

4. C. All breast malignancies that are HER2+ve should be treated with adjuvant Herceptin, a monoclonal antibody targeting the HER2 receptor. Herceptin is associated with significant mortality benefits and disease-free survival. There is a risk of cardiotoxicity and GI upset.

5. C. Red flag features of inflammatory breast cancer include breast pain, peau d'orange, erythema and blood-stained nipple discharge. The speed of onset of symptoms is typical for inflammatory cancer. Mastitis presents with erythema and breast pain, however, is more common in lactating mothers. Paget's disease of the breast presents with a scaly rash and ulceration.

6. A. Cyclical mastalgia presents with bilateral, cyclical breast tenderness and is often associated with premenstrual syndrome. Management is with reassurance, analgesia and a supportive bra.

7. D. A breast abscess presents with severe mastalgia, mass and fever, with purulent nipple discharge. This should be managed with aspiration, fluid culture and antibiotics, typically intravenous flucloxacillin. Warm and cold compresses are useful adjuncts. Evening primrose oil is used by some for cyclical mastalgia, but there is no clear evidence base for its use.

8. E. Paget disease of the breast is a rare malignancy affecting the lactiferous ducts. It presents with a scaly erythematous rash affecting the nipple, nipple retraction and blood-stained nipple discharge. Biopsy will reveal Paget cells. Mastitis presents with acute breast erythema and pain, commonly in lactating mothers. Inflammatory breast cancer is associated with acute breast pain erythema and skin puckering.

9. A. Fibrocystic breast change is suggested by multiple tender nodules in the breast that typically occur with the menstrual cycle. This is the most common cause of benign breast lumps, relating to cyclical fibrosis of breast

tissue. Following breast US to confirm the diagnosis, management involves analgesia and a supportive bra. Evening primrose oil is used by some but there is no evidence to support its use. Warm and cold compresses and antibiotics are used for mastitis.

10. A. A breast cyst is suggested by the sudden appearance of a small lump in the breast that is mobile, soft and mildly tender. They commonly arise in women aged 35–50 as the result of age-related tissue involution. The diagnosis should be confirmed on breast ultrasound, and fine needle aspiration should then be performed if the cyst remains symptomatic.

Chapter 6 Vascular surgery

1. B. A DVT is suggested by symptoms of tenderness, swelling and erythema. Risk factors in the history include recent long-haul travel and smoking. Anticoagulation is warranted, and apixaban is a suitable oral option. Heparin infusions are typically only used in severe renal impairment. There is no evidence of fever to suggest cellulitis, which is treated with flucloxacillin. Emollients are used for venous eczema, which presents with bilateral leg redness and dry skin.

2. A. Abdominal aortic aneurysms are often asymptomatic and detected on screening but can present with abdominal or lower back pain. Abdominal US will detect the aneurysm. There are no urinary symptoms to suggest renal or bladder pathology, and no red flags for cauda equina syndrome to indicate a need for lumbosacral MRI.

3. E. The ulcer is large, irregular and sloughy and over the medial malleolus, a common location for venous ulcers. Large, complicated ulcers can develop with poor wound care and management of comorbidities. Neuropathic and diabetic ulcers typically present with surrounding callous over pressure points and peripheral neuropathy. Arterial ulcers are well-defined, punched out and extremely painful.

4. A. Critical limb ischaemia is suggested by rest pain, ulcers and gangrene. Revascularization can be attempted in minimal tissue necrosis. In this case, the extent of tissue necrosis, ulcers and absence of pedal pulses make successful revascularization unlikely and require early amputation to salvage the remaining limb.

5. D. Intermittent claudication is suggested by cramping left pain on exertion, worse uphill and relieved by rest. There are no skin changes to suggest chronic venous insufficiency, or rest pain, ulcers or gangrene to suggest critical limb ischaemia. Spinal stenosis presents with neurogenic claudication, and leg pain as the result of compression of the spinal nerves in the lumbar spine, which is relieved by bending forward and widening the spinal canal.

6. D. A ruptured abdominal aortic aneurysm is suggested by acute abdominal pain, collapse and hypotension with a pulsatile abdominal mass. The priority is resuscitation, following which transfer to theatre for emergency surgical repair is required. CT angiography is used to confirm the diagnosis in haemodynamically stable patients, before transfer to theatre.

7. C. Intermittent claudication is suggested by cramping leg pain on exertion, relieved by rest, with risk factors including smoking, hypertension and alcohol use. His ABPI is 0.8 and 0.7, confirming a diagnosis of peripheral arterial disease. The management of intermittent claudication is with structured exercise therapy, clopidogrel, atorvastatin and cardiovascular risk modification.

8. A. He has the 6 Ps of peripheral limb ischaemia – pain, pallor, pulselessness, paralysis, paraesthesia and poikilothermia. Atrial fibrillation is a risk factor for acute embolic occlusion of peripheral arteries.

9. B. Those aged 65–75 with a smoking history are eligible for one-off screening for an AAA. Aneurysms >5.5 cm are an indication for surgical repair due to the risk of rupture, even if asymptomatic. Endovascular repair is preferred, involving endoscopic placement of an expandable stent graft at the aneurysm site. There are fewer complications than with open surgical repair, hence this approach is preferred. Surveillance US is indicated for smaller aneurysms.

10. B. A PE is suggested by sudden onset inspiratory chest pain, dyspnoea and cough. Her modified Wells score is 4.5, which makes a PE likely. Both an ECG and chest X-ray would be useful, but a CTPA is required to confirm the diagnosis.

11. B. Chronic venous insufficiency is suggested by lower leg swelling and aching following long periods of standing, worse in the heart and relieved by elevation. This is common in older women. The examination findings indicate haemosiderin deposition and varicosities in the right leg. Cellulitis and thrombophlebitis typically present with unilateral redness and pain.

12. C. Peripheral arterial disease is suggested by cramping leg pain worse on exertion, a pale, cool leg and reduced pedal pulses. Rest pain is suggestive of critical ischaemia. The diagnosis is confirmed on CT, MRI or digital subtraction angiography, but initial testing should involve an ABPI, which will likely be <0.5, and duplex US to detect reduced blood flow.

13. E. Lymphoedema is commonly related to surgery or radiation, where the lymph nodes have been

compromised, and hence lymphatic drainage is reduced. Symptoms include leg swelling, itch and skin changes if severe, including blistering and hyperkeratosis. Lipoedema presents with symmetrical fat deposition in the thighs, buttocks and arms.

14. A. Chronic venous insufficiency is suggested by bilateral leg aching and swelling, haemosiderin deposition and varicosities. Management involves compression bandages and lifestyle measures to improve venous return, including weight loss and leg elevation. Vein ligation can be considered in severe complicated varicosities. Emollients and topical steroids can be considered for stasis dermatitis.

15. C. Lifestyle modifications are an essential element of successful management of PAD to reduce cardiovascular risk and risk of progression. Weight loss and alcohol reduction are all recommended, but smoking cessation is the most important step. Smoking is associated with a high risk of morbidity and mortality, and progression to chronic limb ischaemia. Revascularization attempts are also less likely to be successful. Patients should be counselled about this at every appointment.

Chapter 7 Urology

1. D. Alpha-blockers such as tamsulosin are used in benign prostatic hyperplasia, to alleviate urinary symptoms. 5-alpha reductase inhibitors, such as finasteride, are used to gradually reduce the size of the prostate, but take up to 6 months to work. Oxybutynin and mirabegron are antimuscarinics used to treat overactive bladder.

2. A. Painless haematuria in the older adult, particularly those with a smoking history, is a red flag for bladder cancer. Weight loss, pallor, fatigue and lower limb swelling all suggest urological malignancy.

3. E. First-line management of stress incontinence involves pelvic floor muscle exercises. Most cases result from weakening of the pelvic floor because of pregnancy and childbirth. Difficult labour and delivery or perineal injury increased the risk significantly. After muscle training has been trialled, medical management with duloxetine can be considered. For refractory cases, surgery, including colposuspension, can be considered.

4. B. Dysuria, back pain and fevers, suggest pyelonephritis. Ectopic pregnancy can present similarly, however, there would likely be a history of missed period, vaginal bleeding or shoulder tip pain.

5. D. Testicular torsion is a surgical emergency, with a 6-hour window to save the testes. A tender, fixed testes with a high horizontal lie and an absent cremasteric reflex is the typical presentation. Manual reduction can be attempted

for an incarcerated hernia, and incision and drainage for a hydrocele.

6. C. The initial investigation of erectile dysfunction involves assessment of cardiovascular risk with HbA1c and lipid profile, BMI and blood pressure measurement. Total testosterone may be measured, and if found to be low, FSH, LH and prolactin measured, to assess for hypogonadism, but this is less common. PSA can be measured if the DRE is abnormal. An echocardiogram is only indicated if there is previous cardiac history or cardiac symptoms.

7. C. All these options can cause acute urinary retention. The history of lower back pain suggests a likely prolapsed intervertebral disc as the cause of acute retention. BPH would present with other lower urinary tract symptoms, but is more common in older adults. Ureteric calculi would present with severe loin to groin pain and fever and strictures with a history of urinary tract trauma.

8. D. A firm, painless, irregular, nonfluctuant mass in the testicle of a young man is likely to represent testicular cancer. The lump does not transilluminate or reduce, eliminating hydrocele and hernia. Varicoceles classically feel like a 'bag of worms'. Cysts are soft, small and fluctuant.

9. E. For ureteric colic, management is typically analgesia with strong NSAIDs. PR diclofenac is known to be very effective. For larger stones, lithotripsy can be used to fragment stones and aid passage, and for impacted stones with evidence of infection, antibiotics are indicated and percutaneous nephrostomy can be considered.

10. A. Epididymitis describes inflammation of the epididymis, the cord that connects the testes and vas deferens, which drains into the ejaculatory duct. It presents with LUTS and testicular pain and swelling. Orchitis alone is rare, typically associated with mumps infections and symptoms include acute severe testicular pain and swelling, often with systemic upset.

Chapter 8 Ear, nose and throat

1. C. Otoscopy reveals evidence of acute swelling of the EAC and debris within the canal, associated with itching, hearing loss and discharge from the ear, suggesting OE. OM and OM with effusion both present with changes behind the tympanic membrane, as the pathology is within the middle ear. There is no wax within the canal to suggest impaction. Mastoiditis would present with systemic illness and swelling behind the mastoid process.

2. E. Acute otalgia, hearing loss, inflammation and pus behind the tympanic membrane suggest otitis media. This should be managed conservatively and typically

self-resolves within 3 days. Antibiotics are only indicated if symptoms persist or there is significant systemic disturbance, tympanic membrane perforation or bilateral symptoms.

3. A. The patient describes the characteristic 'drop attacks' of Ménière disease, which present with hours of debilitating rotational vertigo, tinnitus and sensorineural hearing loss. Betahistine is used in the prophylaxis of attacks. Vestibular rehabilitation and prochlorperazine may be used as adjunctive measures if betahistine fails to control symptoms.

4. B. These are typical features of BPPV, with sudden-onset attacks of vertigo with a change in head position, which last seconds to minutes, and spontaneously resolve. Meniere's disease, labyrinthitis and vestibular migraine typically present with hours to days of vertigo. Acoustic neuroma is not associated with vertigo.

5. E. Unilateral nasal polyps are a red flag feature for nasopharyngeal carcinoma. Smoking is a key risk factor for head and neck malignancy – patients with a smoking history who present with symptoms of chronic nasal obstruction, epistaxis or unilateral nasal polyps should be urgently referred to ENT under the two-week-wait pathway for further investigation and treatment.

6. B. These are classic features of chronic rhinosinusitis, with over 3 months of anosmia, nasal congestion and cough with excessive mucus. A history of atopy increases the risk. Allergic rhinitis symptoms are unlikely to be present over this timescale.

7. C. Throat examination reveals unilateral tonsillar enlargement and uvula deviation, associated with trismus, odynophagia and change in vocal resonance, classically described as a 'hot potato voice'. This is the textbook presentation for a peritonsillar abscess.

8. E. Infectious mononucleosis presents with a sore throat, tonsillar exudate, lymphadenopathy, jaundice and splenomegaly. Symptoms typically last longer than standard tonsillitis, and there are often unwell contacts. This should be managed with reassurance and safety netting, with avoidance of contact sports for 6 weeks due to the risk of splenic rupture. Antibiotics are not required, as this is not a bacterial infection.

9. D. New hoarseness of >3 weeks duration in a patient with a smoking history is a red flag for laryngeal malignancy. Laryngitis is typically short-lived; thyroiditis would present with symptoms of thyroid derangement, and vocal cord nodules develop after chronic vocal overuse.

10. D. Excessive daytime somnolence and unrefreshing sleep in the obese patient with a smoking history suggests obstructive sleep apnoea (OSA). OSA should be investigated with polysomnography to detect apnoeic episodes. Other investigations are considered to rule out other differentials if sleep studies are inconclusive.

Chapter 9 Plastics and skin surgery

1. C. The lesion has all the ABCDE criteria for malignant melanoma – asymmetrical, with an irregular border, dark in colour, large and has recently evolved (grown). Excess sun exposure is a risk factor.

2. E. Pressure ulcers are common in older adults, particularly in those with chronic malnutrition and poor skin integrity and develop in pressure areas including the heals. Necrotizing fasciitis is a severe deep-tissue infection, and the patient would be systemically unwell with rapidly spreading tissue necrosis. Neuropathic ulcers also occur on pressure areas, but there would likely be a history of diabetes, or other causes of peripheral neuropathy. Arterial ulcers are small, well-defined, painful lesions.

3. E. Red flag features of necrotizing fasciitis include severe leg pain, swelling, discolouration, skin induration and palpable crepitus. The history of diabetes places him at risk for severe soft tissue infections. The management of necrotizing fasciitis involves urgent surgical debridement and deep tissue MC&S to confirm the diagnosis and remove the necrotic skin. Intravenous antibiotics are given following confirmation of the diagnosis. Amputation may be required if debridement attempts fail.

4. A. These are typical features of basal cell carcinoma, with a raised, pink nodule, with crusty, ulcerated areas, a rolled edge, and superficial telangiectasia and surface sheen. Squamous cell carcinoma, Bowen disease (SCC in situ) and keratoacanthoma present with rapid growth and local destruction. Marjolin's ulcer is a SCC associated with chronic wounds.

5. E. Squamous cell carcinoma is suggested by a painless, slow growing, ulcerating lesion. Immunosuppression is a key risk factor for SCC. All lesions suspicious for SCC should be excised with wide borders, with histological confirmation of the diagnosis. 5-FU and radiotherapy can be used as adjuvant measures. Cryotherapy is used in Bowen disease (SCC in situ).

6. C. Necrotizing fasciitis is a life-threatening soft tissue infection resulting in necrosis of the superficial and deep fascia and subcutaneous fat. Immunosuppressed patients, including intravenous drug users, who are at risk of chronic skin lesions, are particularly high risk. Diagnosis is made following surgical wound debridement and deep tissue biopsy.

7. B. These are red flag features of malignant melanoma, with a changing pigmented lesion, which is asymmetrical in border and colour and large. Melanomas should be managed with full-thickness excisional biopsy with 3 mm margins. Following histological confirmation of the diagnosis, surgical resection with wide local excision is performed.

8. C. Open fractures, particularly those at high risk of wound contamination require antibiotic prophylaxis, even if there is no evidence of active infection, due to the risk of osteomyelitis with communication of the bone with the external environment. Tetanus boosters are given for bites or lacerations. Antiemetics, fluids and analgesia are considered as supportive measures.

9. B. In third-degree circumferential burns, development of a constructive eschar can result in compartment syndrome and limb ischaemia as the skin is hydrated and fluid is returned to the limb compartment. The treatment is with escharotomy or fasciotomy. Amputation may be required if the limb cannot be salvaged. Skin grafting may be used to close the wound following escharotomy and stabilization.

10. C. Necrotizing fasciitis is suggested by severe pain, skin necrosis, exudate and subcutaneous crepitus. Immunosuppression with rheumatoid arthritis and methotrexate use is a risk factor. Osteomyelitis presents with pain, fever and redness of the overlying skin, but does not typically cause skin necrosis and crepitus.

Chapter 10 Cardiothoracic surgery

1. A. For significant stenosis of the left main stem or three-vessel disease, coronary artery bypass grafting remains the management of choice. PCI is reserved for less significant stenosis, or single or double-vessel disease. Bypass grafting typically harvests from the internal thoracic artery, leaving the proximal end attached to the subclavian artery.

2. E. Warfarin remains the anticoagulation therapy of choice in mechanical valve replacement, which is preferred in younger patients due to increased lifespan. Lifelong anticoagulation is required, with a target INR of 2.5–3.5.

3. A. The patient has had a TIA, which indicates a potential underlying diagnosis of carotid artery stenosis. Carotid artery stenosis is diagnosed using ultrasound. In cases of severe (>70%) stenosis, surgical intervention is indicated, which includes endarterectomy, or angioplasty and stenting.

4. B. A ruptured thoracic aortic aneurysm presents with central tearing chest pain, haemodynamic instability, and a widened mediastinum on X-ray. Marfan's syndrome is a significant risk factor for aortic aneurysms. For unruptured cases, TEVAR can be considered, however in acute rupture, open surgery is required.

5. A. CRT, otherwise known as biventricular pacing, synchronizes the contraction of all cardiac chambers. It is used in patients with severe heart failure, with ejection fraction <35%, who remain symptomatic despite optimal medical management. If this fails to control symptoms, LVADs or heart transplant can be considered. ICDs continually monitor the heart rhythm and administer a shock if the patient goes into a shockable arrhythmia, to return the heart to sinus rhythm.

6. E. She has signs of severe aortic stenosis, with the classical SAD triad – syncope, angina, dyspnoea. A slow rising pulse, narrow pulse pressure and ejection systolic murmur radiating to the carotids are typical features. Echocardiogram is required to diagnose the lesion and assess cardiac function.

7. B. He has a spontaneous pneumothorax, which can be seen on the chest X-ray as the area on the right with no lung markings. Large pneumothoraxes in haemodyanmically stable patients should be managed with definitive chest drain placement. In haemodynamic instability, needle aspiration or finger thoracostomy can be considered. Small, asymptomatic pneumothoraxes (<2 cm), can be managed conservatively, with a repeat chest X-ray in 2-4 weeks to confirm resolution.

8. D. These are typical features of pericardial effusion, with shortness of breath, orthopnoea, a feeling of fullness in the chest, quiet heart sounds and a raised JVP. Autoimmune and inflammatory conditions are a risk factor for the development of chronic effusions. The chest X-ray shows the classical 'water bottle sign' of an enlarged, globular heart.

9. E. Chest pain, cough, shortness of breath and dysphagia suggest a thoracic aortic aneurysm with compressive effects. Hiccups occur due to compression of the phrenic nerve. The cardiovascular examination reveals aortic insufficiency, with a wide pulse pressure, diastolic murmur and peripheral oedema.

10. E. A tension pneumothorax is suggested by tracheal deviation and respiratory distress. Emergency management includes needle aspiration, with the insertion of a large bore cannula into the second intercostal space, the midclavicular line. Chest drain can follow for definitive management. Tension pneumothoraxes can deteriorate and arrest rapidly, hence, they are a clinical diagnosis.

Chapter 11 Perioperative management

1. B. 1 L 0.9% NaCl + 40 mmol KCl over 8 hours, 1 L 5% dextrose and 40 mmol KCl over 8 hours, 500 mL 5% dextrose and 20 mmol KCl over 8 hours provides appropriate maintenance electrolyte requirements.

2. B. Oral hypoglycaemic agents such as gliclazide, a sulphonylurea, must be stopped on the day of surgery due to the risk of hypoglycaemia with fasting. Other medications can typically be continued unless there are complications such as AKI.

3. C. Postoperative pyrexia and haemodynamic instability, with tachycardia and hypotension, with rigors when his feed is being changed are suggestive of line infection, a frequent complication of TPN particularly with several days of line use. The Sepsis 6 should be initiated, and the central line removed immediately.

4. E. She has features of opiate overdose, including respiratory depression, reduced GCS, pinpoint pupils and limb twitching. Management is with immediate naloxone to reverse the opiates, and reduction of analgesia. Naloxone has a very short half-life, so multiple injections may be required.

5. B. She has features of a catheter-associated UTI. Urinary tract infections are common in the postoperative period between 3 and 5 days. Management involves immediate catheter removal or replacement, urine sample for MC&S and empirical antibiotics once cultures have been sent. Antibiotics can be tailored once culture results are available.

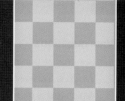

OSCE CASES

Case 1

1. A 66-year-old man has 3 days of colicky abdominal pain and distention, with nausea, vomiting, and constipation. His abdomen is distended. There is a small, painful, firm mass in his right groin and bowel sounds are high-pitched and hyperactive.

Investigations (Fig. 1)

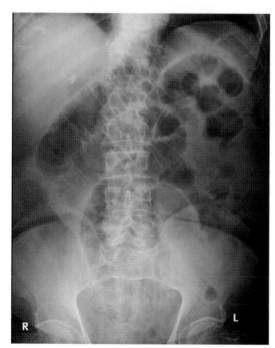

Fig. 1. Abdominal X-ray. (Garden OJ, et al. *Principles and Practice of Surgery*. 8th Edition. Elsevier Ltd. 2023.)

Please present the abdominal X-ray.

Viva questions

1. Summarize the key findings of the abdominal X-ray.
2. Which is the most likely diagnosis?
3. Suggest three other possible causes of the X-ray findings.
4. Which is the most appropriate next step?
5. Which is the most appropriate definitive management?

Case 2

A 42-year-old female has sudden profuse haematemsis.

Please take a focussed gastrointestinal history.

Viva questions

1. What is your differential diagnosis?
2. Which is the most appropriate immediate management?
3. What risk stratification score should be calculated?
4. Which is the most appropriate definitive management?
5. Which medication should be added to her management?

Case 3

A 54-year-old woman has 2 days of fever and colicky upper abdominal pain that became severe and constant this morning, with fever, nausea, and vomiting. She has hypothyroidism and gallstones managed with levothyroxine and over-the-counter paracetamol. Her temperature is 38.1°C, pulse 121 bpm, and BP 105/87 mmHg. There is marked scleral icterus and severe tenderness in the right upper quadrant.

Investigations (Table 1)

Table 1 Blood results

FBC		
Test	Level	Normal range
Hb	120	115–165 g/dL
WCC	18.5	3.6–11.0 × 10⁹/L
Neutrophils	14.1	1.8–7.5 × 10⁹/L
Platelets	280	140–400 × 10⁹/L
CRP	147	<1
LFTs		
Test	Level	Normal range
Bilirubin	50	3–17 μmol/L
Alanine transferase (ALT)	32	3–40 IU/L
Aspartate transaminase (AST)	28	3–30 IU/L
Alkaline phosphatase (ALP)	190	30–100 μmol/L
Gamma glutamyl transferase (γGT)	160	8–60 IU/L

Viva questions

1. Summarize the key findings of the blood results.
2. Which is the likely diagnosis?
3. Which test is most likely to confirm the diagnosis?
4. Which is the most appropriate long-term management?
5. What are the possible complications of this condition?

Case 4

A 32-year-old man has a long history of intermittent diarrhoea and constipation, with abdominal pain relieved by defecation. He has frequent mucus in his stool, but no blood.

Please perform an abdominal examination

The key findings of the abdominal examination include:

- 34-year-old man
- Well at rest
- Cachectic
- Conjunctival pallor
- Multiple oral ulcers
- Multiple abdominal scars

Viva questions

1. Which is the likely diagnosis?
2. What are the key differences between Crohn's disease and ulcerative colitis?
3. What is used to induce remission in IBD?
4. What are some extraintestinal manifestations of Crohn's disease?
5. What are the indications for surgery in IBD?

Case 5

A 64-year-old man has 3 months of a painful lesion on his right lower leg (Fig. 2).

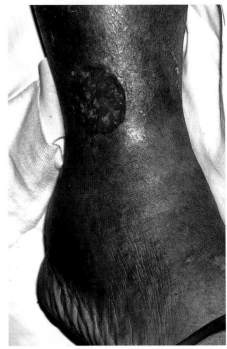

Fig. 2. Arterial Ulcer. (From James WD, Elston DM, Berger TG. *Andrews' Diseases of the skin: clinical dermatology.* 11th Edition, Saunders; 2011.)

Please describe the lesion in question

Viva questions

1. Which is the likely diagnosis?
2. What are the key risk factors for vascular pathology?
3. What ABPI result is diagnostic of peripheral arterial disease?
4. What are the features of critical limb ischaemia?
5. What are the 6 Ps of acute limb ischaemia?

Answers:

Case 1

Abdominal X-ray presentation mark scheme

Step	Introduction	Achieved
1	Confirms patient details	
2	Confirms date and time of film	
3	Check for previous imaging for comparison	
	Image quality	
4	Assesses image projection	
5	Assess image exposure	
	Interpretation	
6	Mentions obvious abnormalities first	
7	Assesses small and large bowel	
8	Assess other organs	
9	Assess bones	
	Final steps	
10	Summarizes findings	
11	Suggests likely diagnosis	
12	Suggests further steps	
	Global score	

Viva question answers

1. Central dilated loops of bowel with muscle bands that cross the entire width of the bowel, indicative of valvulae conniventes, suggesting small bowel obstruction.
2. An obstructed groin hernia (e.g., inguinal, or femoral) causing a small bowel obstruction.
3. Adhesions (most common), tumours (e.g., at the ileocecal valve), strictures.
4. Nil by mouth with nasogastric tube placement with free drainage, and intravenous fluids.
5. Laparotomy, to relieve the obstruction, and to remove any dead bowel, with anastomosis or stoma formation.

Case 2

Haematemesis patient history

Name	Kayla Jones
DOB	8/12/1976 (42 years)
Occupation	Accountant
History	Began vomiting fresh red blood this morning – few tablespoons Happened suddenly, not preceded by retching Associated symptoms: • Some epigastric pain • No swallowing difficulties • Feels lightheaded • Several episodes of dark black stool over last few days • Poor appetite recently, some weight loss due to work-related stress If asked – drank alcohol last night Specifically asked about amount – two bottles of wine Never had anything like this before
PMH	Depression and anxiety
DH	Nil regular Takes paracetamol occasionally
FH	Mum had diabetes
SH	Smokes – 10/day for 10 years Alcohol – several bottles of wine/night for the past few years Drugs – nil Occupation – accountant Lives alone – separated from husband and going through a divorce
ICE	Concerned about bleeding, worried it will happen again Doesn't want to be in hospital

Abdominal history taking mark scheme

Step	Introduction	Achieved
1	Introduces self	
2	Confirms name and age of patient	
3	Explains reason for consultation	
4	Gains consent to proceed	
	History taking	
5	Asks open question – reason for presentation	
6	Asks about previous episodes	
7	Establishes features of hematemesis – onset, timing and frequency of episodes	
8	Assesses features of and quantity of blood lost	
9	Assess for risk factors – NSAIDs, alcohol	
10	Checks for associated symptoms	
11	Asks specifically about GI/ hepatobiliary symptoms and symptoms of shock	
12	Assesses for red flags – dysphagia, loss of appetite, weight loss	
13	Assesses for constitutional features	
14	Past medical history – enquires specifically about GI/bleeding disorders	
15	Drug history – enquires specifically about NSAIDs/anticoagulation/ steroids	
16	Assesses medication compliance	
17	Allergies	
18	Family history – enquires specifically about GI disease	
19	Social history – smokes, drinks or takes recreational drugs, occupation	
20	Takes detailed alcohol history – how much, what, how often, how long for	
21	Asks about foreign travel	
22	Assesses impact of symptoms	
23	Ideas, concerns, expectations	
24	Shows empathy, avoids jargon	
25	Thanks patient	
26	Summarizes key history	
	Global score	

Viva question answers

1. Oesophageal varices secondary to alcohol abuse, gastritis, peptic ulcer, Mallory Weiss tear.
2. Resuscitation with blood products.
3. Glasgow Blatchford score prior to endoscopy, Rockall score after endoscopy.
4. Endoscopy with variceal ligation/banding/clipping.
5. Antibiotics and terlipressin.

Case 3

Viva questions

1. ↑ WBC/neutrophils/CRP – suggests bacterial infection. LFTs – cholestatic picture, with ↑ bilirubin/ALP/yGT
2. Ascending cholangitis – relating to gallstone obstruction of CBD
3. ERCP
4. Cholecystectomy
5. Sepsis, hypovolemic shock, multiorgan dysfunction, death. Biliary strictures, gallstone ileus, cholangiocarcinoma

Case 4

Abdominal examination mark scheme

Step	Introduction	Achieved
	Wash your hands	
	Introduces self, confirmed name and role	
	Confirm patient's name and date of birth	
	Explains what the examination will involve, gains consent to proceed	
	Repositions head of the bed to a 45 degree angle	
	Checks for any pain before proceeding	
	General inspection	
	Inspects for and comments on relevant clinical signs (scars, abdominal distension, pallor, jaundice, cachexia)	
	Inspects around the bed for medication, monitoring devices and mobility aids	
	Hands	
	Inspects for and comments on relevant clinical signs (palmar erythema, koilonychia, leukonychia and Dupuytren's contracture, finger clubbing)	
	Assess for asterixis	
	Assess temperature of hands and CRT	
	Palpate the radial pulse and comments on rate and rhythm	
	Inspects the arms (excoriations, needle track marks)	
	Inspects the axilla (acanthosis nigricans, hair loss)	
	Upper body	
	Eyes – Inspects for and comments on relevant clinical signs (conjunctival pallor, jaundice, corneal arcus, xanthelasma, Kayser-Fleischer rings, perilimbal injection)	
	Mouth – Inspects for and comments on relevant clinical signs (Angular stomatitis, glossitis, oral candidiasis and aphthous ulceration)	
	Neck – Palpate for lymphadenopathy in the supraclavicular fossae (including Virchow's node)	
	Chest – Inspects for and comments on relevant clinical signs (spider naevi, gynaecomastia and hair loss)	

Step	Introduction	Achieved
	Abdominal examination	
	Position the patient lying flat on the bed (arms by their side and legs uncrossed)	
	Inspects for and comments on relevant clinical signs (scars, Cullen's sign, Grey-Turner's sign, striae, abdominal distension, hernias, stomas)	
	Palpation	
	Check for any pain before proceeding	
	Perform light palpation of the abdomen across all nine regions	
	Perform deep palpation of the abdomen across all nine regions	
	Palpate the liver	
	Palpate the gallbladder	
	Palpate the spleen	
	Ballot the kidneys	
	Palpate the aorta	
	Palpate the bladder	
	Abdominal percussion	
	Perform hepatic percussion to identify the liver's borders	
	Perform splenic percussion	
	Perform bladder percussion	
	Assess shifting dullness	
	Abdominal auscultation	
	Auscultate the abdomen to assess bowel sounds	
	Auscultate over the aorta for bruits	
	Auscultate over the renal arteries for bruits	
	Legs – assess for pedal oedema	
	Completing the examination	
	Wash your hands	
	Explain that the examination is now finished to the patient	
	Thank the patient for their time	
	Summarize your findings	
	Suggest further assessments and investigations (e.g., assessment of hernial orifices, digital rectal examination, examination of external genitalia, abdominal imaging)	

Viva question answers

1. Crohn's disease
2. Key differentiating features include (Table 2)

Table 2 Crohn's disease versus ulcerative colitis

Crohn's disease	Ulcerative colitis
From the mouth to the anus	Colon and rectum
Bowel wall thickened – 'cobblestones'	Thin bowel wall
	Continuous disease
'Patchy' disease with skip lesions	Ulcers do not cross the mucosa
Transmural ulceration	Granulomas are uncommon
Granulomas are common	

1. Steroids.
2. Enteropathic arthritis, anterior uveitis, episcleritis, clubbing, erythema nodosum, pyoderma gangrenosum.
3. Failure of medical management to control symptoms, abscess formation and fistulae, obstruction, strictures, toxic megacolon, sepsis, cancer, curative (only UC).

Case 5

Describing a skin lesion mark scheme

Step	Introduction	Achieved
1	Assesses number of lesion(s) (single, multiple)	
2	Assesses location of lesion(s)	
3	Assesses distribution of lesion(s) (vesicular, flexural, extensor, acral)	
4	Assesses lesion(s) size	
5	Provides approximate diameter in centimetres	
6	Assesses lesion(s) configuration	
7	Assesses lesion(s) colour	
8	Assesses lesion(s) structure	
	Pigmented lesions	
9	Assesses for **A**symmetry	
10	Assesses for **B**order irregularity	
11	Assesses **C**olour	
12	Assesses approximate **D**iameter	
13	Comments they would take a history of **E**volution	

Ulcer description

- This is single, large, ulcer approximately 4 cm in diameter on the anterior surface of the lower right shin. The lesion has well-defined borders, is circular and 'punched out' in appearance, and is erythematous with overlying skin loss, but no slough or evidence of infection.

Viva question answers

1. Arterial ulcer
2. Smoking, obesity, male, hypertension, high cholesterol, diabetes
3. <0.9
4. Rest pain, tissue loss (ulcers, gangrene)
5. Pain, pallor, pulselessness, paralysis, paraesthesia, poikilothermia (perishingly cold)

SHORT CLINICAL CASES

Case 1

A 32-year-old man has sudden severe upper abdominal pain radiating to the back, with nausea, vomiting and diarrhoea. He drank two bottles of wine last night. His temperature is 38.1°C, pulse 125 bpm, and BP 129/82 mmHg. There is severe epigastric tenderness and guarding.

a. Which is the most likely diagnosis?
b. What scoring system should be used to assess severity?
c. Which blood test is most suggestive of the diagnosis?
d. The patient is admitted, resuscitated and treated with intravenous fluids, analgesia and nutritional support. Overnight he develops respiratory distress and hypoxia (Fig. 3). Which complication has most likely developed?

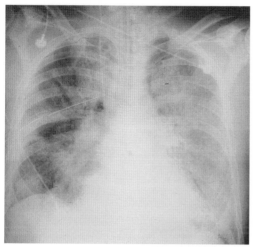

Fig. 3. Chest X-ray. (Louis Vincent J, et al. *Textbook of Critical Care*. 8th Edition. Elsevier Inc. 2024.)

e. The patient recovers and is discharged, however, represents several weeks later with fatigue, abdominal pain, foul smelling diarrhoea, increased thirst and urinary frequency. Which is the likely diagnosis?

Answers

a. Pancreatitis
    - Acute epigastric pain, nausea, vomiting and diarrhoea, with systemic illness and a history of alcohol excess suggests acute pancreatitis.

b. Glasgow score
    - The Glasgow score can be used to assess the severity of pancreatitis. Scores >3 suggest a high mortality risk and a need for ITU consult. The **PANCREAS** mnemonic is used to remember the criteria:
        - **P**aO$_2$ <8 KPa
        - **A**ge >55
        - **N**eutrophils (WBC>15)
        - **C**alcium <2
        - u**R**ea >16
        - **E**nzymes (AST/ALT>200 or LDH >600), **A**lbumin <32
        - **S**ugar (glucose >10).

c. Lipase
    - Both amylase and lipase may be raised in acute pancreatitis. Lipase is more sensitive and specific. Amylase can be raised in other conditions including small bowel obstruction, salivary gland pathology, renal or liver failure, ectopic pregnancy and malignancy. In chronic pancreatitis, both amylase and lipase may be normal.

d. Acute respiratory distress syndrome
    - ARDS is one of the most serius complications of acute pancreatitis. Release of inflammatory mediators from the pancreatitis into the bloodstream results in severe systemic and pulmonary inflammation. A reduced PaO$_2$ and respiratory distress is an indication for immediate HDU/ITU review.

e. Chronic pancreatitis
    - Chronic pancreatitis develops following repeated acute episodes of pancreatitis. Impaired pancreatic exocrine function results in malabsorptive symptoms (steatorrhoea) and impaired endocrine function results in pancreatogenic diabetes. Management includes abstinence from alcohol, replacement pancreatic enzymes and insulin.

Case 2

A 54-year-old man has 3 months of occasional loose, dark stool, that is foul, and tarry in consistency. He has smoked 20 cigarettes a day for 30 years.

a. Which is the most appropriate next step?

b. He is referred for a colonoscopy.

Investigations (Fig. 4)

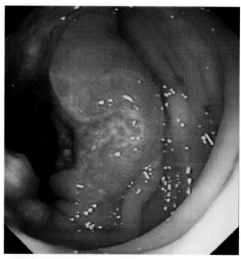

Fig. 4. Colonoscopy findings. (From Garden OJ, et al. *Principles and Practice of Surgery*. 8th Edition. Elsevier Ltd. 2023.

Which is the most likely diagnosis?

c. Histopathology confirms caecal carcinoma. Which is the most appropriate next step in diagnosis?

d. The tumour is staged as T2N0M0. Which is the most appropriate definitive management?

e. A right hemicolectomy is performed, and he is discharged. 6 months later he presents with fatigue, abdominal pain and nausea. Examination reveals a distended abdomen with shifting dullness and cachexia. Which complication has most likely developed?

Answers

a. Urgent colonoscopy
   - The patient has red flag features of colorectal carcinoma, with change in bowel habit in an adult >50 with a smoking history. Any patient with suspicious features should be urgently referred for colonoscopy.
b. Colorectal cancer
   - The colonoscopy reveals a large ulcerated colonic mass. A biopsy is required to confirm the diagnosis, but this lesion is highly suspicious for cancer.
c. CT Thorax, abdomen and pelvis
   - Following a diagnosis of cancer, staging should be performed, using CTTAP to assess for local and distant spread. CEA levels are used as a prognostic marker and cannot aid diagnosis or guide management
d. Right hemicolectomy
   - A caecal carcinoma with no evidence of regional or distant metastasis is suitable for curative resection, with a right hemicolectomy.
e. Peritoneal carcinomatosis
   - Colorectal carcinoma has a risk of peritoneal seeding, and the development of peritoneal carcinomatosis. This is often a terminal feature, with poor 5-year survival rates. Cytoreductive surgery can be performed to aid prognosis.

Case 3

1. A 45-year-old woman has 2 months of unintentional weight gain, fatigue, low mood, and generalized muscle aches. Her pulse is 92 bpm and BP 167/109 mmHg.
   Examination: in (Fig. 5)

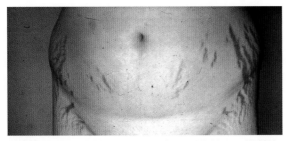

Fig. 5. Examination findings. (From Qureshi Z, Hotton E, Mak S. *The Unofficial Guide to Passing OSCEs*. 4th Edition. UGTM (Unofficial Guide to Medicine). Elsevier Ltd. 2024.)

a. Which is the most appropriate immediate investigation?
b. A dexamethasone suppression test is performed, which reveals suppression of both cortisol and ACTH. Which is the most likely location of the lesion?
c. Which is the most appropriate next step in diagnosis?
d. An MRI Sella is performed, which demonstrates a pituitary microadenoma. Which is the most appropriate management?
e. Several months after surgery, she presents with excessive thirst and frequent urination. Which complication has most likely developed?

Answers

a. Dexamethasone suppression test
   - The patient has features of Cushing syndrome, including weight gain, mood disturbance, osmotic symptoms relating to hyperglycaemia, and examination findings of central adiposity and abdominal striae. The dexamethasone suppression test determines whether excess circulating glucocorticoid relates to autonomous adrenal secretion or excess pituitary or ectopic ACTH release.
b. The pituitary gland
   - Suppression of both cortisol and ACTH indicates negative pituitary feedback, reducing ACTH release and subsequent adrenal cortisol release. In adrenal adenomas, ACTH is suppressed but cortisol will remains high, as the adenoma is releasing cortisol independently of pituitary regulation. In ectopic ACTH release, neither ACTH nor cortisol will be suppressed.
c. MRI Sella
   - MRI Sella is the investigation of choice to diagnose a pituitary adenoma.
d. Transsphenoidal hypophysectomy
   - Transsphenoidal hypophysectomy is indicated to remove the adenoma. Patients may develop hypopituitarism afterwards and require pituitary hormone replacement.
e. Cranial diabetes insipidus
   - Hypopituitarism can develop after pituitary surgery. In this case, reduced ADH release has resulted in cranial diabetes insipidus, presenting with thirst and frequent urination. In this case, reduced ADH release has resulted in cranial diabetes insipidus, with symptoms of thirst and frequent urination.

Case 4

1. A 72-year-old man has 6 months of painless difficulty initiating his urinary stream, poor flow, terminal dribbling, increased frequency and nocturia. He is increasingly fatigued and has lost several kilos of weight over this

period. He has hypertension, managed with amlodipine. He has a palpable bladder. Digital rectal examination reveals an enlarged prostate with loss of the central sulcus, and a firm nodule on the left lobe.

a. Which is the most likely diagnosis?
b. Which is the most appropriate next step in diagnosis?
c. Given a diagnosis of prostate cancer, which scoring system should be used for staging?
d. The patient undergoes brachytherapy to treat his cancer. He presents several weeks later with rectal pain and bloody diarrhoea. Which complication of treatment has most likely developed? Which complication has most likely developed?
e. A year later he presents with chest and shoulder pain. Investigations (Fig. 6)

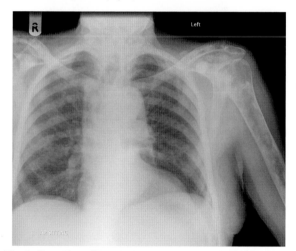

Fig. 6. Chest X-ray. (From Au-Yong I, Au-Yong A, Broderick, N. *On-Call X-Rays Made Easy.* Churchill Livingstone, Elsevier Ltd. 2010.)

What complication of cancer has he developed?

Answers
a. Prostate cancer
  • Painless lower urinary tract symptoms, fatigue and weight loss with a firm nodule on DRE suggest prostate cancer.
b. Multiparametric MRI
  • Multiparametric MRIs are used to first line for diagnosis of prostate cancer, following which, transrectal or transperineal prostate biopsy will confirm the diagnosis. PSA is notoriously unreliable and can be raised for a variety of reasons, including BPH, prostatitis or sexual intercourse.
c. Gleason score
  • The Gleason score is the grading system to classify the aggressiveness of prostate cancer. Cancer cells are scored 1 to 5 based on differentiation from normal tissue, and the two highest tissue scores are added together to indicate the level of aggression.

d. Radiation proctitis
  • Complications of brachytherapy include proctitis and cystitis, relating to local inflammation from radioactive seeds implanted in the prostate. Long term, there is an increased risk of bladder or rectal cancer.
e. Bone metastases
  • Prostate cancer typically metastasises to bone, with widespread sclerotic lesions. Multiple areas of increased density can be seen in the ribs, clavicles, and humerus. Gynaecomastia has developed, which can relate to antiandrogen therapy used as an adjunctive treatment.

Case 5

1. A 38-year-old woman presents has 3 months of a gradually enlarging, painless neck lump. There is a 6 cm, firm, nonfluctuant midline neck mass, which is painless, and moves on swallowing, but not on tongue protrusion. Examination (Fig. 7)

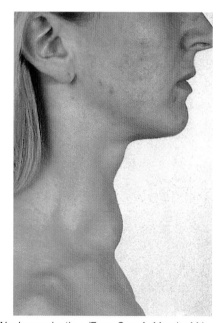

Fig. 7. Neck examination. (From Gaw A, Murphy MJ, Srivastava R, Cowan RA, O'Reilly DSJ. *Clinical Biochemistry: An Illustrated Colour Text. 5th Edition*. Churchill Livingstone, Elsevier; 2013.)

a. Which is the most likely diagnosis?
b. Which is the most appropriate next step in diagnosis?
c. Thyroid ultrasound confirms the mass is a thyroid nodule. How would malignancy be excluded?
d. Histology confirms thyroid malignancy. Which subtype is most likely in this case?

e. A diagnosis of papillary carcinoma is made. Which is the most appropriate management?

Answers

a. Thyroid nodule
   - A small, gradually enlarging, painless neck lump, which moves on swallowing but not on tongue protrusion, suggests a thyroid nodule.

b. Thyroid ultrasound
   - A thyroid US will confirm the lesion arises from the thyroid, to guide further diagnostic investigations. TFTs will be useful to determine if the lesion is hormone-producing or impairing thyroid function but will not aid the diagnosis of the mass.

c. Fine needle aspiration and cytology
   - Fine needle aspiration and cytology will provide a histological diagnosis.

d. Papillary carcinoma
   - Papillary carcinomas are the most common subtype of thyroid malignancy, occurring in 75-80% of cases, typically in young women. They are slow growing and are often initially asymptomatic. There is an excellent prognosis, with a 99% 5-year survival rate.

e. Thyroidectomy
   - Most papillary cancers are treated with thyroidectomy +/− radical neck dissection in nodal involvement. Small nodules confined to one lobe may be managed with lobectomy. Treatment after surgery may include radioactive iodine therapy for advanced cancers or in metastasis. After a thyroidectomy, thyroid replacement therapy is required lifelong.

Case 6

1. A 60-year-old man has 3 weeks of a dry cough and shortness of breath, after 3 months of fatigue, with several stones of unintentional weight loss and loss of appetite. He is an ex-smoker of 40-pack-years.
   a. Which is the most appropriate next step?
   b. A chest X-ray suggests a lesion in the left lung. Which test is most likely to confirm the diagnosis?
   c. Bronchoscopy and biopsy reveal an adenocarcinoma confined to the left upper lobe. Which is the most appropriate treatment?
   d. Following lobectomy, the patient develops a fever, with purulence and persistent bubbling of the chest drain. Chest X-ray reveals a new air-fluid level in the pleural cavity. What complication of surgery has he likely developed? Which complication has most likely developed?
   e. Several months later, he presents with left hip pain (Fig. 8)

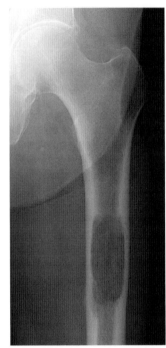

Fig. 8. Hip X-ray. (From Silverman PM. *Oncologic Imaging: A Multidisciplinary Approach.* 2nd Edition. Saunders, Elsevier Inc. 2022.)

What complication of his cancer has he likely developed?

Answers

a. Chest X-ray
   - In patients with a smoking history, an unexplained cough, shortness of breath and weight loss are red flags for lung cancer, warranting an an urgent CXR.

b. Bronchoscopy and biopsy
   - Bronchoscopy with endobronchial ultrasound enables detailed assessment of and biopsy of the mass for histology.

c. Lobectomy
   - Surgery is first line for patients with non-small cell lung cancer isolated to a single lobe. Lobectomy involves removing the entire lobe containing the tumour and is the most common method.

d. Bronchopleural fistula
   - A bronchopleural fistula is a pathological connection between the bronchus and the pleural space and is common in patients following lung resection. The connection can result in persistent air leak, purulent drainage, empyema and pleural effusion.

e. Lytic bony metastases
   - Non-small cell lung cancer commonly metastasises to bone. Here, you can see lucency in the left hip, suggesting bony metastases.

Abstract

Abbreviations

AAA Abdominal aortic aneurysm

ABPI Ankle brachial pressure index

ACL Anterior cruciate ligament

ACS Acute chest syndrome

AF Atrial fibrillation

AIDS Acquired immune deficiency syndrome

AKI Acute kidney injury

ALI Acute limb ischaemia

ALL Acute lymphoblastic leukaemia

ALS Advanced life support

ALT Alanine aminotransferase

AMI Acute mesenteric ischaemia

AMTS Abbreviated Mental Test Score

APTT Activated partial thromboplastin time

ASO Antistreptolysin O

ATN Acute tubular necrosis

'AVPU' Alert, voice, pain, unconscious

AXR Abdominal X-ray

BD Bis die; twice a day

BLS Basic life support

BMI Body mass index

BNF British National Formulary

BNP Brain natriuretic peptide

BP Blood pressure

BPH Benign prostatic hyperplasia

BPPV Benign paroxysmal positional vertigo

bpm Beats per minute (for pulse only)

Ca^{2+} Calcium

CAD Coronary artery disease

CAH Congenital adrenal hyperplasia

CAP Community acquired pneumonia

CBD Common bile duct

CBG Capillary blood glucose

CES Cauda equina syndrome

CF Cystic fibrosis

CK Creatine kinase

CKD Chronic kidney disease

CLI Critical limb ischaemia

CMN Congenital melanocytic nevus

COPD Chronic obstructive pulmonary disease

CO$_2$ Carbon dioxide

CPAP Continuous positive airway pressure

CPR Cardiopulmonary resuscitation

Creat Creatinine

CRP C-reactive protein

CRT Capillary refill time

CSF Cerebrospinal fluid

CT Computerised tomography

CTA CT angiography

CTCAP CT chest, abdomen, pelvic

CTPA Computed tomography pulmonary angiogram

CVP Central venous pressure

CXR Chest X-ray

DIC Disseminated intravascular coagulation

DIP Distal interphalangeal

DKA Diabetic ketoacidosis

DMARD Disease modifying anti-rheumatic drug

DRE Digital rectal examination

DVT Deep vein thrombosis

EAC External auditory canal

EBV Epstein–Barr virus

ECG Electrocardiogram

eGFR Glomerular filtration rate

ERCP Endoscopic retrograde cholangiopancreatography

ESR Erythrocyte sedimentation rate

ESWL Extracorporeal shock wave lithotripsy

EUS Endoscopic ultrasound

FAST Focussed assessment with sonography for trauma

FBC Full blood count

FEV Forced expiratory volume

FFP Fresh-frozen plasma

FSH Follicle stimulating hormone

FSGS Focal segmental glomerulosclerosis

FVC Forced vital capacity

FVIII Factor VIII

GAS Group A beta-hemolytic streptococcus

GCS Glasgow Coma Scale

GIT Gastrointestinal tract

GORD Gastroesophageal reflux disease

GUM Genitourinary medicine

HBA1c Glycated haemoglobin

HCG (or hCG) Human chorionic gonadotropin

HIV Human immunodeficiency virus

HRCT High resolution computed tomography

HSV Herpes simplex virus

HUS Haemolytic uraemic syndrome

IBD Inflammatory bowel disease

IBS Irritable bowel syndrome

ICP Intracranial pressure

ICU Intensive care unit

IDA Iron deficiency anaemia

IHD Ischaemic heart disease

IM Intramuscular

IO Intraosseous

ITP Immune thrombocytopenia

IV Intravenous

IVDU Intravenous drug use

IVF In vitro fertilisation

JIA Juvenile idiopathic arthritis

JVP Jugular venous pressure

K Potassium

LBO Large bowel obstruction

LDH Lactate dehydrogenase

LFT Liver function tests

LH Luteinising hormone

LLQ Left lower quadrant

LUQ Left upper quadrant

LUTS Lower urinary tract symptoms

MCA Middle cerebral artery

MCD Minimal change disease

MCL Medial collateral ligament

MCP Metacarpophalangeal joints

MCV Mean cell volume

mmHg Millimetres of mercury (for blood pressure only)

MRI Magnetic resonance imaging

MSU Mid-stream urine

Na Sodium

NAAT Nucleic acid amplification test

NEC Necrotising enterocolitis

NEWS National Early Warning System

NG Nasogastric

NHS National Health Service

NICE The National Institute for Health & Clinical Excellence

NOF Neck of femur

NSAIDs Nonsteroidal anti-inflammatory drugs

OE Otitis externa

OM Otitis media

OME Otitis media with effusion

ORIF Open reduction and internal fixation

OSA Obstructive sleep apnoea

PAD Peripheral arterial disease

PCR Polymerase chain reaction

PE Pulmonary embolism

PEFR Peak expiratory flow rate

PIP Proximal interphalangeal

PPV Positive pressure ventilation

PR Per rectum

PRN Pro re nata; as needed

PSA Prostate specific antigen

PSGN Post-streptococcal glomerulonephritis

PT Prothrombin time

PUD Peptic ulcer disease

QDS Quarter in die; four times a day

O$_2$ Oxygen

OGD Oesophagogastroduodenoscopy

OSA Obstructive sleep apnoea

Plt Platelet count

RAPD Relative afferent pupillary defect

RBC Red blood cell count

RLQ Right lower quadrant

RR Respiratory rate

RSV Respiratory syncytial virus

RUQ Right upper quadrant

SAH Subarachnoid haemorrhage

SBO Small bowel obstruction

SBP Spontaneous bacterial peritonitis

SJS Stevens–Johnson syndrome

SLE Systemic lupus erythematosus

SNHL Sensorineural hearing loss

SP Spontaneous pneumothorax

SpO$_2$ Oxygen saturation (in %)

STI Sexually transmitted infection

SVC Superior vena cava

SVCO Superior vena cava obstruction

T4 Thyroxine

TAVR Transcatheter aortic valve replacement

TB Tuberculosis

TBSA Total body surface area

TCA Tricyclic antidepressant

TDS ter die sumendus; three times a day

TIA Transient ischaemic attack

TFT Thyroid function tests

TM Tympanic membrane

TOF Tetralogy of Fallot

TSH Thyroid stimulating hormone

TSS Toxic shock syndrome

TURP Transurethral resection of the prostate

U&E Urea and electrolytes

UGIB Upper gastrointestinal bleed

UPSI Unprotected sexual intercourse

Ur Urea

URTI Upper respiratory tract infection

US Ultrasound

UTI Urinary tract infection

VDRL Venereal disease research laboratory

VEGF Vascular endothelial growth factor

VP Ventriculoperitoneal

VSD Ventricular septal defect

VTE Venous thromboembolism

WBC White blood cell count